T0195450

Look for these other volumes in the *Mosby Physiology Series:*

Blaustein, Kao, & Matteson: *CELLULAR PHYSIOLOGY AND NEUROPHYSIOLOGY*

Cloutier: *RESPIRATORY PHYSIOLOGY*

Koeppen & Stanton: *RENAL PHYSIOLOGY*

Johnson: *GASTROINTESTINAL PHYSIOLOGY*

Pappano & Weir: *CARDIOVASCULAR PHYSIOLOGY*

Hudnall: *HEMATOLOGY: A PATHOPHYSIOLOGIC APPROACH*

Endocrine and Reproductive Physiology

5TH EDITION

Bruce A. White, PhD
Professor
Department of Cell Biology
Co-Director of Histopathology Labs
UConn Health
Farmington, Connecticut

John R. Harrison, PhD
Director, Human and Virtual Anatomy Labs
Program Director, Fabric of Anatomy and Biology Labs
Basic Science Principal
UConn Health
Farmington, Connecticut

Lisa M. Mehlmann, PhD
Associate Professor, Department of Cell Biology
UConn Health
Farmington, Connecticut

ELSEVIER

ELSEVIER

3251 Riverport Lane
St. Louis, Missouri 63043

ENDOCRINE AND REPRODUCTIVE PHYSIOLOGY:
MOSBY PHYSIOLOGY SERIES, FIFTH EDITION

ISBN: 978-0-323-59573-5

Copyright © 2019, Elsevier Inc. All rights reserved.

Previous editions copyrighted 2013, 2007, 2000, and 1997.

No part of this publication may be reproduced or transmitted in any form or by any means, electronic or mechanical, including photocopying, recording, or any information storage and retrieval system, without permission in writing from the publisher. Details on how to seek permission, further information about the Publisher's permissions policies and our arrangements with organizations such as the Copyright Clearance Center and the Copyright Licensing Agency, can be found at our website: www.elsevier.com/permissions.

This book and the individual contributions contained in it are protected under copyright by the Publisher (other than as may be noted herein).

Notices

Practitioners and researchers must always rely on their own experience and knowledge in evaluating and using any information, methods, compounds or experiments described herein. Because of rapid advances in the medical sciences, in particular, independent verification of diagnoses and drug dosages should be made. To the fullest extent of the law, no responsibility is assumed by Elsevier, authors, editors or contributors for any injury and/or damage to persons or property as a matter of products liability, negligence or otherwise, or from any use or operation of any methods, products, instructions, or ideas contained in the material herein.

Library of Congress Control Number: 2018951176

Content Strategist: Marybeth Thiel
Senior Content Development Specialist: Marybeth Thiel
Publishing Services Manager: Shereen Jameel
Senior Project Manager: Umarani Natarajan
Design Direction: Ryan Cook

Printed in the United States of America

Last digit is the print number: 9 8 7 6 5 4 3

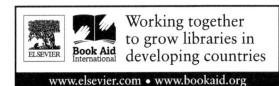

PREFACE

In a recent article in the *New Yorker* entitled "Bodies At Rest and In Motion," Dr. Siddhartha Mukherjee, physician, faculty member at the Columbia University Medical Center, and the Pulitzer Prize-winning author of *The Emperor of All Maladies: A Biography of Cancer,* makes us think about how much effort goes into the maintenance of our bodies and how much that effort is taken for granted until systems start to fail. He reminds us of Walter Cannon, who in the 1920s defined our bodies' ability to maintain a relatively constant internal environment in the face of a changing external environment as "homeostasis," a concept that was built on Claude Bernard's emphasis on the constancy of the "milieu interior."

Modern biologists and medical researchers continue to perform studies into the mechanisms by which homeostasis is maintained, and the etiologies and pathogenesis related to the breakdown of such mechanisms. The endocrine system represents an organ system that is essentially devoted to the maintenance of homeostasis. The endocrine system continually monitors circulating levels of key nutrients, ions, and metabolites, and integrates the function of multiple organ systems to keep levels within a normal range. Also, in connection with the central nervous system (CNS), the endocrine system monitors the time of day, nutritional status and levels of stress, and adjusts metabolism, sleep/awake cycles, the immune system, physical activity and other functions accordingly. Both the CNS and endocrine systems also monitor the energy stores and age of our bodies, critical information that guides the large investment by our bodies into pubertal awakening and continued function of the reproductive systems, as largely orchestrated by the endocrine system.

This 5th edition of *Endocrine and Reproductive Physiology* is designed to provide the student with the basics, with limited discussion of endocrine and reproductive pathologies as a means to emphasize normal physiology. The 5th edition has been updated by the efforts of two new authors. Dr. John Harrison has revised the chapters on calcium/phosphate regulation, hypothalamus-pituitary function, and the thyroid gland, and Dr. Lisa Mehlmann has revised the chapters on the life cycle of the reproductive systems, the female reproductive system, and pregnancy and lactation. We have strived for clarity and simplicity that hopefully will confer a basic understanding of these remarkably complex systems.

We wish to thank Marybeth Thiel at Elsevier for her patience and assistance in developing the 5th edition.

Bruce A. White

v

CONTENTS

Introduction to the Endocrine System

OBJECTIVES

1. List the main endocrine glands of the body.
2. List the chemical nature of the major hormones.
3. Describe how the chemical nature influences hormone synthesis, storage, secretion, transport, clearance, mechanism of action, and appropriate route of exogenous hormone administration.
4. Explain the significance of hormone binding to plasma proteins.
5. Describe the major signal transduction pathways, and their mechanism for termination, for different classes of hormones and provide a specific example of each.

Endocrine glands secrete chemical messengers, called hormones (Box 1.1), into the extracellular fluid in a highly regulated manner. Secreted hormones gain access to the circulation, often via fenestrated capillaries, and regulate target organs throughout the body. The endocrine system is composed of the pituitary gland, the thyroid gland, parathyroid glands, and adrenal glands (Fig. 1.1). The endocrine system also includes the ovary and testis, which carry out a gametogenic function that is absolutely dependent on their endogenous endocrine function. In addition to dedicated endocrine glands, endocrine cells reside as a minor component (in terms of mass) in other organs, either as groups of cells (the islets of Langerhans in the pancreas) or as individual cells spread throughout several glands, including the gastrointestinal (GI) tract, kidney, heart, adipose tissue, and liver. In addition, there are several types of hypothalamic neuroendocrine neurons that produce hormones. The placenta serves as a transitory exchange organ, but also functions as an important endocrine structure of pregnancy.

The endocrine system also encompasses a range of specific enzymes, either cell-associated or circulating, that perform the function of peripheral conversion of hormonal precursors (see Box 1.1). For example, angiotensinogen from the liver is converted in the circulation to angiotensin I by the renal-derived enzyme renin, followed by conversion to the active hormone angiotensin II by the transmembrane ectoenzyme angiotensin I–converting enzyme (ACE) that is enriched in the endothelia of the lungs (see Chapter 7). Another example of peripheral conversion of a precursor to an active hormone involves the two sequential

hydroxylations of vitamin D in hepatocytes and renal tubular cells.

Numerous extracellular messengers, including prostaglandins, growth factors, neurotransmitters, and cytokines, also regulate cellular function. However, these messengers act predominantly within the context of a microenvironment in an autocrine or paracrine manner, and thus are discussed only to a limited extent where needed.

To function, hormones must bind to specific receptors expressed by specific target cell types within target organs. Hormones are also referred to as ligands, in the context of ligand receptor binding, and as agonists, in that their binding to the receptor is transduced into a cellular response. Receptor antagonists typically bind to a receptor and lock it in an inactive state, unable to induce a cellular response. Drugs that bind to and alter the activity of steroid hormone receptors are referred to as selective receptor modulators. For example, Tamoxifen is a mixed estrogen receptor agonist/antagonist, and thus is referred to as a "selective estrogen receptor modulator" or SERM. Loss or inactivation of a receptor leads to hormonal resistance. Constitutive activation of a receptor leads to unregulated, hormone-independent activation of cellular processes.

The widespread delivery of hormones in the blood makes the endocrine system ideal for the functional coordination of multiple organs and cell types in the following contexts:

1. Allowing normal development and growth of the organism
2. Maintaining internal homeostasis

BOX 1.1   A List of Most Hormones and Their Sites of Production

Hormones Synthesized and Secreted by Dedicated Endocrine Glands

Pituitary Gland
  Growth hormone (GH)
  Prolactin
  Adrenocorticotropic hormone (ACTH)
  Thyroid-stimulating hormone (TSH)
  Follicle-stimulating hormone (FSH)
  Luteinizing hormone (LH)

Thyroid Gland
  Tetraiodothyronine (T_4; thyroxine)
  Triiodothyronine (T_3)
  Calcitonin

Parathyroid Glands
  Parathyroid hormone (PTH)

Islets of Langerhans (Endocrine Pancreas)
  Insulin
  Glucagon
  Somatostatin

Adrenal Gland
  Epinephrine
  Norepinephrine
  Cortisol
  Aldosterone
  Dehydroepiandrosterone sulfate (DHEAS)

Hormones Synthesized by Gonads
  Ovaries
    Estradiol-17β
    Progesterone
    Inhibin
  Testes
    Testosterone
    Antimüllerian hormone (AMH)
    Inhibin

Hormones Synthesized in Organs with a Primary Function Other Than Endocrine

Brain (Hypothalamus)
  Antidiuretic hormone (ADH; vasopressin)
  Oxytocin
  Corticotropin-releasing hormone (CRH)
  Thyrotropin-releasing hormone
  Gonadotropin-releasing hormone (GnRH)
  Growth hormone–releasing hormone (GHRH)
  Somatostatin

  Dopamine

Brain (Pineal Gland)
  Melatonin

Heart
  Atrial natriuretic peptide (ANP)

Kidney
  Erythropoietin

Adipose Tissue
  Leptin
  Adiponectin

Stomach
  Gastrin
  Somatostatin
  Ghrelin

Intestines
  Secretin
  Cholecystokinin
  Glucagon-like peptide-1 (GLP-1)
  Glucagon-like peptide-2 (GLP-2)
  Glucose-dependent insulinotropic peptide (GIP; gastrin inhibitory peptide)
  Motilin

Liver
  Insulin-like growth factor-I (IGF-I)

Hormones Produced to a Significant Degree by Peripheral Conversion

Lungs
  Angiotensin II

Kidney
  1α,25-dihydroxyvitamin D

Adipose, Mammary Glands, Other Organs
  Estradiol-17β

Liver, Other Organs
  Testosterone

Genital Skin, Prostate, Sebaceous Gland, Other Organs
  5-Dihydrotestosterone (DHT)

Many Organs
  T_3

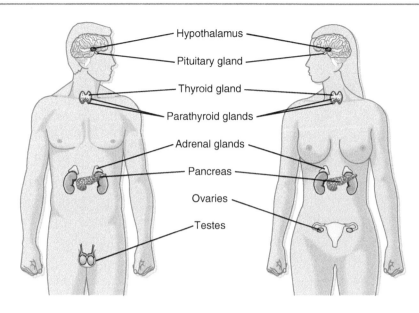

Fig. 1.1 Major glands of the endocrine system. (From Koeppen BM, Stanton BA, editors: *Berne and Levy Physiology*, 6th ed., Philadelphia, 2010, Mosby.)

3. Regulating the onset of reproductive maturity at puberty and the function of the reproductive system in the adult

In the adult, endocrine organs produce and secrete their hormones in response to **feedback control systems** that are tuned to **set-points**, or set ranges, of the levels of circulating hormones. These set-points are genetically determined but may be altered by age, circadian rhythms (24-hour cycles or diurnal rhythms), seasonal cycles, the environment, stress, inflammation, and other influences.

Major forms of endocrine disease are caused by lack of hormone (e.g., hypothyroidism), excess of hormone (e.g., hyperparathyroidism) or dysfunction of receptor (hormonal resistance). It is important to appreciate that hormones often stimulate both the differentiated function and growth of target tissues and organs. This underlies the role of hormones in driving neoplastic transformation and cancer progression (i.e., the existence of hormonally responsive cancers). The pathogenesis of these and other forms of endocrine disease are discussed in the subsequent chapters.

The material in this chapter covers generalizations common to all hormones or to specific groups of hormones. The chemical nature of the hormones and their mechanisms of action are discussed. This presentation provides the generalized information necessary to categorize the hormones and to make predictions about the most likely characteristics of a given hormone. Some of the exceptions to these generalizations are discussed later.

BOX 1.2 Characteristics of Protein/Peptide Hormones

- Synthesized as prehormones or preprohormones
- Stored in membrane-bound secretory vesicles (sometimes called *secretory granules*)
- Regulated at the level of secretion (regulated exocytosis) and synthesis
- Often circulate in blood unbound
- Usually administered by injection
- Hydrophilic and signal through transmembrane receptors

CHEMICAL NATURE OF HORMONES

Hormones are classified biochemically as **proteins/peptides, catecholamines, steroid hormones,** and **iodothyronines.** The chemical nature of a hormone determines the following:
1. How it is synthesized, stored, and released in a regulated manner
2. How it is carried in the blood
3. Its biologic half-life ($t_{1/2}$) and mode of clearance
4. Its cellular mechanism of action

Proteins/Peptides

The **protein and peptide hormones** can be grouped into structurally related molecules that are encoded by gene families (Box 1.2). Protein/peptide hormones gain their specificity from their primary amino acid sequence, which

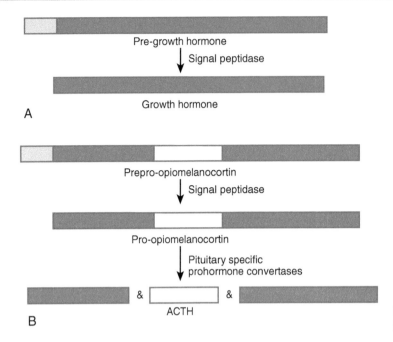

Fig. 1.2 Prehormone (A) and preprohormone (B) processing with specific examples.

confers specific higher-order structures, and from post-translational modifications, such as glycosylation.

Protein/peptide hormones are synthesized on the polyribosome as larger **preprohormones**. The nascent peptides have at their N terminus a group of 15 to 30 amino acids called the **signal peptide**, which directs the growing polypeptide through the endoplasmic reticular membrane into the cisternae. The signal peptide is enzymatically removed, and the protein is then transported from the cisternae to the Golgi apparatus, where it is packaged into a membrane-bound secretory vesicle that buds off into the cytoplasm. Posttranslational modification occurs in the endoplasmic reticulum, Golgi apparatus, and secretory vesicle.

The original gene transcript is called either a **prehormone** or a **preprohormone** (Fig. 1.2). Removing the signal peptide produces either a hormone or a prohormone. A **prohormone** is a polypeptide that requires further cleavage before the mature hormone is produced. Often this final cleavage occurs while the prohormone is within the Golgi apparatus or the secretory vesicle. Sometimes prohormones contain the sequence of multiple hormones. For example, the protein, proopiomelanocortin (POMC), contains the amino acid sequences of adrenocorticotropic hormone (ACTH) and α-melanocyte-stimulating hormone (αMSH). However, the pituitary corticotrope produces ACTH only, whereas keratinocytes and specific hypothalamic neurons produce αMSH, but not ACTH. The ability of cells to process the same prohormone into different peptides is due to cell type expression of **prohormone convertases**, resulting in cell-specific processing of the prohormone.

Protein/peptide hormones are stored in the gland as membrane-bound **secretory vesicles** and are released by exocytosis through the **regulated secretory pathway**. This means that hormones are not continually secreted, but rather that they are secreted in response to a stimulus, through a mechanism of **stimulus-secretion coupling**. Regulated exocytosis is induced by an elevation of **intracellular Ca^{2+}** along with activation of other components (e.g., small G proteins), which interact with vesicular and cell membrane components. This ultimately leads to the fusion of the secretory vesicular membrane with the cell membrane and exocytosis of the vesicular contents.

Protein/peptide hormones are soluble in aqueous solvents and, with the notable exceptions of the insulin-like growth factors (IGFs) and growth hormone (GH), circulate in the blood predominantly in an unbound form; therefore they tend to have short biologic half-lives ($t_{1/2}$). Protein hormones are removed from the circulation by receptor-mediated endocytosis and lysosomal turnover of hormone receptor complexes (see later). Many protein hormones are small enough to appear in the urine in a

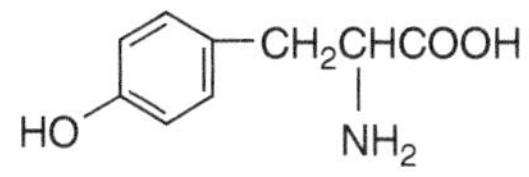

Tyrosine

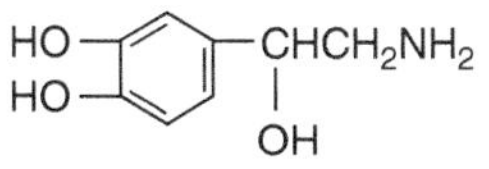

Norepinephrine

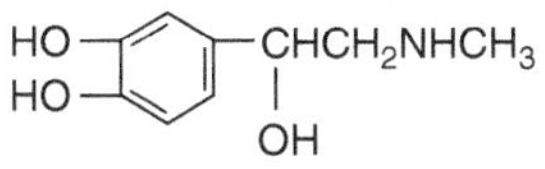

Epinephrine

Fig. 1.3 Structure of the catecholamines, norepinephrine and epinephrine, and their precursor, tyrosine.

physiologically active form. For example, follicle-stimulating hormone (FSH) and luteinizing hormone (LH) are present in urine. Pregnancy tests using human urine are based on the presence of the placental LH-like hormone, human chorionic gonadotropin (hCG).

Proteins/peptides are readily digested if administered orally. Hence, they must be administered by injection or, in the case of small peptides, through a mucous membrane (sublingually or intranasally). Because proteins/peptides do not cross cell membranes readily, they signal through transmembrane receptors.

Catecholamines

Catecholamines are synthesized by the adrenal medulla and neurons and include norepinephrine, epinephrine, and dopamine (Fig. 1.3; Box 1.3). The primary hormonal product of the adrenal medulla is epinephrine, and to a lesser extent, norepinephrine. Epinephrine is produced by enzymatic modifications of the amino acid tyrosine. Epinephrine and other catecholamines are ultimately stored in secretory vesicles that are part of the regulated secretory pathway. Epinephrine is hydrophilic and circulates either unbound or loosely bound to albumin. Epinephrine and norepinephrine are similar to protein/peptide hormones in that they signal through membrane receptors, called adrenergic receptors. Catecholamines have short biologic half-lives (a few minutes) and are inactivated by intracellular enzymes. Inactivated forms diffuse out of cells and are excreted in the urine.

BOX 1.3   Characteristics of Catecholamines

- Derived from enzymatic modification of tyrosine
- Stored in membrane-bound secretory vesicles
- Regulated at the level of secretion (regulated exocytosis) and through the regulation of the enzymatic pathway required for their synthesis
- Transported in blood free or only loosely associated with proteins
- Often administered as an aerosol puff for opening bronchioles, and several specific analogs (agonists and antagonists) can be taken orally
- Hydrophilic and signal through transmembrane G-protein-coupled receptors called *adrenergic receptors*

BOX 1.4   Characteristics of Steroid Hormones

- Derived from enzymatic modification of cholesterol
- Cannot be stored in secretory vesicles because of lipophilic nature
- Regulated at the level of the enzymatic pathway required for their synthesis
- Transported in the blood bound to transport proteins (binding globulins)
- Signal through intracellular receptors (nuclear hormone receptor family)
- Can be administered orally

Steroid Hormones

Steroid hormones are made by the adrenal cortex, ovaries, testes, and placenta (Box 1.4). Steroid hormones from these glands fall into five categories: progestins, mineralocorticoids, glucocorticoids, androgens, and estrogens (Table 1.1). Progestins and the corticoids are 21-carbon steroids, whereas androgens are 19-carbon steroids and estrogens are 18-carbon steroids. Steroid hormones also include the active metabolite of vitamin D, which is a secosteroid (see Chapter 4).

Steroid hormones are synthesized by a series of enzymatic modifications of cholesterol (Fig. 1.4). The enzymatic modifications of cholesterol are of three general types: hydroxylations, dehydrogenations/hydrogenations, and breakage of carbon-carbon bonds. The purpose of these modifications is to produce a cholesterol derivative that is sufficiently unique to be recognized by a specific receptor. Thus progestins bind to the progesterone receptor (PR), mineralocorticoids bind to the mineralocorticoid receptor (MR), glucocorticoids bind to the glucocorticoid

TABLE 1.1	Steroid Hormones			
Family	**No. of Carbons**	**Specific Hormone**	**Primary Site of Synthesis**	**Primary Receptor**
Progestin	21	Progesterone	Ovary placenta	Progesterone receptor (PR)
Glucocorticoid	21	Cortisol, Corticosterone	Adrenal cortex	Glucocorticoid receptor (GR)
Mineralocorticoid	21	Aldosterone, 11-Deoxycorticosterone	Adrenal cortex	Mineralocorticoid receptor (MR)
Androgen	19	Testosterone, Dihydrotestosterone	Testis	Androgen receptor (AR)
Estrogen	18	Estradiol-17β, Estriol	Ovary placenta	Estrogen receptor (ER)

receptor (GR), androgens bind to the **androgen receptor (AR)**, estrogens bind to the **estrogen receptor (ER)**, and the active vitamin D metabolite binds to the **vitamin D receptor (VDR)**.

The complexity of steroid hormone action is increased by the expression of multiple forms of each receptor. Additionally, there is some degree of nonspecificity between steroid hormones and the receptors they bind to. For example, glucocorticoids bind to the MR with high affinity, and progestins, glucocorticoids, and androgens can all interact with the PR, GR, and AR to some degree. An appreciation of this "cross-talk" is important to the physician who is prescribing synthetic steroids. For example, medroxyprogesterone acetate (a synthetic progesterone given for hormone replacement therapy in postmenopausal women) binds well to the AR as well as the PR. As discussed subsequently, steroid hormones are lipophilic and pass through cell membranes easily. Accordingly, classic steroid hormone receptors are localized intracellularly and act by regulating gene expression. More recently, membrane and juxtamembrane receptors have been discovered that mediate rapid, nongenomic actions of steroid hormones.

Steroidogenic cell types are defined as cells that can convert **cholesterol** to **pregnenolone**, which is the first reaction common to all steroidogenic pathways. Steroidogenic cells have some capacity for cholesterol synthesis but often obtain cholesterol from circulating **cholesterol-rich lipoproteins** (low-density lipoproteins and high-density lipoproteins; see Chapter 3). Pregnenolone is then further modified by six or fewer enzymatic reactions. Because of their hydrophobic nature, steroid hormones and precursors can leave the steroidogenic cell easily and so are not stored. Thus steroidogenesis is regulated at the level of uptake, storage, and mobilization of cholesterol and at the level of steroidogenic enzyme gene expression and activity. Steroids are *not* regulated at the level of secretion of the preformed hormone. A clinical implication of this mode of secretion is that high levels of **steroid hormone precursors**

are easily released into the blood when a *downstream* steroidogenic enzyme within a given pathway is inactive or absent (Fig. 1.5). In comparing the ultrastructure of a protein hormone–producing cell to that of a steroidogenic cell, protein hormone–producing cells store the product in secretory granules and have extensive rough endoplasmic reticula. In contrast, steroidogenic cells store the precursor (cholesterol esters) in the form of lipid droplets, but do not store the product. Steroidogenic enzymes are localized to smooth endoplasmic reticulum membrane and within mitochondria, and these two organelles are numerous in steroidogenic cells.

An important feature of steroidogenesis is that steroid hormones often undergo further modifications (apart from those involved in deactivation and excretion) after their release from the original steroidogenic cell. This is referred to as **peripheral conversion**. For example, estrogen synthesis by the ovary and placenta requires at least two cell types to complete the pathway of cholesterol to estrogen (see Chapters 10 and 11). This means that one cell secretes a precursor, and a second cell converts the precursor to estrogen. There is also considerable peripheral conversion of active steroid hormones. For example, the testis secretes sparingly little estrogen. However, adipose, muscle, and other tissues express the enzyme for converting testosterone (a potent androgen) to estradiol-17β. Peripheral conversion of steroids plays an important role in several endocrine disorders (e.g., see Fig. 1.5).

Steroid hormones are hydrophobic, and a significant fraction circulates in the blood bound to transport proteins (see later). These include albumin, but also the specific transport proteins, **sex hormone–binding globulin (SHBG)** and **corticosteroid-binding globulin (CBG)** (see later). Excretion of hormones typically involves inactivating modifications followed by glucuronide or sulfate conjugation in the liver. These modifications increase the water solubility of the steroid and decrease its affinity for transport proteins, allowing the inactivated steroid

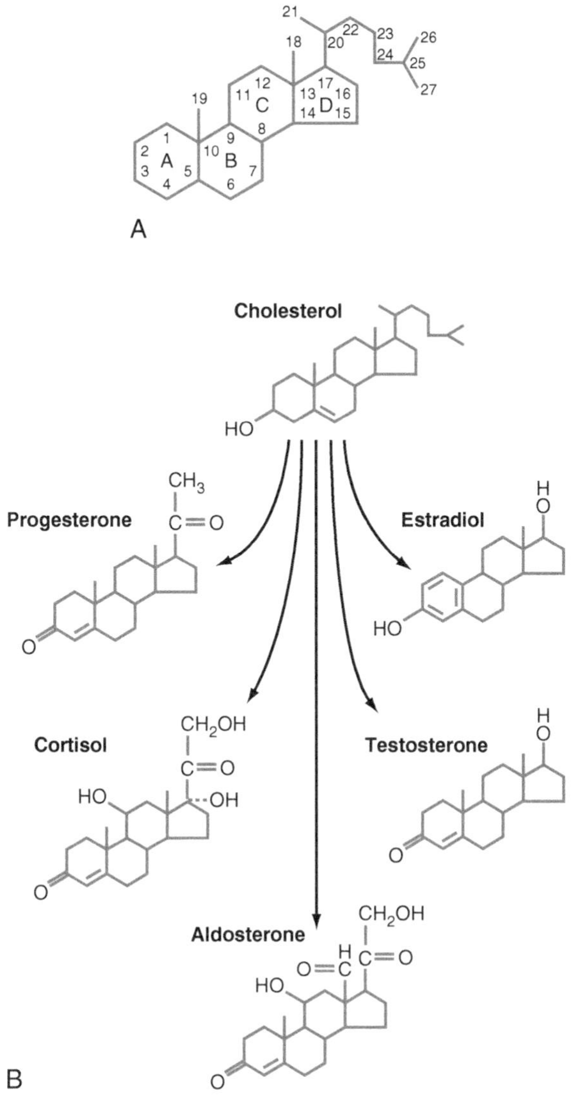

Fig. 1.4 Cholesterol (A) and steroid hormone derivatives (B). (From Koeppen BM, Stanton BA, editors: *Berne and Levy Physiology*, 6th ed., Philadelphia, 2010, Mosby.)

hormone to be excreted by the kidney. Steroid compounds are absorbed fairly readily in the GI tract and therefore often may be administered orally.

Thyroid Hormones

Thyroid hormones are classified as iodothyronines (Fig. 1.6) that are made by the coupling of iodinated tyrosine residues through an ether linkage (Box 1.5; also see Chapter 6). Their specificity is determined by the thyronine structure, but also by exactly where the thyronine is iodinated. Normally,

the predominant iodothyronine released by the thyroid is T_4 (3,5,3′,5′-tetraiodothyronine, also called **thyroxine**), which acts as a circulating precursor of the active form, T_3 (3,5,3′-triiodothyronine). Thus peripheral conversion through specific 5′-deiodination plays an important role in thyroid function (see Chapter 6). Thyroid hormones cross cell membranes by both diffusion and transport systems. They are stored extracellularly in the thyroid as an integral part of the glycoprotein molecule thyroglobulin (see Chapter 6). Thyroid hormones are sparingly soluble in blood and are transported in blood bound to **thyroid hormone–binding globulin (TBG)**. T_4 and T_3 have long half-lives of 7 days and 24 hours, respectively. Thyroid hormones are similar to steroid hormones in that the **thyroid hormone receptor (TR)** is intracellular and acts as a transcription factor. In fact, the TR belongs to the same gene family that includes steroid hormone receptors and VDRs. Thyroid hormones can be administered orally and sufficient hormone is absorbed intact to make this an effective mode of therapy.

TRANSPORT OF HORMONES IN THE CIRCULATION

A significant amount of steroid and thyroid hormones is transported in the blood bound to plasma proteins that are produced in a regulated manner by the liver. Protein and polypeptide hormones are generally transported free in the blood. There exists an equilibrium among the concentrations of bound hormone, free hormone, and plasma transport protein.

The **free hormone** is the biologically active form for target organ action, feedback control, and clearance by uptake and metabolism. Consequently, in evaluating hormonal status, one must sometimes determine free hormone levels rather than total hormone levels alone. This is particularly important because hormone transport proteins themselves are regulated by altered endocrine and disease states.

Protein binding serves several purposes. It prolongs the circulating $t_{1/2}$ of the hormone. The bound hormone represents a "reservoir" of hormone and as such can serve to buffer acute changes in hormone secretion. In addition, steroid and thyroid hormones are lipophilic and hydrophobic. Binding to transport proteins prevents these hormones from simply partitioning into the cells near their site of secretion and allows them to be transported throughout the circulation.

CELLULAR RESPONSES TO HORMONES

Hormones regulate essentially every major aspect of cellular function in every organ system. Hormones control the growth and proliferation of cells. Hormones regulate the differentiation of cells through genetic and epigenetic

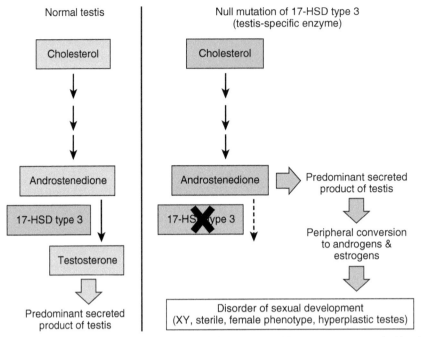

Fig. 1.5 Example of the effect of an enzyme defect on steroid hormone precursors in blood.

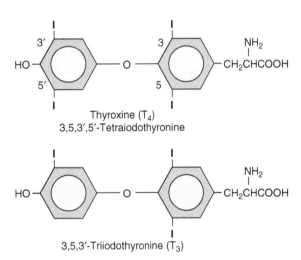

Thyroxine (T₄)
3,5,3′,5′-Tetraiodothyronine

3,5,3′-Triiodothyronine (T₃)

Fig. 1.6 Structure of thyroid hormones, which are iodinated thyronines.

BOX 1.5 **Characteristics of Thyroid Hormones**

- Derived from the iodination of tyrosines, which are coupled to form iodothyronines
- Lipophilic, but stored in thyroid follicle cells by covalent attachment to thyroglobulin
- Regulated at the level of synthesis, iodination, and secretion
- Transported in blood tightly bound to proteins
- Signal through intracellular receptors (nuclear hormone receptor family)
- Can be administered orally

changes and their ability to survive or undergo programmed cell death. Hormones influence cellular metabolism, ionic composition, and transmembrane potential. Hormones orchestrate several complex cytoskeletal-associated events, including cell shape, migration, division, exocytosis, recycling/endocytosis, and cell-cell and cell-matrix adhesion.

Hormones regulate the expression and function of cytosolic, membrane, and secreted proteins, and a specific hormone may determine the level of its own receptor, or the receptors for other hormones.

Although hormones can exert coordinated, pleiotropic control on multiple aspects of cell function, any given hormone does not regulate every function in every cell type. Rather, a single hormone controls a subset of cellular functions in only the cell types that express **receptors** for that hormone (i.e., the **target cells**). Thus selective receptor expression determines which cells will respond to a given hormone. Moreover, the differentiated epigenetic state of a specific cell will determine how it will respond to a hormone. Thus the specificity of hormonal responses resides in the structure of the hormone itself, the receptor for the hormone, and the cell type in which the receptor is expressed. Serum hormone concentrations are extremely low (picomolar to nanomolar range). Therefore a receptor must have a high affinity, as well as specificity, for its cognate hormone.

Hormone receptors fall into two general classes: transmembrane receptors and intracellular receptors that belong to the nuclear hormone receptor family.

Transmembrane Receptors

Most hormones are proteins, peptides, or catecholamines that cannot pass through the cell membrane. Thus these hormones must interact with transmembrane protein receptors. Transmembrane receptors are proteins that contain three domains (proceeding from outside to inside the cell): (1) an extracellular domain that harbors a high-affinity binding site for a specific hormone; (2) one or more hydrophobic, transmembrane domains that span the cell membrane; and (3) a cytosolic domain that is linked to signaling proteins.

Hormone binding to a transmembrane receptor induces a conformational shift in all three domains of the receptor protein. This hormone receptor binding–induced conformational change is referred to as a signal. The signal is transduced into the activation of one or more intracellular signaling molecules. Signaling molecules then act on effector proteins, which, in turn, modify specific cellular functions. The combination of hormone receptor binding (signal), activation of signaling molecules (transduction), and the regulation of one or more effector proteins is referred to as a signal transduction pathway (also called simply a signaling pathway), and the final integrated outcome is referred to as the cellular response.

Signaling pathways linked to transmembrane receptors are usually characterized by the following:

A. Receptor binding followed by a conformational shift that extends to the cytosolic domain. The conformational shift may result in one or more of the following:
   1. Activation of a guanine exchange function of a receptor.
   2. Homodimerization and/or heterodimerization of receptors to other receptors or coreceptors within the membrane.
   3. Recruitment and activation of signaling proteins by the cytosolic domain.

B. Multiple, hierarchal steps in which *downstream* effector proteins are dependent on and driven by *upstream* receptors and signaling molecules and effector proteins. This means that loss or inactivation of one or more components within the pathway leads to hormonal resistance, whereas constitutive activation or overexpression of components can provoke a cellular response in a hormone-independent, unregulated manner.

C. Amplification of the initial hormone receptor binding–induced signal, usually by inclusion of an enzymatic step within a signaling pathway. Amplification can be so great that maximal response to a hormone is achieved upon hormone binding to a fraction of available receptors.

D. Activation of multiple divergent or convergent pathways from one hormone receptor–binding event. For example, binding of insulin to its receptor activates three separate signaling pathways.

E. Antagonism by constitutive and regulated negative feedback reactions. This means that a signal is dampened or terminated by opposing pathways. Gain of function of opposing pathways can result in hormonal resistance.

Signaling pathways use several common modes of informational transfer (i.e., intracellular messengers and signaling events). These include the following:

1. Conformational shifts. Many signaling components are proteins and have the ability to toggle between two (or more) conformational states that alter their activity, stability, or intracellular location. As discussed previously, signaling begins with hormone receptor binding that induces a conformational change in the receptor (Fig. 1.7). The other modes of informational transfer discussed later either regulate or are regulated by conformational shifts in transmembrane receptors and in downstream signaling proteins.

2. Covalent phosphorylation of proteins and lipids (Fig. 1.8). Enzymes that phosphorylate proteins or lipids are called kinases, whereas those that catalyze dephosphorylation are called phosphatases. Protein kinases and phosphatases can be classified as either tyrosine-specific kinases and phosphatases or serine/threonine-specific kinases and phosphatases. There are also *mixed function* kinases and phosphatases that recognize all three residues. An important lipid kinase is phosphatidylinositol-3-kinase (PI3K; see later). The phosphorylated state of a signaling component can alter the following:
   a. Activity. Phosphorylation can activate or deactivate a substrate, and proteins often have multiple sites of phosphorylation that induce quantitative and/or qualitative changes in the protein's activity.
   b. Stability. For example, phosphorylation of proteins can induce their subsequent ubiquitination and proteasomal degradation.
   c. Subcellular location. For example, the phosphorylation of some nuclear transcription factors induces their translocation to and retention in the cytoplasm.

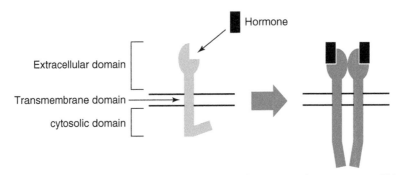

Fig. 1.7 Example of hormone-induced conformational change in transmembrane receptor. This often promotes dimerization of receptors as well as conformational changes in the cytosolic domain that unmasks a specific activity (e.g., guanine nucleotide exchange factor activity, tyrosine kinase activity).

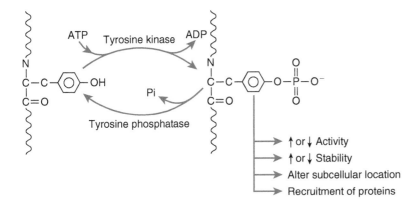

Fig. 1.8 Phosphorylation/dephosphorylation in signal transduction pathways. In this case phosphotyrosine is shown.

d. **Recruitment and clustering of other signaling proteins.** For example, phosphorylation of the cytosolic domain of a transmembrane receptor often induces the recruitment of signaling proteins to the receptor where they are phosphorylated. Recruitment happens because the recruited protein harbors a domain that specifically recognizes and binds to the phosphorylated residue. Another important example of recruitment by phosphorylation is the recruitment of the protein kinase Akt/PKB to the cell membrane, where it is phosphorylated and activated by the protein kinase, PDK1. In this case Akt/PKB and PDK1 are recruited to the cell membrane by the phosphorylated membrane lipid, phosphatidylinositol 3,4,5-triphosphate (PIP$_3$).

3. **Covalent acetylation/deacetylation of proteins.** Acetylation (as well as phosphorylation) of histones and other chromatin proteins imparts **epigenetic regulation** by altering chromatin structure and accessibility in a regulated and, in some cases, heritable manner. Many extranuclear proteins are also regulated by their degree of acetylation. **Acetyl transferases** drive acetylation, whereas **deacetylases** drive deacetylation. A major deacetylase family is comprised of the seven **sirtuins (SIRTs)**.

4. **Noncovalent guanosine nucleotide triphosphate (GTP) binding to GTP-binding proteins (G proteins).** G proteins represent a large family of molecular switches, which are latent and inactive when bound to GDP, and active when bound to GTP (Fig. 1.9). G proteins are activated by **guanine nucleotide exchange factors (GEFs)**, which promote the dissociation of GDP and binding of GTP. G proteins have intrinsic **GTPase** activity. GTP is normally hydrolyzed to GDP within seconds by the G protein, thereby terminating the transducing activity of the G protein. Another G-protein termination mechanism (which represents a target for drug development to treat certain endocrine diseases) is the family of proteins called **regulators of G-protein signaling (RGS proteins)**, which bind to active G proteins and increase their intrinsic GTPase activity.

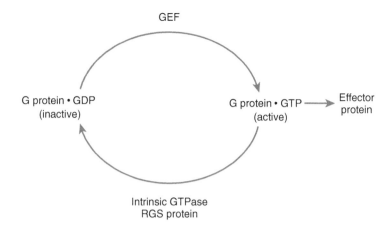

Fig. **1.9** G proteins in signal transduction pathways. *GEF,* Guanine nucleotide exchange factor; *RGS,* regulator of G-protein signaling.

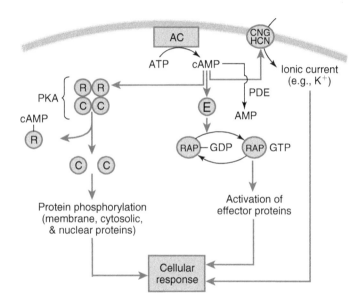

Fig. **1.10** Cyclic AMP/PKA in signal transduction pathways. *AC,* Adenylyl cyclase; *PDE,* phosphodiesterase; *R & C,* regulatory and catalytic subunits, respectively, of protein kinase A (PKA); *E,* Epac (exchange protein activated by cAMP); *CNG,* cyclic nucleotide–gated channel; *HCN,* hyperpolarization-induced cyclic nucleotide–modulated channel.

5. **Noncovalent binding of cyclic nucleotide monophosphates to their specific effector proteins (Fig. 1.10).** Cyclic adenosine monophosphate (cAMP) is generated from adenosine triphosphate (ATP) by **adenylyl cyclase,** which is primarily a membrane protein. Adenylyl cyclase is activated and inhibited by the G proteins, Gs-α and Gi-α, respectively (see later). There are three general intracellular effectors of cyclic AMP (cAMP):

a. cAMP binds to the regulatory subunit of **protein kinase A (PKA;** also called **cAMP-dependent protein kinase).** Inactive PKA is a heterotetramer composed of two catalytic subunits and two regulatory subunits. cAMP binding causes the regulatory subunits to dissociate from the catalytic subunits, thereby generating two molecules of active catalytic PKA subunits (PKA$_c$). PKA$_c$ phosphorylates numerous proteins on serine and threonine residues.

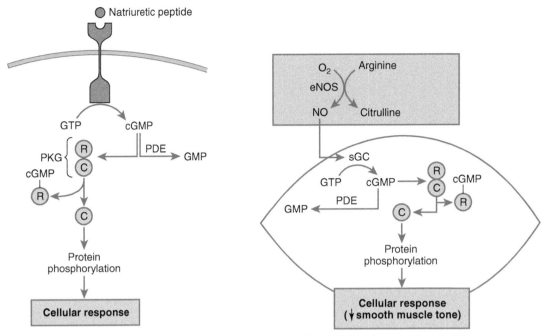

Fig. 1.11 Membrane-bound and soluble guanylyl cyclases. *R* and *C*, Regulatory and catalytic subunits, respectively, of protein kinase G (PKG). *eNOS*, endothelial nitric oxide synthase; *NO*, nitric oxide; *sGC*, soluble guanylyl cyclase.

Substrates of PKA$_c$ include numerous cytosolic proteins as well as transcription factors, most notably **cAMP-responsive element–binding protein (CREB protein)**.

b. A second effector of cAMP is **Epac (exchange protein activated by cAMP)**, which has two isoforms. Epac proteins act as GEFs (see earlier) for small G proteins (called Raps). Raps in turn control a wide array of cell functions, including formation of cell-cell junctional complexes and cell-matrix adhesion, Ca^{2+} release from intracellular stores (especially in cardiac muscle), and in the augmentation of glucose-dependent insulin secretion by glucagon-like peptide-1 in pancreatic islet β cells (see Chapter 3).

c. cAMP (and cyclic guanosine monophosphate [cGMP], discussed later) also binds directly to and regulates **ion channels**. These are of two types: **cyclic nucleotide gated (CNG) channels** and **hyperpolarization-activated cyclic nucleotide modulated (HCN) channels**. For example, norepinephrine, which acts through a Gs-coupled receptor, increases heart rate in part through increasing a depolarizing inward K$^+$ and Na$^+$ current via an HCN at the sinoatrial node.

cGMP is produced from GTP by **guanylyl cyclase**, which exists in both transmembrane and soluble forms (Fig. 1.11). The transmembrane form of guanylyl cyclase is a hormone receptor, **natriuretic peptide receptor (NPR-A and NPR-B)**, for the **natriuretic peptides (atrial = ANP; brain = BNP; C-type = CNP)**. The soluble form of guanylyl cyclase is activated by another messenger, **nitric oxide (NO)**. Nitric oxide is produced from molecular oxygen and arginine by the enzyme **nitric oxide synthase (NOS)**. In vascular endothelial cells, endothelial NOS (eNOS) activity is the target of vasodilatory neuronal signals (e.g., acetylcholine) and certain hormones (estrogen). NO then diffuses into vascular smooth muscle and activates soluble guanylyl cyclase to produce cGMP. cGMP activates **protein kinase G (PKG)**, which phosphorylates and regulates numerous proteins. In vascular smooth muscle, this leads to relaxation and vasodilation. As discussed earlier, cGMP also regulates ion channels. cAMP and cGMP are degraded to AMP and GMP, respectively, by **phosphodiesterases** (see Figs. 1.10 and 1.11), thereby terminating their signaling function. Phosphodiesterases represent a large family of proteins and display cell-specific expression. cAMP phosphodiesterases are inhibited by caffeine and other methylxanthines. cGMP is degraded by cGMP phosphodiesterases, of which one isoform is inhibited by sildenafil

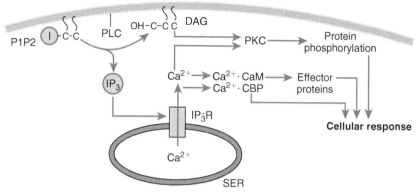

Fig. 1.12 IP_3 (inositol 1,4,5-triphosphate) and DAG (diacylglycerol) in signaling pathways. *CaM,* Calmodulin; *CBP,* calcium-binding proteins; *IP$_3$R,* IP$_3$ receptor; *PIP$_2$,* phosphatidylinositol 4,5-bisphosphate; *PLC,* phospholipase C; *SER,* smooth endoplasmic reticulum.

(Viagra). In some contexts, cAMP and cGMP can modulate each other (a phenomenon called **cross-talk**) through the regulation of phosphodiesterases. For example, oocyte arrest is maintained by high levels of cAMP. The LH surge decreases cGMP in surrounding follicle cells by decreasing the local production of a natriuretic peptide. This results in lowered oocyte cyclic GMP. Because cGMP inhibits the oocyte cAMP-specific phosphodiesterase, lowered cGMP leads to decreased cAMP, thereby allowing the oocyte to complete the first meiotic division (see Chapter 10).

6. Generation of lipid informational molecules, which act as intracellular messengers. These include diacylglycerol (DAG) and inositol 1,4,5-triphosphate (IP_3), which are cleaved from phosphatidylinositol 4,5-bisphosphate (PIP$_2$) by membrane-bound phospholipase C (PLC). DAG activates certain isoforms of protein kinase C (Fig. 1.12). IP_3 binds to the IP_3 receptor, which is a large complex forming a Ca^{2+} channel, on the endoplasmic reticulum membrane, and promotes Ca^{2+} efflux (see later) from the endoplasmic reticulum into the cytoplasm. Some isoforms of DAG-activated PKC are also Ca^{2+} dependent, so the actions of IP_3 converge on and reinforce those of DAG. The DAG signal is terminated by lipases, whereas IP_3 is rapidly inactivated by dephosphorylation.

7. **Noncovalent Ca^{2+} binding** (see Fig. 1.12). Cytosolic levels of Ca^{2+} are maintained at very low levels (i.e., 10^{-7} to 10^{-8} M), by either active transport of Ca^{2+} out of the cell, or into intracellular compartments (e.g., endoplasmic reticulum). As discussed earlier, IP_3 binding to the IP_3 receptor increases the flow of Ca^{2+} into the cytoplasm from the endoplasmic reticulum. Ca^{2+} can also enter the cytoplasm through the regulated opening of Ca^{2+} channels in the cell membrane.

This leads to an increase in Ca^{2+} binding directly to numerous specific effector proteins, which leads to a change in their activities. Additionally, Ca^{2+} regulates several effector proteins indirectly, through binding to the signaling protein, calmodulin. Several of the Ca^{2+}/calmodulin targets are enzymes, which amplify the initial signal of increased cytosolic Ca^{2+}. The Ca^{2+}-dependent signal is terminated by the lowering of cytosolic Ca^{2+} by cell membrane and endoplasmic reticular Ca^{2+} ATPases (i.e., Ca^{2+} pumps).

Transmembrane Receptors Using G Proteins

The largest family of hormone receptors is the **G-protein-coupled receptor (GPCR)** family. These receptors span the cell membrane seven times and are referred to as *7-helix transmembrane receptors.* The G proteins that directly interact with GPCRs are termed **heterotrimeric G proteins** and are composed of an α subunit (Gα), and a β/γ subunit dimer (Gβ/γ). The Gα subunit binds GTP and functions as the primary G-protein signal transducer. GPCRs are, in fact, ligand-activated GEFs (see earlier). This means that on hormone binding, the conformation of the receptor shifts to the active state. Once active, the GPCR induces the exchange of GDP for GTP, thereby activating Gα. One hormone-bound receptor activates 100 or more G proteins. GTP-bound Gα then dissociates from Gβ/γ and binds to and activates one or more effector proteins (Fig. 1.13).

How do G proteins link specific hormone receptor–binding events with specific downstream effector proteins? There are at least 16 Gα proteins that show specificity with respect to cell-type expression, GPCR binding, and effector protein activation. A rather ubiquitous Gα protein is called **Gs-α**, which stimulates the membrane enzyme, adenylyl cyclase, and increases the levels of another messenger,

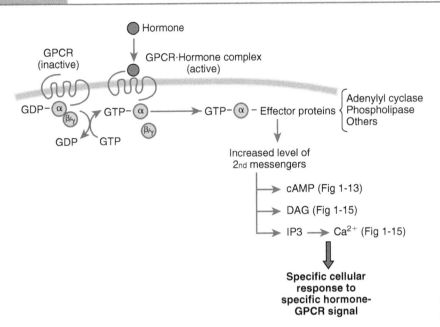

Fig. 1.13 Signaling pathway for hormones that bind to GPCRs.

cAMP (see earlier). Some GPCRs couple to Gi-α, which inhibits adenylyl cyclase. A third major hormonal signaling pathway is through Gq-α, which activates phospholipase C (PLC). As discussed previously, PLC generates two lipid messengers, DAG and IP$_3$, from PIP$_2$. Defects in G-protein structure and expression are linked to endocrine diseases such as pseudohypoparathyroidism (loss of Gs activity) or pituitary tumors (loss of intrinsic GTPase activity in Gs, thereby extending its time in the active state).

GPCR-dependent signaling pathways regulate a broad range of cellular responses. For example, the pancreatic hormone, glucagon, regulates numerous aspects of hepatic metabolism (see Chapter 3). The glucagon receptor is linked to the Gs-cAMP-PKA pathway, which diverges to regulate enzyme activity at both posttranslational and transcriptional levels. PKA phosphorylates and thereby activates phosphorylase kinase. Phosphorylase kinase phosphorylates and activates glycogen phosphorylase, which catalyzes the release of glucose molecules from glycogen. Catalytic subunits of PKA also enter the nucleus, where they phosphorylate and activate the transcription factor, CREB protein. Phospho-CREB then increases the transcriptional rate of genes encoding specific enzymes (e.g., phosphoenolpyruvate carboxykinase).

In summary, signaling from one GPCR can regulate a number of targets in different cellular compartments with different kinetics (Fig. 1.14).

As mentioned, G-protein signaling is terminated by intrinsic GTPase activity, converting GTP to GDP. This returns the G protein to an inactive state (bound to GDP). Another termination mechanism involves desensitization and endocytosis of the GPCR (Fig. 1.15). Hormone binding to the receptor increases the ability of GPCR kinases (GRKs) to phosphorylate the intracellular domain of GPCRs. This phosphorylation recruits proteins called β-arrestins. GRK-induced phosphorylation and β-arrestin binding inactivate the receptor, and β-arrestin couples the receptor to clathrin-mediated endocytotic machinery. Some GPCRs are dephosphorylated and rapidly recycled back to the cell membrane (without hormone), whereas others are degraded in lysosomes. GRK/β-arrestin-dependent inactivation and endocytosis is an important mechanism for hormonal desensitization of a cell after exposure to excessive hormone. Hormone receptor endocytosis (also called *receptor-mediated endocytosis*) is also an important mechanism for clearing protein and peptide hormones from the blood.

Receptor Tyrosine Kinases

Receptor tyrosine kinases (RTKs) can be classified into two groups: the first acting as receptors for several growth factors (e.g., epidermal growth factor, platelet-derived growth factor), and the second group for insulin and IGFs. The former group of RTKs comprises transmembrane glycoproteins with an intracellular domain containing intrinsic tyrosine kinase activity. Growth factor binding induces dimerization of the RTK within the cell membrane, followed by transphosphorylation of tyrosine residues, generating phosphotyrosine (pY). The phosphotyrosines

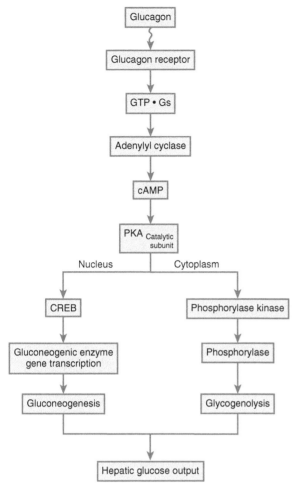

Fig. 1.14 Coordinated regulation of cytoplasmic and nuclear events by PKA to produce a general cellular response.

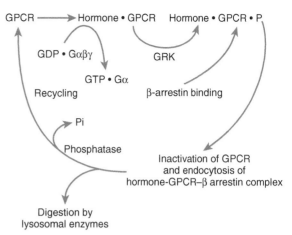

Fig. 1.15 GPCR inactivation and endocytosis to lysosomes (desensitization) and/or recycling back to the cell membrane in a dephosphorylated form (resensitization).

function to recruit proteins. One recruited protein is phospholipase C, which is then activated by phosphorylation and generates the messengers DAG and IP_3 from PIP_2 (see earlier). A second critically important protein that is recruited to pY residues is the adapter protein, Grb2, which is complexed with a GEF named SOS. Recruitment of SOS to the membrane allows it to activate a small, membrane-bound monomeric G protein called Ras. Ras then binds to its effector protein, Raf. Raf is a serine-specific kinase that phosphorylates and activates the dual-function kinase, MEK. MEK then phosphorylates and activates a mitogen-activated protein kinase (MAP kinase, also called ERK). Activated MAP kinases then enter the nucleus and phosphorylate and activate several transcription factors. This signaling pathway is referred to as the *MAP kinase cascade,* and it transduces and amplifies a growth factor–RTK

signal into a cellular response involving a change in the expression of genes encoding proteins involved in proliferation and survival.

The insulin receptor (IR) differs from growth factor RTKs in several respects. First, the latent IR is already dimerized by Cys-Cys bonds, and insulin binding induces a conformational change that leads to transphosphorylation of the cytoplasmic domains (Fig. 1.16). A major recruited protein to pY residues is the insulin receptor substrate (IRS), which is then phosphorylated on tyrosine residues by the IR. The pY residues on IRS recruit the Grb2-2/SOS complex, thereby activating growth responses to insulin through the MAP kinase pathway (see Fig. 1.16). The pY residues on the IRS also recruit the lipid kinase, PI3K, activating and concentrating the kinase near its substrate, PIP_2, in the cell membrane. As discussed earlier, this ultimately leads to activation of Akt/PKB, which is required for the metabolic responses to insulin (Fig. 1.17). The IR also activates a pathway involving the small G protein, TC-10 (see Fig. 1.17). The small G-protein-dependent pathway and the Akt/PKB pathway are both required for the actions of insulin on glucose uptake (see Chapter 3).

RTKs are downregulated by ligand-induced endocytosis. Additionally, the signaling pathways from RTKs, including IR and IRS, are inhibited by serine/threonine phosphorylation, tyrosine dephosphorylation, and the suppressor of cytokine signaling proteins (see next section).

Receptors Associated with Cytoplasmic Tyrosine Kinases

Another class of membrane receptor falls into the cytokine receptor family and includes receptors for GH, prolactin, erythropoietin, and leptin. These receptors, which

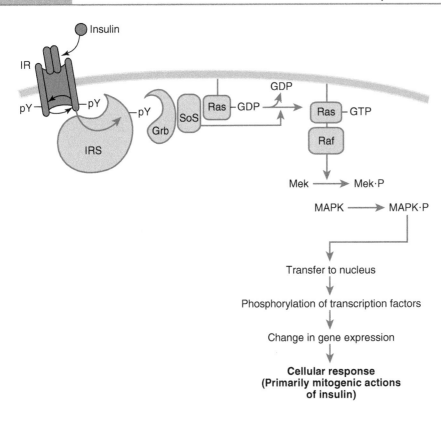

Fig. 1.16 Signaling from the insulin receptor (a receptor tyrosine kinase) through the MAPK pathway. *pY*, Phosphorylated tyrosine residue in protein.

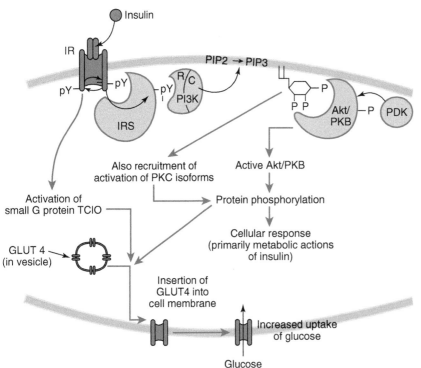

Fig. 1.17 Signaling from the insulin receptor through the phosphatidylinositol-3-kinase (PI3K)/Akt/PKB pathway. PIP_2, Phosphatidylinositol 4,5-bisphosphate; PIP_3, Phosphatidylinositol 3,4,5 trisphosphate; *PKC*, protein kinase C; *pY*, phosphorylated tyrosine residue in protein; *R* and *C*; regulatory and catalytic subunits, respectively, of PI3K.

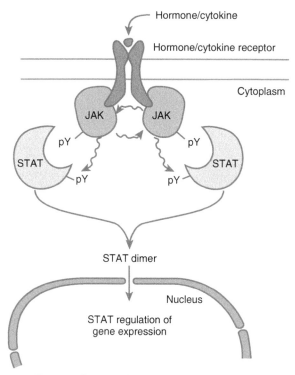

Fig. 1.18 Signaling from cytokine receptor family.

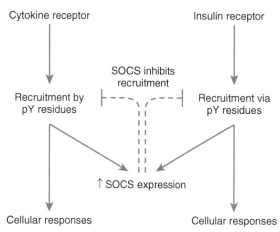

Fig. 1.19 Role of suppressor of cytokine signaling (SOCS) protein in terminating signals from cytokine family and insulin receptors.

exist as dimers, do not have intrinsic protein kinase activity. Instead, the cytoplasmic domains are stably associated with members of the JAK kinase family (Fig. 1.18). Hormone binding induces a conformational change, bringing the two JAKs associated with the dimerized receptor closer together and causing their transphosphorylation and activation. JAKs then phosphorylate tyrosine residues on the cytoplasmic domains of the receptor. The pY residues recruit latent transcription factors called STAT (signal transducers and activators of transcription) proteins. STATs become phosphorylated by JAKs, which causes them to dissociate from the receptor, dimerize, and translocate into the nucleus, where they regulate gene expression.

A negative feedback loop has been identified for JAK/STAT signaling. STATs stimulate expression of one or more suppressors of cytokine signaling (SOCS) proteins. SOCS proteins compete with STATs for binding to the pY residues on cytokine receptors (Fig. 1.19). This terminates the signaling pathway at the step of STAT activation. Recent studies show that a SOCS protein is induced by insulin signaling. SOCS 3 protein plays a role in terminating the signal from the IR, but also in reducing insulin sensitivity in hyperinsulinemic patients.

Receptor Serine/Threonine Kinase Receptors

One group of transmembrane receptors are bound and activated by members of the transforming growth factor (TGF)-β family, which includes the hormones antimüllerian hormone and inhibin. Unbound receptors exist as dissociated heterodimers, called RI and RII (Fig. 1.20). Hormone binding to RII induces dimerization of RII with RI, and RII activates RI by phosphorylation. RI then activates latent transcription factors called Smads. Activated Smads heterodimerize with a Co-Smad, enter the nucleus, and regulate specific gene expression.

Membrane Guanylyl Cyclase Receptors

As discussed previously, the membrane-bound forms of guanylyl cyclase constitute a family of a receptors for natriuretic peptides (see Fig. 1.11). The hormonal role of atrial natriuretic peptide (ANP) will be discussed in Chapter 7.

Signaling from Intracellular Receptors

Steroid hormones, thyroid hormones, and 1,25-dihydroxyvitamin D act primarily through intracellular receptors. These receptors are structurally similar and are members of the nuclear hormone receptor superfamily that includes receptors for steroid hormones, thyroid hormone, lipid-soluble vitamins, peroxisome proliferator–activated receptors (PPARs), and other metabolic receptors (liver X receptor, farnesyl X receptor).

Nuclear hormone receptors act as transcriptional regulators. This means that the signal of hormone receptor binding is transduced ultimately into a change in the transcriptional rate of a subset of the genes that are expressed within a differentiated cell type. One receptor binds to a specific DNA sequence, called a hormone response element,

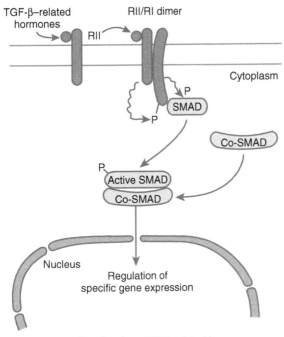

TGF-β–related
hormones

RII/RI dimer

RII

Cytoplasm

P

SMAD

P

Co-SMAD

P

Active SMAD

Co-SMAD

Nucleus

Regulation of
specific gene expression

Fig. 1.20 Signaling from TGF-β-related hormones.

often close to the promoter of one gene, and influences the rate of transcription of that gene in a hormone-dependent manner (see later). However, multiple hormone receptor–binding events are collectively transduced into the regulation of several genes. Moreover, regulation by one hormone usually includes activation and repression of the transcription of many genes in a given cell type. Note that we have already discussed examples of signaling to transcription factors by transmembrane receptors. Table 1.2 summarizes the four general modes of hormonal regulation of gene transcription.

Nuclear hormone receptors have three major structural domains: an **amino terminus domain (ATD), a middle DNA-binding domain (DBD), and a carboxyl terminus ligand-binding domain (LBD)** (Fig. 1.21). The amino terminus domain contains a hormone-independent transcriptional activation domain. The DNA-binding domain contains two zinc finger motifs, which represent small loops organized by Zn^{2+} binding to four cysteine residues at the base of each loop. The two zinc fingers and neighboring amino acids confer the ability to recognize and bind to specific DNA sequences, which are called **hormone-response elements (HREs)**. The **carboxyl terminal ligand-binding domain** contains several subdomains:

TABLE 1.2	Mechanisms by Which Hormones Regulate Gene Expression			
Hormone Type	**Steroid Hormones**	**Thyroid Hormones**	**Catecholamines, Peptides, Proteins**	**Catecholamines, Peptides, Proteins**
Cell membrane	Passes through cell membrane	Passes through cell membrane, possibly use transporter	Binds to extracellular domain of trans-membrane receptor	Binds to extracellular domain of transmembrane receptor
Cytoplasm	Binds to receptor, HRC translocates to nucleus	Moves through cytoplasm directly to nucleus to bind receptor	Ultimately activates cytoplasmic protein kinase, translocates to the nucleus	Activates a latent transcription factor in cytoplasm, TF translocates to the nucleus
Nucleus	HRC binds to response elements (often as dimer), recruits coregulatory proteins and alters gene expression	Hormone binds to receptor already bound to response elements, HRC induces exchange of coregulatory proteins, alters gene expression	Phosphorylates TF, which binds to DNA and recruits coregulatory proteins, alters gene expression	TF binds to DNA and recruits coregulatory proteins, alters gene expression
Examples	Cortisol	T_3	Glucagon	Growth hormone

HRC, Hormone-receptor complex; *TF,* transcription factor.

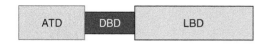

ATD (Amino Terminus Domain)
• Ligand-independent association with coregulatory proteins
• Ligand-independent phosphorylation sites

DBD (DNA Binding Domain)
• DNA binding via zinc finger domains
• Dimerization

LBD (Ligand Binding Domain)
• Ligand-binding
• Ligand-dependent association with coregulatory proteins
• Dimerization
• Nuclear translocation
• Association with chaperone proteins

Fig. 1.21 Domains of nuclear hormone receptor.

1. Site of hormone recognition and binding
2. Hormone-dependent transcriptional activation domain
3. Nuclear translocation signal
4. Binding domain for heat-shock proteins
5. Dimerization subdomain

There are numerous variations in the details of nuclear receptor mechanisms of action. Two generalized pathways by which nuclear hormone receptors increase gene transcription are the following (Fig. 1.22):

Pathway 1: Unactivated receptor is cytoplasmic or nuclear and binds DNA and recruits coactivator proteins on hormone binding. This mode is observed for the ER, PR, GR, MR, and AR (i.e., steroid hormone receptors). In the absence of hormone, some of these receptors are held in the cytoplasm through an interaction with **chaperone proteins** (so-called **heat-shock proteins** because their levels increase in response to elevated temperatures and other stresses). Chaperone proteins maintain the stability of the nuclear receptor in an inactive configuration. Hormone binding induces a conformational change in the receptor, causing its dissociation from heat-shock proteins. This exposes the nuclear localization signal and dimerization domains, so receptors dimerize and enter the nucleus. Once in the nucleus, these receptors bind to their respective HREs. The HREs for the PR, GR, MR, and AR are inverted repeats with the recognition sequence, AGAACANNNTGTTCT. Specificity is conferred by neighboring base sequences and possibly by receptor interaction with other transcriptional factors in the context of a specific gene promoter. The ER usually binds to an inverted repeat with the recognition sequence, AGGTCANNNTGACCT. The specific HREs are also referred to as an **estrogen-response element (ERE)**, progesterone-response element (PRE), glucocorticoid-response element (GRE), mineralocorticoid-response element (MRE), and **androgen-response element (ARE)**. Once bound to their respective HREs, these receptors recruit other proteins, called **coregulatory proteins**, which are either **coactivators** or **corepressors**. Coactivators act to recruit other components of the transcriptional machinery and probably activate some of these components. Coactivators also possess intrinsic histone acetyltransferase (HAT) activity, which acetylates histones in the region of the promoter. Histone acetylation relaxes chromatin coiling, making that region more accessible to transcriptional machinery. Although the mechanistic details are beyond the scope of this chapter, the student should appreciate that steroid receptors can also repress gene transcription through recruitment of corepressors that possess **histone deacetylase (HDAC)** activity and that transcriptional activation and repression pathways are induced concomitantly in the same cell. HDAC inhibitors are being studied in the context of treating some cancers because they restart the expression of silenced tumor suppressor genes.

Pathway 2: Receptor is always in nucleus and exchanges corepressors with coactivators on hormone binding. This pathway is used by the **thyroid hormone receptors (THRs)**, VDRs, **PPARs**, and **retinoic acid receptors**. For example, the THR is bound, usually as a heterodimer, with the retinoic acid X receptor (RXR). In the absence of thyroid hormone, the THR/RXR recruits corepressors. As stated earlier, corepressors recruit proteins with histone deacetylase (HDAC) activity. In contrast to histone acetylation, histone deacetylation allows tighter coiling of chromatin, which makes promoters in that region less accessible to the transcriptional machinery. Thus THR/RXR heterodimers are bound to **thyroid hormone response elements (TREs)** in the absence of hormone and maintain the expression of neighboring genes at a "repressed" level. Thyroid hormone (and other ligands of this class) readily move into the nucleus and bind to their receptors. Thyroid hormone binding induces dissociation of corepressor proteins, thereby increasing gene expression to a *basal* level. The hormone receptor complex subsequently recruits coactivator proteins, which further increase transcriptional activity to the "stimulated" level.

Termination of steroid hormone receptor signaling is poorly understood but appears to involve phosphorylation, ubiquitination, and proteasomal degradation. Circulating steroid and thyroid hormones are cleared as described previously.

In summary, hormones signal to cells through membrane or intracellular receptors. Membrane receptors have rapid effects on cellular processes (e.g., enzyme activity, cytoskeletal arrangement) that are independent of new

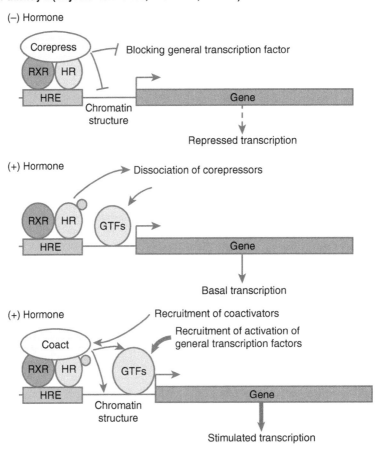

Fig. 1.22 Two general mechanisms by which nuclear receptor and hormone complexes increase gene transcription. *Coact*, Coactivator proteins; *corepress*, corepressor proteins; *GTFs*, general transcription factors; *HR*, hormone receptor; *HRE*, hormone response element; *RXR*, retinoid X receptor.

protein synthesis. Membrane receptors can also rapidly regulate gene expression through either mobile kinases (e.g., PKA, MAPKs) or mobile transcription factors (e.g., STATs, Smads). Steroid hormones have slower, longer-term effects that involve chromatin remodeling and changes in gene expression. Increasing evidence points to rapid, nongenomic effects of steroid hormones as well, but these pathways are still being elucidated.

The presence of a functional receptor is an absolute requirement for hormone action, and loss of a receptor produces essentially the same symptoms as loss of hormone. In addition to the receptor, there are fairly complex pathways involving numerous intracellular messengers and effector proteins. Accordingly, endocrine diseases can arise from abnormal expression or activity of any of these signal transduction pathway components.

Overview of the Termination Signals

Most of what has been discussed in this chapter describes the stimulatory arm of signal transduction. As noted earlier, all signal transduction of hormonal signals must have termination mechanisms to avoid sustained and uncontrolled stimulation of target cells. Part of this stems from the cessation of the original stimulus for increasing a hormone's level, and mechanisms to clear the hormone (i.e., removal of signal). However, there exists a wide array of intracellular mechanisms that terminate the signaling pathway within the target cells. Some of these are listed in Table 1.3. Note that overactivity of terminating mechanisms can lead to hormonal resistance.

TABLE 1.3 Some Modes of Signal Transduction Termination

Mechanism of Signal Transduction Termination	Example
Receptor-mediated endocytosis linked to lysosomal degradation	Many transmembrane receptors
Phosphorylation/dephosphorylation of receptor or "downstream" components of signaling pathway	Serine phosphorylation of insulin receptor and insulin receptor substrate by other signaling pathways
Ubiquitination/proteasomal degradation	Steroid hormone receptors
Binding of an inhibitory regulatory factor	Regulatory subunit of PKA
Intrinsic terminating enzymatic activity	GTPase activity of G proteins

SUMMARY

1. The **endocrine system** is composed of:
   - Dedicated hormone-producing glands (pituitary, thyroid, parathyroid, and adrenal)
   - Hypothalamic neuroendocrine neurons
   - Scattered endocrine cells that exist as clusters of endocrine-only cells (islets of Langerhans) or as cells within organs that are have a nonendocrine primary function (pancreas, GI tract, kidney)
   - **Testes** and **ovaries**, whose intrinsic endocrine function is absolutely necessary for gametogenesis
2. Endocrine signaling involves the secretion of a chemical messenger, called a **hormone**, that circulates in the blood and reaches an equilibrium with the extracellular fluid. Hormones alter many functions of their target cells, tissues, and organs through specific, high-affinity interactions with their **receptors**.
3. Protein/peptide hormones:
   - Are produced on ribosomes, become inserted into the cisternae of the endoplasmic reticulum, transit the Golgi apparatus, and finally are stored in membrane-bound secretory vesicles. The release of these vesicles represents a **regulated mode of exocytosis**. Each hormone is first made as a **prehormone**, containing a signal peptide that guides the elongating polypeptide into the cisternae of the endoplasmic reticulum.
   - Are frequently synthesized as **preprohormones**. After removal of the signal peptide, the **prohormone** is processed by **prohormone convertases**.
   - Typically do not cross cell membranes and act through **transmembrane receptors** (see later).
   - Mostly circulate as **free hormones**, and are excreted in the urine or cleared by **receptor-mediated endocytosis** and lysosomal degradation.
4. Catecholamine hormones:
   - Include the hormones, **epinephrine (Epi)** and **norepinephrine (Norepi)**. Epi and Norepi are derivatives of tyrosine, which is enzymatically modified by several reactions. Ultimately, Epi and Norepi are stored in a secretory vesicle and are released through regulated exocytosis.

- Act through transmembrane GPCRs receptors called **adrenergic receptors**.
5. Steroid hormones:
   - Include cortisol (glucocorticoid), aldosterone (mineralocorticoid), testosterone, and dihydrotestosterone (androgens), estradiol (estrogen), progesterone (progestin), and 1,25 dihydroxyvitamin D_3 (secosteroid).
   - Are derivatives of cholesterol, which is modified by a series of cell-specific enzymatic reactions.
   - Are lipophilic and cross membranes readily. Thus steroid hormones cannot be stored in secretory vesicles. Steroid production is regulated at the level of synthesis. Several steroid hormones are produced to a significant extent by peripheral conversion of precursors.
   - Circulate bound to transport proteins. Steroid hormones are cleared by enzymatic modifications that increase their solubility in blood and decrease their affinity for transport proteins. Steroid hormones and their inactive metabolites are excreted in the urine.
   - Act through intracellular receptors, which are members of the nuclear hormone receptor family. Most steroid hormone receptors reside in the cytoplasm and are translocated to the nucleus after ligand (hormone) binding. Each steroid hormone regulates the expression of numerous genes in their target cells.
6. Thyroid hormones are:
   - Iodinated derivatives of thyronine. The term *thyroid hormone* typically refers to 3,5,3′,5′-tetraiodothyronine (T_4 or thyroxine) and 3,5,3′-triiodothyronine (T_3). T_4 is an inactive precursor of T_3, which is produced by 5′-deiodination of T_4.
   - Synthesized and released by the **thyroid epithelium** (see Chapter 6 for more detail)
   - Circulate tightly bound to **transport proteins**
   - Lipophilic and cross cell membranes. T_3 binds to one of several isoforms of **thyroid hormone receptors** (THRs), which form heterodimers with retinoid X receptor (RXR) and reside bound to their response elements in the nucleus in the absence of hormone. Hormone binding induces an exchange in the coregulatory proteins that interact with the THRs.
7. Protein, peptide, and catecholamine hormones signal through transmembrane receptors and use several common forms of informational transfer:
   - Conformational change
   - Binding by activated G proteins
   - Binding by Ca^{2+} or Ca^{2+}-calmodulin. IP_3 is a major lipid messenger that increases cytosolic Ca^{2+} levels through binding to the IP_3 receptor.
   - Phosphorylation and dephosphorylation, using kinases and phosphatases, respectively. The phosphorylation state of a protein affects activity, stability, subcellular localization, and recruitment binding of other proteins. Note that phosphorylated lipids such as PIP_3 also play a role in signaling.
8. Transmembrane receptor families:
   - **G-protein-coupled receptors (GPCRs)** act as **guanine nucleotide exchange factors (GEFs)** to activate the Gα subunit of the heterotrimeric α/β/γ G-protein complex. Depending on the type of Gα subunit that is activated, this will **increase cAMP levels, decrease cAMP levels**, or **increase protein kinase C activity and Ca^{2+} levels**. All catecholamine receptors (adrenergic receptors) are **GPCRs**. GPCRs are internalized by a receptor-mediated endocytosis that involves **GRK** and β-arrestin. Endocytosis results in the lysosomal clearance of the hormone. The receptor may be digested in the lysosome or may be recycled to the cell membrane.
   - The **insulin receptor** is a **tyrosine kinase receptor** that activates the **Akt/PKB pathway**, the **G-protein TC10-related pathway**, and the **MAPK pathway**. The insulin receptor uses the scaffolding protein **insulin receptor substrate (IRS; four isoforms)** as part of its signaling to these three pathways.
   - Some protein hormones (e.g., growth hormone, prolactin) bind to transmembrane receptors that belong to the **cytokine receptor family**. These are constitutively dimerized receptors that are bound by **janus kinases (JAKs)**. Hormone binding interacts with both extracellular domains and induces JAK-JAK cross-phosphorylation, followed by recruitment and binding of **STAT proteins**. Phosphorylation of STATs activates them and induces their translocation to the nucleus, where they act as transcription factors.
   - Hormones that are related to **transforming growth factor-β (TGF-β)**, such as **antimüllerian hormone**, signal through a **coreceptor (receptor I and receptor II) complex** that ultimately signals to the nucleus through activated **Smad** proteins.
   - **Atrial natriuretic peptide (and related peptides)** bind to a transmembrane receptor that contains a **guanylyl cyclase** domain within the cytosolic domain. These receptors signal by **increasing cGMP**, which activates **protein kinase G (PKG)** and **cyclic nucleotide-gated channels**. cGMP also regulates selective **phosphodiesterases**.
9. Intracellular Receptors
   - **Steroid hormones** bind to members of the **nuclear hormone transcription factor family**. Steroid

hormone receptors usually reside in the cytoplasm. Hormone binding induces **nuclear translocation, dimerization,** and **DNA binding.** Steroid hormone receptor complexes regulate many genes in a target cell.

10. **Thyroid hormone (T$_3$) receptors (THRs)** are related to steroid hormone receptor, but they constitutively remain in the nucleus bound to thyroid hormone response DNA elements. T$_3$ binding typically induces an exchange of coregulatory proteins and altered gene expression.

SELF-STUDY PROBLEMS

1. How do protein hormones differ from steroid hormones in terms of their storage within an endocrine cell?
2. How does binding to serum transport proteins influence hormone metabolism and hormone action?
3. How would a large increase in the GTPase activity of Gs-α affect signaling through GPCRs linked to Gs-α?
4. What role does the IRS protein play in transducing insulin receptor signaling into a growth response? A metabolic response?
5. Name an example of a transmembrane receptor–associated transcription factor that translocates to the nucleus.
6. Explain the mechanism of receptor-mediated endocytosis of a hormone that binds to a GPCR.
7. What is the importance of the GEF activity of a GPCR to its ability to signal?
8. Explain how PLC generates two second messengers.

KEY WORDS AND CONCEPTS

7-Helix transmembrane receptors
Adenylyl cyclase
Adrenal cortex
Agonist
Androgen
Androgen receptor
Androgen response element (ARE)
Antagonist
β-Arrestins
Ca^{2+}
Ca^{2+} ATPases
Ca^{2+} channels
Calmodulin
cAMP phosphodiesterase
cAMP response element–binding protein (CREB)
Catecholamine
Cellular response
cGMP phosphodiesterase
Circadian (diurnal) rhythms
Coactivator proteins
Corepressors
Corticosteroid-binding globulin
Covalent phosphorylation of proteins and lipids
Cyclic AMP
Cyclic GMP
Cyclic nucleotide monophosphates
Cycloperhydrophenanthrene ring
Cytokine receptor family
Diacylglycerol (DAG)
Docking protein
Effector proteins
Eicosanoids

Endocrine gland
Endocrine system
Epinephrine
Estrogen
Estrogen receptor
Estrogen response element (ERE)
Exocrine gland
Exocytosis
G-protein exchange factor (GEF)
Gα
Gi-α
Glucocorticoid
Glucocorticoid receptor
Glucocorticoid response element (GRE)
Glucuronide conjugation
GPCR kinase (GRK)
G-protein-coupled receptor (GPCR)
Gq-α
Grb2/SOS
Gs-α
GTP-binding proteins (G proteins)
Guanylyl cyclase
Gβ/γ
Heterotrimeric G proteins
High-affinity receptor
Histone acetyltransferase (HAT)
Histone deacetylase (HDAC)
Hormonal desensitization
Hormonal resistance
Hormone
Hormone response elements (HREs)
Inositol 1,4,5-triphosphate (IP$_3$)

Insulin receptor (IR)
Insulin receptor substrate (IRS)
Intracellular messengers
Intrinsic GTPase activity
Iodothyronine
JAK kinase family
Leukotrienes
Ligand
Ligand-activated GEF
Ligand-induced endocytosis
MEK
Mineralocorticoid
Mineralocorticoid receptor
Mineralocorticoid response element (MRE)
Mitogen-activated protein kinase (MAPK)
Mixed-function kinases and phosphatases
Nitric oxide (NO)
Norepinephrine
Nuclear receptor superfamily
Ovary
Peripheral conversion
Phosphatidylinositol 3,4,5-triphosphate (PIP_3)
Phosphatidylinositol-3-kinase (PI3K)
Phospholipase C
Phosphotyrosine (pY)
PKA catalytic subunit
PKA regulatory subunit
Placenta
Prehormone
Preprohormone
Progesterone receptor
Progesterone response element (PRE)
Progestin
Prohormone convertase
Prostacyclin
Prostaglandins
Protein kinase A (PKA)
Protein kinase B (PKB/Akt)

Protein kinase G (PKG)
Protein/peptide hormone
Raf
Ras
Receptor
Receptor serine/threonine kinases
Receptor tyrosine kinases (RTKs)
Regulated secretory pathway
Regulators of G-protein signaling (RGS proteins)
Second messenger hypothesis
Serine/threonine-specific kinases and phosphatases
Set-point
Sex hormone–binding globulin
Signal peptidase
Signal peptide
Signal recognition complex
Signal transduction pathway
Smads
STAT
Steroid hormone
Steroidogenic cells
Stimulus-secretion coupling
Sulfate conjugation
Suppressors of cytokine signaling (SOCS) proteins
Target cell
Target organ
Testis
Thromboxanes
Thyroid hormone receptor
Thyroid hormone–binding globulin
Thyroid hormone–response element (TRE)
Transforming growth factor (TGF)-β family
Transport proteins
Tyrosine kinases and phosphatases
Ultradian rhythms
Vitamin D
Vitamin D receptor
Vitamin D response element (VRE)

Endocrine Function of the Gastrointestinal Tract

OBJECTIVES

1. List the members of the three enteroendocrine hormone families: gastrin, secretin, and motilin.
2. Describe how autonomic innervation and gastric and duodenal hormones regulate gastric acid secretion and gastric motility.
3. Diagram the regulation of secretion from the exocrine pancreas and the gallbladder and their associated ducts from autonomic innervation and duodenal hormones.
4. Explain how motilin regulates gastric and small intestinal contractions during the interdigestive period.

5. Explain the role of enteroendocrine hormones in the regulation of gastrointestinal (GI) tract growth (an enterotropic action).
6. Describe the role of glucagon-like peptide-1 (GLP-1) and gastric inhibitory polypeptide (GIP) as incretin hormones.

Note: A fifth general function of GI hormones, the effect on appetite, is discussed in the context of energy homeostasis in Chapter 3.

We begin our discussion of endocrine physiology with the hormonal function and regulation of the gastrointestinal (GI) tract. The discovery of secretin in 1902 by Bayliss and Starling represented the first characterization of a *hormone* as a blood-borne chemical messenger, released at one site and acting at multiple other sites. Indeed, the epithelial layer of the mucosa of the GI tract harbors numerous enteroendocrine cell types, which collectively represent the largest endocrine cell mass in the body.

The diffuse enteroendocrine system is perhaps the most basic example of endocrine tissue in that it is composed of unicellular *glands* situated within a simple epithelium. Most enteroendocrine cells, called open cells, extend from the basal lamina of this epithelium to the apical surface (Fig. 2.1), although there are also closed enteroendocrine cells, which do not extend to the luminal surface. The apical membranes of open enteroendocrine cells express either receptors or transporters that allow the cell to *sample* the contents of the lumen. Luminal contents, called secretogogues, stimulate specific enteroendocrine cell types to secrete their hormones. This *sampling* or *nutrient tasting* is independent of osmotic and mechanical forces. The secretogogue mechanisms involved are poorly understood, but some appear to require the absorption of the nutrient. There is also evidence for the luminal secretion of paracrine peptide factors from the surrounding

absorptive epithelial cells that stimulate hormonal release from enteroendocrine cells. As part of their response to luminal contents, specific enteroendocrine cell types display distinct localizations along the GI tract (Table 2.1). We will see that these localizations are central to the regulation and function of each cell type.

In the simplest model of enteroendocrine cell function, a hormone is released from the basolateral membrane in response to the presence of a secretogogue at the luminal side of the cell. The secreted hormone diffuses into blood vessels in the underlying lamina propria, thereby gaining access to the general circulation. Circulating GI hormones regulate GI tract functions by binding to specific receptors at one or more sites within the GI tract and its extramural glands. In the classic model, the secretion of the hormone by an enteroendocrine cell is subsequently terminated when the luminal concentration of its secretogogue diminishes, thereby terminating the secretion of the hormone.

This simple model of the enteroendocrine system does not fully account for the integration with other systemic responses to a meal. Both *open* and *closed* enteroendocrine cells are regulated by the enteric nervous system (ENS) and paracrine factors secreted by neighboring epithelial cells (intrinsic regulators of enteroendocrine cell function). Additionally, there are extrinsic regulators of enteroendocrine cells, most notably the autonomic

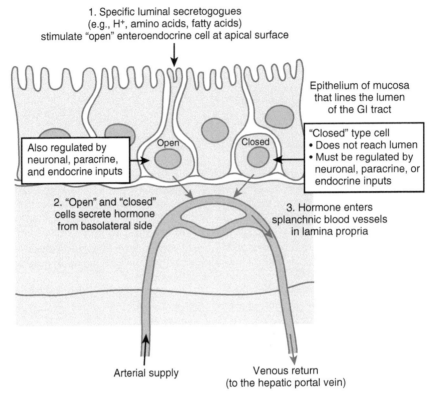

1. Specific luminal secretogogues
(e.g., H⁺, amino acids, fatty acids)
stimulate "open" enteroendocrine cell at apical surface

Epithelium of mucosa
that lines the lumen
of the GI tract

Open   Closed

Also regulated by
neuronal, paracrine,
and endocrine inputs

"Closed" type cell
• Does not reach lumen
• Must be regulated by
  neuronal, paracrine, or
  endocrine inputs

2. "Open" and "closed"
cells secrete hormone
from basolateral side

3. Hormone enters
splanchnic blood vessels
in lamina propria

Arterial supply

Venous return
(to the hepatic portal vein)

Fig. 2.1 Closed and open enteroendocrine cells. Enteroendocrine cells sit within the simple epithelium of the GI tract. "Open" cells extend from the basal lamina to the lumen. "Closed" cells do not reach the lumen. Both cells secrete hormones that enter capillaries in the lamina propria beneath the epithelium.

TABLE 2.1	Distribution of Enteroendocrine Cells Along the GI Tract				
	Stomach	**Duodenum**	**Jejunum**	**Ileum**	**Colon**
G cell (gastrin)	x	(x)			
S cell (secretin)		x	x		
I cell (CCK)		x	x	(x)	
K cell (GIP)		x	x		
L cell (GLP-1)				x	x
L cell (GLP-2)				x	x
M cell (motilin)		x	x		
Ghrelin-secreting cell	x	(x)	(x)	(x)	(x)

x, Primary location of concentration; *(x)*, less concentrated.

nervous system and endocrine glands that reside outside of the GI tract. Conversely, GI hormones can have local (i.e., paracrine) actions on the **afferent nerves of autonomic or enteric reflexes**, so the response to a GI hormone can be mediated by a neurotransmitter. Thus GI tract function is orchestrated through a complex interplay of neural and endocrine responses and actions. It is not surprising,

therefore, that GI function is often perturbed in patients with psychiatric disorders (e.g., depression) and endocrine disorders (e.g., hyperthyroidism).

The hormones secreted by the enteroendocrine system function to maintain the health of the GI tract and its extramural glands and provide an integrated response to the acquisition of nutrients. This integrated response to GI

TABLE 2.2 Enteroendocrine Hormone Families and Their Receptors

Hormone family	Members of family	Receptor and primary signaling pathway	Primary distribution of the receptor (related to GI function)
Gastrin	Gastrin (G cell)	CCK2 receptor Gq - ↑ in Ca²⁺ and PKC	Gastric ECL cell and parietal cell
	CCK (I cell)	CCK1 receptor Gq - ↑ in Ca²⁺ and PKC	Gallbladder muscularis and sphincter of hepatopancreatic ampulla Pancreatic acinar cells Pancreatic ducts Vagal afferents and enteric neurons Stomach muscularis and pyloric sphincter Gastric D cells
Secretin	Secretin (S cell)	Secretin receptor Gs - ↑ in cAMP	Pancreatic ducts and biliary ducts Pancreatic acinar cells G cells and pancreatic cells
	GLP-1 (L cell)	GLP-1 receptor Gs - ↑ in cAMP	β Cells of pancreatic islets
	GLP-2 (L cell)	GLP-2 receptor Gs - ↑ in cAMP	GI tract, especially small intestine
	GIP (K cell)	GIP receptor Gs - ↑ in cAMP	β Cells of pancreatic islets Gastric mucosa and muscularis
Motilin	Motilin (M cell)	Motilin receptor Gq - ↑ in Ca²⁺ and PKC (also binds erythromycin)	Stomach and small intestines, especially in smooth muscle cells and enteric neurons
	Ghrelin (P/D1 cell)	GHS receptor type 1a (GHS-RIa) Gq - ↑ in Ca²⁺ and PKC	Pituitary and hypothalamus

hormones is due, in part, to their ability to regulate multiple functions of the GI tract.

ENTEROENDOCRINE HORMONE FAMILIES AND THEIR RECEPTORS

All established GI hormones are peptides and bind to G-protein-coupled receptors (GPCRs; see Chapter 1) located on the plasma membrane of target cells. GI hormones, as well as their cognate GPCRs, can be organized into gene families based on structural homologies. In this chapter, we discuss members of three enteroendocrine hormone families: gastrin, secretin, and motilin (Table 2.2).

The gastrin family includes gastrin and cholecystokinin (CCK), which share a common stretch of 5 amino acids at the C-terminus. Gastrin binds with high affinity to the CCK-2 receptor (previously called the CCK-B/gastrin receptor). CCK binds with high affinity to the CCK-1 receptor. Receptors of this family are Gq-coupled receptors that are linked to Ca²⁺ and diacylglycerol (DAG)/PKC-signaling pathways.

The secretin family includes the hormones secretin, glucagon, and glucagon-like peptides (including GLP-1 and GLP-2) and gastric inhibitory polypeptide (GIP; more recently referred to as glucose-dependent insulinotropic peptide—see later). This family also includes the neurocrine factor, vasoactive intestinal peptide (VIP). The corresponding GPCRs for each member of the secretin family of peptides are also structurally related. These receptors are all primarily coupled to Gs signaling pathways that increase intracellular cyclic adenosine monophosphate (cAMP) in target cells.

The motilin family includes the hormones motilin and ghrelin. Ghrelin was originally identified as a growth hormone secretogogue (GHS) but is most abundant in the fundus of the stomach. The receptors for motilin and ghrelin are GPCRs that are linked to Gα-q/phospholipase/IP₃ pathways, which, in turn, stimulate protein kinase C- and Ca²⁺-dependent signaling pathways (see Chapter 1).

Many GI peptides are also expressed by tissues outside of the GI tract. Pathophysiologically, GI peptides can be secreted in an uncontrolled manner from tumors. Other physiologic sites of production include other endocrine glands (e.g., the pituitary gland) and reproductive structures. Several peptides are produced by the central (CNS) and peripheral (PNS) nervous systems, where they are used as neurotransmitters or neuromodulatory factors. For example, CCK is expressed in the neocortical region of the CNS and the genitourinary-associated nerves of the PNS. As for its role in the CNS, CCK has been linked to anxiety and panic disorders. This also means that receptors for these peptides also reside within the CNS, the PNS, and probably other nonneural tissues. Thus a pharmacologic agent (agonist or antagonist) related to a specific GI peptide can potentially have a wide range of effects, depending on its stability and whether it can cross the blood-brain barrier. The possibility also exists that extra-GI sites of synthesis can "spill over" into the general circulation and affect GI function.

GASTRIN AND THE REGULATION OF GASTRIC FUNCTION

The **stomach** acts as a food reservoir. People eat discontinuously and typically eat more at one sitting than their GI tract can process immediately. Thus the stomach holds the ingested food and gradually releases partially digested food (chyme) into the first part of the small intestine, the duodenum. The layers of the stomach wall carry out two basic functions: secretion and contraction/relaxation.

Overview of Regulation of Gastric Secretion and Motility

The innermost layer of the stomach wall, the **gastric mucosa**, contains glandular and surface mucus-producing epithelia and can be divided into proximal and distal segments. Two of the proximal portions of the stomach (**fundus and body**) contain the main gastric mucosal glands (Fig. 2.2). Within these glands, the **parietal cells** secrete "hydrochloric acid"(**HCl**), which is important for hydrolysis of macromolecules, activation of proenzymes, and the sterilization of ingested food. Parietal cells also secrete **intrinsic factor**, which is a glycoprotein required for the efficient absorption of vitamin B_{12}.

The glands of the fundus and body also contain the **chief cells**, which secrete digestive enzymes (e.g., pepsinogen, gastric lipase). A third cell type, the **mucous cell**, is found in the neck of the gastric glands and on the surface throughout the stomach. Mucous cells secrete mucigens, which buffer and protect the lining of the stomach, particularly in the vicinity of the main gastric glands. Because gastric enzyme and mucus production is primarily under nervous control, with little endocrine input, we focus here on gastric acid secretion and motility.

The distal part of the gastric mucosa, the **pyloric antrum**, has an important enteroendocrine function. This part of the stomach contains two types of "open" enteroendocrine cells. The **G cells** secrete **gastrin**, a hormone, and the **D cells** secrete **somatostatin**, a paracrine factor. These

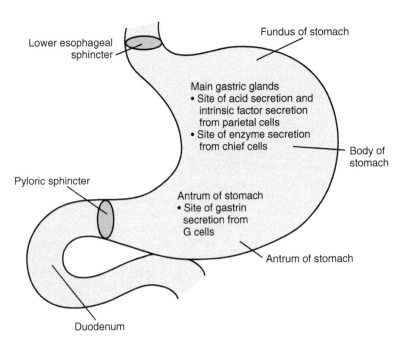

Fundus of stomach

Lower esophageal sphincter

Main gastric glands
• Site of acid secretion and intrinsic factor secretion from parietal cells
• Site of enzyme secretion from chief cells

Body of stomach

Pyloric sphincter

Antrum of stomach
• Site of gastrin secretion from G cells

Antrum of stomach

Duodenum

Fig. 2.2 Anatomy of the stomach.

two peptides act antagonistically in a negative feedback loop to regulate gastric blood flow, cell growth, secretion, and motility (see later). D cells are also found within the fundus and body region, where they directly inhibit parietal cell secretion.

An outer layer of the stomach wall, the muscularis externa, is composed of smooth muscle. The relaxation of this muscle allows distention and storage, and its contractions ultimately move the partially digested food (chyme) into the duodenum. There are two gateways into and out of the stomach. These are the lower esophageal sphincter (LES) and the pyloric sphincter, respectively. The LES allows swallowed food particles to enter the stomach and protects the esophagus from the reflux of acidic chyme. The pyloric sphincter operates in conjunction with the muscularis externa to allow only small particles of digested chyme to escape the stomach and enter the duodenum. The pyloric sphincter also prevents backflow of chyme into the stomach.

In general, regulation of gastric function involves the stimulation of secretion and motility as needed (i.e., in the presence of food), and the inhibition of gastric secretion and motility as acidic chyme reduces the pH of the stomach, or as chyme moves into the small intestine and colon. In this way, the stomach avoids excessive acid secretion in the absence of buffering foodstuffs. Further, the portion of the GI tract below the stomach protects itself from exposure to excessive amounts of acid, which is both damaging to the intestinal lining and inhibitory to the activity of intestinal enzymes. Additionally, the small intestine, in which the majority of digestion and absorption occurs, controls the flow rate of food into and through the small intestine to optimize digestion and absorption of nutrients, salts, and water. The inability to properly regulate acid secretion and its flow into the intestine usually gives rise to duodenal ulcers, although patients with a gastrin-producing tumor (Zollinger-Ellison syndrome) can present with ulceration of the esophagus, stomach, and duodenum.

The general model of gastric control in response to a meal can be organized into three phases. The cephalic phase, which accounts for about 20% of the response to a meal during the digestive period, is activated by the actual or imagined smell and sight of food, or by the presence of food in the mouth. The cephalic phase is associated with increased gastric secretion but decreased motility, in anticipation of the need to store and start digesting food. The gastric phase, which accounts for about 10% of the postprandial response, is activated by the presence of food in, and mechanical distention of, the stomach. During the gastric phase, secretion is strongly stimulated, and this is accompanied by an increase in peristaltic contractions and gastric emptying. The third phase is the intestinal phase, during which an acidic mixture of partially digested food (chyme) moves in a regulated manner through the pyloric sphincter into the small intestine and ultimately into the colon. The processes of enzymatic digestion and absorption that occur during the digestive phase account for 70% of the digestive period. The movement of food into the lower GI tract generally moderates both gastric secretion and emptying.

Gastrin and the Stimulation of Gastric Function

Gastric HCl secretion from parietal cells is stimulated by three pathways:
- Paracrine stimulation by histamine, which is secreted by neighboring enterochromaffin-like (ECL) cells that reside within the lamina propria of the mucosa
- ENS and vagal parasympathetic nervous system stimulation via gastrin-releasing peptide (GRP) and acetylcholine
- Direct and indirect hormonal stimulation by the peptide hormone gastrin

Gastrin is produced by the G cells of the stomach antrum and proximal duodenum. In humans, the term *gastrin* refers to a 17-amino acid peptide that has modifications at both termini (G-17). In fact, the production of G-17 is an excellent example of how a peptide-encoding gene gives rise to multiple, larger precursors, which are also secreted into the blood. G-17 is the product of sequential posttranslational processing of preprogastrin, which can be generally characterized in three phases (Fig. 2.3). In the first phase, sulfation and proteolysis generate a mixture of gastrin precursors, called *progastrins*. The second phase involves proteolysis within secretory granules that generates C-termini peptides. Processing of these intermediates also includes the cyclization of the glutaminyl to a pyroglutamyl residue. The third stage involves the amidation of the C-terminus to produce amidated gastrins. The primary secreted bioactive product of human G cells is G-17 (i.e., 17 amino acids). The pyroglutamyl residue at the amino terminus and the amidation of the C-terminus protect G-17 from digestion by circulating aminopeptidases and carboxypeptidases. G-17 binds with high affinity to the CCK2 receptor and is responsible for all of the gastrin effects on the stomach. The last four amino acids assign gastrin-like biologic activity to G-17. A synthetic, clinically used form of gastrin, pentagastrin, contains the last four amino acids, plus an alanine at the amino terminus that confers increased stability.

During the cephalic phase, gastric HCl secretion is stimulated by vagal (parasympathetic) inputs. Preganglionic vagal efferents activate enteric neurons that directly stimulate the parietal cells and stimulate the release of histamine from ECL cells (Fig. 2.4). These actions are mediated

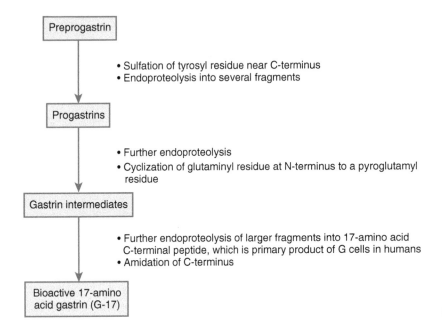

Fig. 2.3 Processing of preprogastrin.

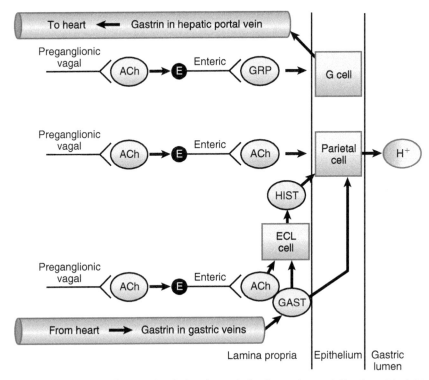

Fig. 2.4 Regulation of gastric HCl secretion during the cephalic phase of a meal. The thought, sight, or smell of food, or the presence of food in the mouth, stimulates acid secretion through the vagal preganglionic para-sympathetic nerves, which stimulate the release of acetylcholine *(ACh)* from postganglionic enteric nerves. Enteric nerve fibers secreting ACh stimulate parietal cells directly and through the release of histamine from enterochromaffin-like *(ECL)* cells. Gastrin is also stimulated by enteric neuronal fibers that release gastrin-releasing peptide *(GRP)*. As a hormone, gastrin levels increase in the general circulation. Gastrin stimulates gastric HCl secretion by binding to CCK2 receptors on ECL cells (and, to a lesser extent, on parietal cells).

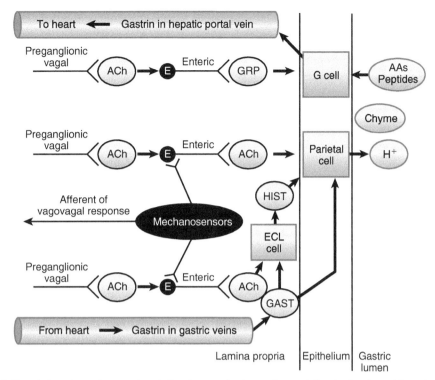

Fig. 2.5 Regulation of gastrin secretion during the gastric phase of a meal. Luminal amino acids and peptides strongly stimulate G cells in the antrum to secrete gastrin. Gastrin secretion and HCl secretion are also stimulated by stomach distention through local and autonomic (vagovagal) reflexes.

by **acetylcholine**, which binds to the **muscarinic receptor**. Vagal stimulation of gastrin is mediated by the neurocrine factor, **GRP**, released from **enteric neurons**.

During the gastric phase, gastrin secretion from G cells is primarily stimulated by the presence of peptides and amino acids in the lumen of the antrum (Fig. 2.5). Gastrin secretion can also be stimulated by **stomach distention** as detected by **mechanosensors** during the gastric phase, acting through local neuronal pathways, and through a **vagovagal reflex**. Circulating gastrin levels increase by severalfold within 30 to 60 minutes after ingestion of a meal.

The primary action of gastrin is the stimulation of HCl secretion by the parietal cells of the gastric glands within the fundus and body of the stomach. To accomplish this, gastrin must enter and circulate through the general circulation and then exit capillaries and venules within the lamina propria of the gastric mucosa in the body and fundus (i.e., *upstream* of where gastrin is released within the stomach).

Gastrin evokes HCl secretion primarily through binding to the **CCK2 receptor** on **ECL cells**. ECL cells, which reside in the lamina propria of the gastric mucosa, produce **histamine** in response to gastrin (see Fig. 2.5). Gastrin

binding to the Gq-coupled CCK2 receptor on ECL cells increases intracellular Ca^{2+}, which leads to exocytosis of histamine-containing secretory vesicles. Gastrin also increases histamine synthesis and storage by increasing the expression of histidine decarboxylase, which generates histamine from histidine, and type 2 vesicular monoamine transporter (VMAT-2), which transports and concentrates histamine into the secretory vesicles. Thus gastrin coordinates both the secretion and synthesis of histamine in ECL cells. Histamine, in turn, stimulates HCl secretion in a paracrine manner by binding to the **H2 receptor** on nearby epithelial parietal cells. Gastrin also has a direct, although less important, effect on parietal cells.

During the **intestinal phase** of a meal, the decrease in gastric contents relieves the stimulation of G cells by amino acids and peptides, and by distention-induced vagovagal pathways. The decrease in gastric contents also reduces the buffering capacity of the gastric lumen. Thus during the intestinal phase and the interdigestive period, the acidity of the stomach decreases. When the pH falls below 3, acid stimulates the **D cells** to secrete the paracrine peptide, **somatostatin**. Somatostatin acts through its receptors (SS-R) to inhibit gastrin secretion from neighboring G cells (Fig. 2.6).

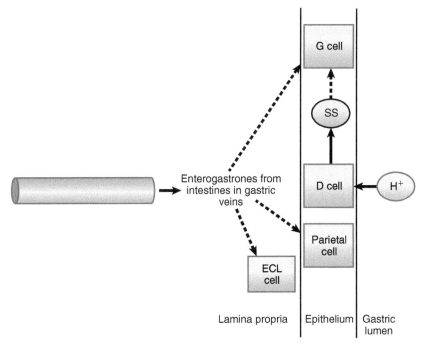

Fig. 2.6 Regulation of gastrin secretion during the intestinal phase of a meal. The exit of food (chyme) from the stomach lumen reduces buffering of HCl. A low pH stimulates D cells to release the paracrine factor, somatostatin (SS), which inhibits gastrin secretion from neighboring G cells. The exact nature of physiologic enterogastrones in humans is not well established. Candidates include secretin and gastric-inhibitory peptide (gip) from the small intestine, and peptide yy from the ileum and colon.

Gastrin release and gastric emptying are also inhibited during the intestinal phase by the release of hormones and neural signals from the small intestine and colon in response to acidity, hypertonicity, distention, and specific molecules (e.g., fatty acids). These hormones are collectively referred to as enterogastrones. The identity of the physiologic enterogastrones in humans that inhibit gastric acid secretion remains uncertain but includes candidates such as secretin and GIP from the duodenum and jejunum and peptide YY and GLP-1 from the distal ileum and colon. CCK is a well-established inhibitor of gastric motility and emptying. CCK is released from the duodenum and jejunum in response to the presence of luminal fatty acids (see Fig. 2.6).

ENTEROENDOCRINE REGULATION OF THE EXOCRINE PANCREAS AND GALLBLADDER

The exocrine pancreas is an extramural gland that empties its secretory products through a main excretory duct into the GI tract at the duodenum (Fig. 2.7). The acini of the exocrine pancreas produce enzymes necessary to digest macromolecules in the small intestine. Pancreatic enzymes

have optimal activities at a neutral pH. Accordingly, the cells that line the pancreatic ducts secrete a bicarbonate-rich fluid, which serves to neutralize acidic chyme in the duodenum. The gallbladder is also an extramural organ. It receives bile that is secreted by the liver. Bile is both stored and concentrated in the gallbladder. Bile is released into small intestine through the common bile duct, which usually joins the main pancreatic duct to form the hepatopancreatic ampulla just before opening into the duodenum (see Fig. 2.7). A major function of bile is the emulsification of triglycerides to increase their accessibility to pancreatic lipase. To perform this function, aggregates (called *micelles*) of bile acids and other lipids are required. Micelle formation requires neutral or slightly alkaline conditions. Accordingly, the epithelial cells of the common bile duct secrete a bicarbonate-rich fluid.

Pancreatic and gallbladder functions are primarily regulated by the autonomic nervous system during the interdigestive period (pancreatic secretion occurs in phase with the migrating myoelectric complex [MMC] in humans), and during the cephalic and gastric phases of the digestive period. However, during the intestinal phase, when these glands are most active, they are predominantly under

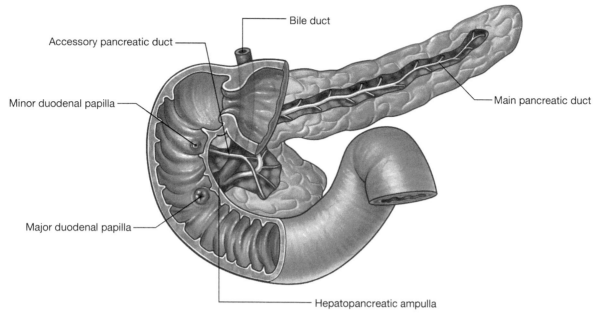

Bile duct

Accessory pancreatic duct

Minor duodenal papilla

Main pancreatic duct

Major duodenal papilla

Hepatopancreatic ampulla

Fig. 2.7 Anatomy of the common bile duct, pancreas, pancreatic duct, and duodenum. The gallbladder (not shown) stores and concentrates bile from the liver. Contraction of the gallbladder and relaxation of the sphincter of Oddi (surrounds the hepatopancreatic ampulla) allows bile to flow down the common bile duct into the duodenum. Pancreatic enzymes and bicarbonate reach the duodenum via larger and larger ducts that eventually form the main pancreatic duct. This duct joins the common bile duct just before it reaches the duodenum, to form the hepatopancreatic ampulla. The termini of the secretory units are the pancreatic acini, which secrete enzymes. The ductal epithelium secretes a bicarbonate-rich fluid. Note that the ductal epithelium of the common bile duct also secretes a bicarbonate-rich fluid. (© Churchill Livingstone Elsevier. Drake et al: *Gray's Anatomy for Students*, second edition, 2010.)

endocrine control by two GI hormones, secretin and CCK. Secretin primarily regulates ductal secretion of a bicarbonate-rich fluid from both pancreatic and bile ducts. CCK primarily stimulates enzyme secretion from pancreatic acinar cells and gallbladder contraction. This dual regulation allows for fine-tuning of the qualitative nature of the product (e.g., in terms of the percentage of bicarbonate and protein in pancreatic juice) that is finally secreted into the duodenum.

The classic model for secretin and CCK action on the pancreas is that the appearance of acid, long-chain fatty acids, and glycine-containing dipeptides and tripeptides in the duodenum stimulates the *open* enteroendocrine cells to secrete the two hormones. Secretin and CCK then circulate in the blood and bind to their specific receptors on either ductal or acinar cells, respectively (Fig. 2.8).

However, there is evidence that secretin has permissive effects on CCK actions, and vice versa. Moreover, it is also clear that the autonomic and ENSs have a permissive effect on the secretin and CCK actions. The neurotransmitter, ACh, and a secretin-related enteric neurocrine

peptide, VIP, stimulate pancreatic ductal and acinar cells and synergize with secretin and CCK. Patients who have a VIPoma (i.e., a tumor producing high levels of VIP) suffer from pancreatic diarrhea because of a constant high level of pancreatic secretion into the gut.

Secretin

Secretin is produced by S cells in the duodenum and jejunum. Similar to gastrin, secretin is produced by posttranslational processing of a larger preprosecretin molecule. Most secretin is a carboxyl-amidated 27-amino acid peptide.

The primary stimulus for secretin release is a decrease in duodenal pH. The threshold pH value for secretin release is 4.5. Circulating secretin levels increase rapidly (approximately 10 minutes) after acidified chyme passes through the pyloric sphincter into the duodenum. The exact mechanism by which H^+ induces secretin release from S cells is unclear. There is evidence for a direct action of H^+ on S cells as well as evidence for indirect actions through enteric neurons and through a phospholipase A_2-like secretin-releasing factor.

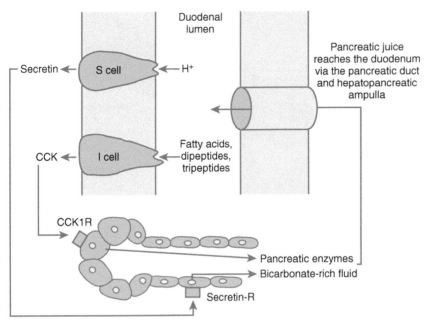

Fig. 2.8 Hormonal regulation of pancreatic secretion by secretin and CCK.

The primary short-term action of secretin is the stimulation of the secretion of a **bicarbonate-rich fluid** from the **pancreatic** and **biliary ducts** during the **intestinal phase** of the digestive period (see Fig. 2.8). Secretin acts through the **secretin receptor**, which is linked to cAMP-dependent pathways. Signaling from the secretin receptor opens apical Cl^- channels (**cystic fibrosis transmembrane conductance regulator** or **CFTR**) thereby increases the flow of transport Cl^- (and, through paracellular osmotic drag, water) into the lumen. Cl^- is then exchanged for bicarbonate anion. Upregulation of this process by secretin can occur through the opening of preexisting CFTR transporters in the apical membrane and through the exocytotic insertion of transporter-containing vesicles into the membrane. The importance of the CFTR channel to pancreatic function underlies the dysfunction of pancreatic secretion observed in patients with **cystic fibrosis**.

Secretin also binds to its receptor on the pancreatic acinar cells. Although secretin has a minimal effect on acinar cells by itself, secretin synergizes with the hormone CCK to further enhance pancreatic enzyme secretion over that achieved by CCK alone. Secretin may also function as an **enterogastrone** by inhibiting stomach acid secretion.

Cholecystokinin

CCK is a 33-amino acid peptide produced by the **I cells** of the duodenum and jejunum. CCK is structurally similar to gastrin, with the 5 amino acids at the carboxyl terminus identical to both hormones. CCK is also sulfated on a tyrosine that is the seventh amino acid from the carboxy terminus. CCK binds primarily to the **CCK1 receptor** (formerly called the *CCKA receptor*), whereas gastrin preferentially binds to the CCK2 receptor. Both hormones can weakly interact with the other's receptor, and desulfation of CCK increases its affinity for the CCK2 receptor. The CCK1 receptor is linked to protein kinase C–dependent and Ca^{2+}-dependent pathways.

The primary stimulus for CCK secretion is the presence of **long-chain fatty acids** or **monoglycerides** in the small intestine (see Fig. 2.8). CCK secretion is also induced by glycine-containing dipeptides and tripeptides. The mechanism by which any of these act to stimulate CCK release is obscure, although there is some evidence for a postabsorptive effect of lipids after their assembly into chylomicrons. There is also evidence for a CCK-releasing peptide (CCK-RP) that is released luminally from enterocytes and stimulates CCK release through binding to a CCK-RP receptor on the apical membrane of I cells. Like secretin, CCK primarily regulates **pancreatic** and **biliary function**. In the pancreas, CCK stimulates enzyme secretion from the acinar cells (see Fig. 2.8). The CCK1 receptor increases intracellular DAG and Ca^{2+}, which results in the exocytosis of enzyme-containing secretion granules. CCK also has a permissive effect on the ability of secretin to stimulate bicarbonate secretion.

CCK is a strong stimulator of gallbladder contraction, and CCK deficiency disorders have been linked to impairment of gallbladder contraction and cholelithiasis (gallstones). CCK induces gallbladder contraction both directly and indirectly through activation of vagal afferent neurons. CCK also stimulates bile secretion into the duodenum through promoting relaxation of the sphincter of the hepatopancreatic ampulla (sphincter of Oddi). This latter action on hepatobiliary function is likely due to the CCK-dependent release of inhibitory neurotransmitters, such as nitric oxide, from enteric neurons. As mentioned, CCK also inhibits gastric emptying, which reduces duodenal acidity and allows emulsification, digestion, and absorption of lipids.

Motilin and Stimulation of Gastric and Small Intestinal Contractions During the Interdigestive Period

Motilin is a 22-amino acid peptide produced from a 114-amino acid prepromotilin and secreted by the M cells of the small intestine. Motilin secretion is inhibited by the presence of food or acid in the small intestine and is stimulated by alkalinization of the small intestine.

Circulating motilin levels peak every 1 to 2 hours in fasting individuals, in phase with the MMC. The MMC is a set of organized contractions that move aborally from the stomach to the ileum and clean the stomach and small intestines of indigestible particles. The MMC may also prevent the colonic bacteria from migrating into the small intestine. Motilin may function to either initiate or integrate the MMC.

The motilin receptor is a GPCR that activates the phospholipase C signaling pathway. The motilin receptor also binds and is activated by the macrolide antibiotic, erythromycin (see Table 2.2). Erythromycin and other motilin receptor agonists are used in the treatment of delayed gastric emptying (gastroparesis), which is common in patients with diabetes mellitus and in some postsurgical patients.

INSULINOTROPIC ACTIONS OF GASTROINTESTINAL PEPTIDES (INCRETIN ACTION)

Elevated circulating levels of nutrients, particularly blood glucose, are strong stimuli of insulin secretion from the pancreatic β cells (see Chapter 3). The possibility that GI hormones also regulate the secretion of insulin was revealed by observations that oral administration of glucose caused a greater rise in insulin than did glucose administered by an intravenous route. This enteroinsular response gave rise to the concept of incretins. In this model, an enteroendocrine

cell type senses nutrients in the GI tract and releases a hormone (an incretin), which, in turn, prepares the pancreatic β cells for the impending rise in blood nutrients (primarily blood glucose). There are two incretins in humans, gastric inhibitory peptide (GIP; also referred to as glucose-dependent insulinotropic peptide), and glucagon-like peptide-1 (GLP-1). These peptides (or analogs thereof) are currently being investigated for the treatment of type 2 diabetes mellitus (see Chapter 3). An important feature of incretins is that their ability to increase insulin secretion is strongly dependent on glucose levels. This means that incretin analogs pose a low risk for inducing severe hypoglycemia (low blood sugar) because once blood glucose falls, the effect of incretins is terminated.

In general, GIP and GLP-1 act through Gs-coupled receptors on β cells, which increase cAMP. This acts in a permissive or synergistic manner with the main glucose/adenosine triphosphate (ATP)-dependent pathway that leads to an increased intracellular Ca^{2+} and the release of insulin. For example, cAMP-EPAC signaling (see Chapter 1) may promote the docking and regulated exocytosis of secretory vesicles in β cells. Incretins also enhance the synthesis of insulin and of proteins that sensitize the β cells to glucose levels, such as the glucose transporter, GLUT-2, and hexokinase.

Gastric Inhibitory Peptide/Glucose-Dependent Insulinotropic Peptide

GIP is a 42-amino acid peptide secreted by the K cells of the small intestine and is a member of the secretin gene family. The primary stimulus for GIP release is the presence of long-chain fatty acids, triglycerides, glucose, and amino acids in the lumen of the small intestine.

GIP was first discovered as an enterogastrone in animal models, in which it inhibited gastric acid secretion and intestinal motility. However, physiologic levels of GIP have only a modest effect on stomach function in humans. In contrast, GIP has an important physiologic role as an incretin. GIP knockout mice display a reduced ability to maintain normal blood glucose levels after an oral glucose load (impaired glucose tolerance).

In rare cases, the GIP receptor is inappropriately expressed on cells of the zona fasciculata of the adrenal cortex (see Chapter 7). These patients display enlarged adrenals and food-induced hypercortisolism. In these patients, food in the small intestine stimulates the release of GIP, which then stimulates cortisol production by the adrenal cortex (see Chapter 7).

Glucagon-like Peptide-1

The glucagon gene is an example of a gene that encodes a large precursor protein (preproglucagon), which is proteolytically processed to form active and inactive peptides

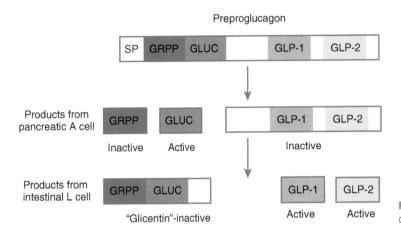

Fig. 2.9 Cell-specific processing of preproglucagon.

(Fig. 2.9). Furthermore, the **prohormone convertases** that digest preproglucagon display cell-specific expression, so different products are released from different cell types. In the α cells of the endocrine pancreas, the active product is **glucagon** (see Chapter 3). In contrast, **intestinal L cells** express preproglucagon but secrete **GLP-1** and **GLP-2** as biologically active peptides. GLP-1 is stimulated by the presence of **free fatty acids and glucose** in the lumen of the ileum and colon. GLP-1 secretion is also increased by neuronal pathways stimulated by free fatty acids and glucose in the upper small intestine. GLP-1 is cosecreted with the other glucagon-derived peptide, **GLP-2**, and **peptide YY** (which is not structurally related to glucagon). The tropic effect of GLP-2 is discussed later.

Like GIP, GLP-1 acts as an incretin. GLP-1 knockout mice have impaired glucose tolerance. GLP-1, along with peptide YY, also appears to be a component of the **ileal brake**, in which free fatty acids and carbohydrates in the ileum inhibit gastric emptying through increased secretion of GLP-1 and peptide YY. This enterogastrone action of GLP-1 further enhances the ability of the organism to control excessive blood glucose excursions. A problem with the therapeutic use of native GLP-1 is the fact that it is rapidly degraded. The use of more stable analogs, called **exendins**, and inhibitors of enzymatic degradation are currently under investigation for enhancing pancreatic β-cell function in type 2 diabetic patients.

ENTEROTROPIC ACTIONS OF GASTROINTESTINAL HORMONES

An important characteristic of many hormones is their ability to promote the growth of their target tissues. This tropic effect helps maintain the health and integrity of the target tissues and optimizes the ability of target tissues to

perform their differentiated functions. In addition to the actions of GI hormones on the maintenance of healthy GI structure and physiology, the tropic actions of GI hormones are of current clinical interest for several reasons, including the following:

- The promotion of hypertrophy and hyperplasia of GI tissues, which sometimes progress to cancer, by the excessive secretion of a GI hormone (usually from a tumor)
- The ability of the GI tract to adapt to a diseased portion of the tract, and/or corrective surgery that involves resection or bypass of a GI segment
- The ability to grow new pieces of GI tissue in vitro (i.e., tissue-engineered neointestine) from pluripotential or stem cells, which can be used for replacement of diseased or resected portions
- The ability to promote pancreatic islet growth and neogenesis in diabetic patients

Gastrin

In addition to its well-established role in the regulation of gastric acid secretion, gastrin exerts several other effects on the stomach and GI tract. The second most important action of gastrin is its **developmental and trophic effect** on the **gastric mucosa**. Gastrin knockout mice display poorly differentiated gastric mucosa, with a reduced number of ECL and parietal cells. In contrast, patients suffering from Zollinger-Ellison syndrome (see earlier) exhibit hypertrophy and hyperplasia of the gastric mucosa, as well as enlarged submucosal rugal folds. Overgrowth is particularly true for the ECL cell population. Although ECL cell proliferation can progress to **carcinoid tumor** formation, this is rare and usually requires other abnormalities. As discussed earlier, progastrin and glycine-extended gastrin (G-Gly) appear to promote the proliferation of colonic mucosa.

Gastric acid, through its effects on D cells and somatostatin release, inhibits the growth of G cells. Thus long-term inhibition of gastric acid production (e.g., with pharmacologic proton pump inhibitors or H$_2$ receptor blockers) can lead to an overgrowth of antral G cells.

Secretin and Cholecystokinin

CCK has a direct effect on **pancreatic acinar cells** that **promotes their maintenance and growth. Secretin inhibits pancreatic ductal cell growth** through binding to the secretin receptor. In contrast, the secretin-related neurotransmitter, **VIP, stimulates ductal growth** through the **VIP receptor** (called **VPAC$_1$ receptor**). In some **ductal pancreatic adenocarcinomas, the secretin receptor is defective, but the VPAC$_1$ receptor is intact. Thus loss of secretin receptor function may shift the cell toward net proliferation.

Glucagon-like Peptide-1

One of the most exciting and promising aspects of enterotropic actions of GI hormones is the **tropic effect that GLP-1 has on pancreatic islet development and growth,** particularly with respect to the β cells. GLP-1 has been shown to induce differentiation of human islet stem cells into β cells in vitro. In mice and rats, GLP-1 and

exendin-4 have protected against surgically and chemically induced diabetes, increased β-cell mass and neogenesis, and inhibited β-cell apoptosis. Further, GLP-1 receptor knockout mice do not display exendin-4-induced regeneration of islets after partial pancreatectomy. Thus GLP-1 or analogs may become valuable reagents in the treatment of diabetic patients whose β-cell mass has been compromised.

Glucagon-like Peptide-2

GLP-2 is cosecreted with GLP-1 by the **intestinal L cells.** Unlike GLP-1, GLP-2 does not have an insulinotropic action. GLP-2 binds to its own receptor (the GLP-2 receptor) and has **potent trophic effects on the intestines.** In fact, evidence of this effect was first discovered in a patient who presented with a massive overgrowth of the small intestine. The patient was also found to have a tumor in the kidney that was producing large amounts of glucagon-related peptides. **GLP-2 has been used to prevent mucosal atrophy** in patients receiving total parenteral nutrition, and it **promotes intestinal growth and adaptation** in patients undergoing resection of bowel. GLP-2 also has positive effects on hexose transport and **may enhance other absorptive functions of intestinal villi.**

SUMMARY

1. Gastrointestinal (GI) hormones are produced by enteroendocrine cells. GI hormones are peptides or proteins and bind to G-protein-coupled receptors on their target cells. GI hormones are produced by specific cell types that reside in specific regions of the GI tract. The secretion of GI hormones is stimulated primarily by luminal secretogogues and by neuronal (enteric and autonomic) and paracrine signals.

2. Gastrin plays a major role in the stimulation of gastric acid secretion. Gastrin is secreted by G cells in the stomach antrum in response to amino acids and peptides in the antral lumen and in response to neuronal stimulation. The primary secreted form of gastrin by the stomach is the 17-amino acid G-17 form. G-17 has a cyclized glutaminyl residue at its N-terminus and an amidated glycine at its C-terminus, which increase the biologic half-life of secreted gastrin. Gastrin binds to the CCK2 receptor and acts primarily by stimulating enterochromaffin-like cells (ECL cells) to secrete histamine. Histamine then stimulates the parietal cells of the stomach to secrete HCl.

3. The major enteroendocrine cells of the duodenum and jejunum are the S cells and I cells, which secrete secretin and cholecystokinin (CCK), respectively. Secretin is released primarily during the *intestinal* phase of a

meal in response to increased acidity in the duodenum. Secretin promotes the secretion of a bicarbonate-rich fluid from the bile and pancreatic ducts, which empty into the duodenum. CCK promotes the contraction of the gallbladder and relaxation of the sphincter of the hepatopancreatic ampulla, thus promoting the emptying of bile into the duodenum. CCK also stimulates enzyme secretion from pancreatic acinar cells.

4. Motilin is secreted by the M cells of the small intestine during the interdigestive phase (i.e., between meals), in phase with the migrating myoelectric complex. Motilin promotes emptying of the stomach and small intestine. The motilin receptor is activated by erythromycin, which can be used to treat delayed gastric emptying (gastroparesis).

5. GI hormones called incretins are secreted in response to luminal nutrients (especially glucose) and increase the ability of blood glucose to stimulate insulin secretion from the pancreatic islets of Langerhans. Incretins include gastric inhibitory peptide (GIP), which has been named more recently for its incretin effect as glucose-dependent insulinotropic peptide. GIP is secreted from the K cells of the small intestine. Another important incretin is glucagon-like peptide-1 (GLP-1), which is secreted by the intestinal L cells. Because of their

ability to sensitize insulin-producing β cells to glucose, incretins are being tested for the treatment of type 2 diabetes mellitus (T2DM; see Chapter 3).

6. GI hormones also have important trophic effects. Gastrin stimulates the growth of the gastric mucosa, especially the ECL cells and submucosa. Secretin and CCK promote the growth of exocrine pancreas tissue. GLP-1 promotes β-cell proliferation, which may prove

an important function of GLP-1 in the treatment of T2DM. GLP-2, which is related to, but is a separate hormone from, GLP-1, promotes GI mucosal growth and is used to treat patients at risk for GI mucosal atrophy.

7. Zollinger-Ellinger syndrome is caused by a gastrin-producing tumor. Patients have ulcerations of the esophagus, stomach, and duodenum, and overgrowth of the stomach mucosa and rugal submucosal folds.

SELF-STUDY PROBLEMS

1. What are the three phases of the digestive period? Which one has the greatest release of gastrin? Why?
2. When administered during the interdigestive period, what are the predicted effects on gastrin secretion of the following experimental agents?
   a. A somatostatin antagonist
   b. A mix of amino acids in the antral lumen
   c. Increased acidity in the antral lumen
   d. A muscarinic agonist
   e. Gastrin-releasing peptide
3. What is the relation between gastric emptying and gastrin secretion from duodenal S and I cells?

4. What are the effects of CCK on the following?
   a. Pancreatic bicarbonate secretion
   b. Pancreatic enzyme secretion
   c. Biliary bicarbonate secretion
   d. Contraction of the gallbladder muscularis
   e. Contraction of the sphincter of Oddi
5. What is the relation between GLP-1 and glucagon?
6. Define *incretin.* Name two incretins.
7. What enterotropic effect is observed in patients with Zollinger-Ellison syndrome?
8. Why does erythromycin promote gastric emptying?

KEYWORDS AND CONCEPTS

Acetylcholine
Amidated gastrins
Autonomic nervous system
CCK
CCK1 receptor
Cephalic phase
Chief cells
Cholecystokinin (CCK)
Chyme
Duodenum
Endocrine glands
Enteric nervous system
Enteroendocrine cell
Enterogastrones
Enterochromaffin-like (ECL) cells
Enterotropic action
Erythromycin
Exendins
Exocrine pancreas
Extrinsic regulators
Food-induced hypercortisolism
Fundus and body
G-17
Gallbladder
Gastric phase
Gastrin

Gastrin-releasing peptide (GRP)
Gastroparesis
Ghrelin
Glucose-dependent/insulinotropic peptide
G-protein-coupled receptors
Growth hormone secretogogue
HCl
Hormone
I cells
Impaired glucose tolerance
Incretins
Incretion action
Intestinal phase
Intrinsic factor
Intrinsic regulators
Migrating myoelectric complex (MMC)
Motilin
Mucigens
Oxyntic cells
Paracrine
Parietal cells
Pentagastrin
Peptide YY
Preprogastrin
Pyloric antrum
S cells

Secretin
Secretin-releasing factor
Secretogogues
Somatostatin
Stomach

Vagal parasympathetic nervous system
Vagovagal reflex
Vasoactive intestinal peptide
Vitamin B_{12}
Zollinger-Ellison syndrome

3

Energy Metabolism

OBJECTIVES

1. Explain energy metabolism in general and how the challenges to provide adequate energy to all cells change during the digestive phase versus the fasting phase.
2. List the primary hormones involved in the regulation of energy metabolic homeostasis, and describe their site of synthesis, regulation of production, and receptor signaling pathways.
3. Diagram the hormonal regulation of specific enzymatic pathways in the hepatocyte, skeletal muscle fiber, and adipocyte during the digestive phase.
4. Diagram the hormonal regulation of specific enzymatic pathways in the hepatocyte, skeletal muscle fiber, and adipocyte during the fasting phase.
5. Explain the role of adipose tissue as an endocrine organ.
6. Explain imbalances in energy metabolism and their consequences in type 1 and type 2 diabetes mellitus.

OVERVIEW OF ENERGY METABOLISM

Absolute, Continuous, and Universal Requirement for Adenosine Triphosphate

Cells continually perform work to grow, proliferate, and migrate; to maintain their structural integrity and internal environment; to respond to stimuli; and to perform their differentiated functions such as contraction, secretion, phagocytosis and propagation of an action potential. For example, while reading the previous sentence, your heart contracted and relaxed about 16 times, and about 3.5 million red blood cells entered your blood from bone marrow. Indeed, the resting metabolic rate (as when sitting and reading) constitutes about 60% to 70% of total potential energy expenditure.

Cells derive their energy to perform this nonstop work primarily from the universal energy carrier, adenosine triphosphate (ATP). The enzymatic hydrolysis of the terminal one or two phosphate groups releases a significant amount of energy that is coupled to and drives many energetically unfavorable reactions. However, ATP cannot be stored. Rather, cells need a continually renewable supply of ATP, which is achieved by continually oxidizing carbon-based fuels (Figs. 3.1A and B). The primary, monomeric fuels are monosaccharides (primarily glucose), free fatty acids (FFAs; also called nonesterified fatty acids),

amino acids (AAs), and ketone bodies. Certain cells can store some of these fuels as polymers and access them as needed (e.g., skeletal muscle stores glucose as glycogen to be used during exercise). However, most cell types continually import monomeric fuels that are delivered to the extracellular microenvironment from the circulation and then enter cells via specific transporters.

Because cells depend on the continuous delivery of monomeric fuels from the circulation, the body as a whole must (1) maintain adequate circulation to all cells and (2) maintain adequate levels of primary fuels and O_2 within the circulation at all times. Inability to do so results in reversible cell injury and, ultimately, irreversible cell injury and cell death. Conversely, while inadequate levels of fuels can lead to cell dysfunction and death, excessive levels of fuels, both extracellularly and intracellularly, can also lead to serious injury (see later). *Thus the regulation of whole body energy metabolism serves to maintain adequate levels of intracellular ATP in all cell types at all times, while keeping the concentrations of intracellular and circulating fuels below critical thresholds.* The amount and type of circulating fuels available to cells change during the day, as well as during exercise, fasting, or starvation. Consequently, whole body metabolism needs to be dynamic and flexible. This is achieved through regulation of metabolism by endocrine, paracrine, and neuronal signaling, and by intracellular components that act as sensors of specific nutrients, metabolites, ions, or the adenosine monophosphate (AMP)/ATP ratio.

Cell-Specific Metabolism of Primary Fuels

For a specific fuel to be utilized by a specific cell type, that cell must express (1) cell membrane–associated transporters and, in some cases, intracellular organelle–associated transporters, that can import and export a specific fuel; and (2) the enzymes and cofactors that comprise specific metabolic pathways for a given fuel. Key components of these are regulated by hormones, metabolites, and intracellular energy sensors during the digestive versus fasting phases.

The cell types that play major roles in the coordination of fuel utilization and are major targets of hormonal and neuronal regulation are (1) the hepatocyte, (2) skeletal muscle fiber, and (3) the adipocyte (see Fig. 3.1A and B).

After the introduction of insulin and glucagon synthesis and regulation, this chapter will discuss the metabolic function and its regulation for each of these cell types in the context of the digestive phase and the fasting phase.

Nutrient Partitioning: The Digestive Phase

The digestive phase (or fed state) refers to the period of about 2 to 3 hours after the ingestion of a meal. Circulating fuels typically rise to levels that exceed the metabolic needs of the body. Because human metabolism has evolved to be very thrifty, excessive fuels are not wasted, but rather partitioned into various storage depots. The storage form of glucose is glycogen, the storage form of FFAs is triglyceride (TG), and the storage form of AAs is protein, especially skeletal muscle proteins (see Fig. 3.1A).

A major challenge associated with the digestive phase is to prevent prolonged excessive circulating and intracellular levels of nutrients. Insulin is the primary digestive

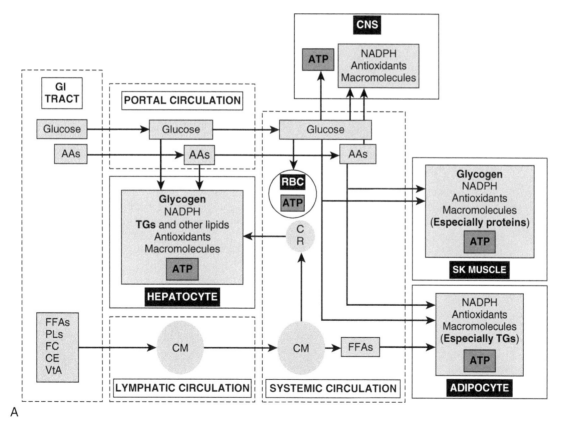

A

Fig. 3.1 (A) Use and partitioning of free fatty acids *(FFAs)*, amino acids *(AAs)*, and glucose during the digestive phase. *CM,* Chylomicron; *CR,* Chylomicron remnant. Bolded polymers in gray boxes represent storage forms. (B) Use and partitioning of fuels during the fasting phase. *KBs,* Ketone bodies.*VLDL,* very-low-density lipoprotein.

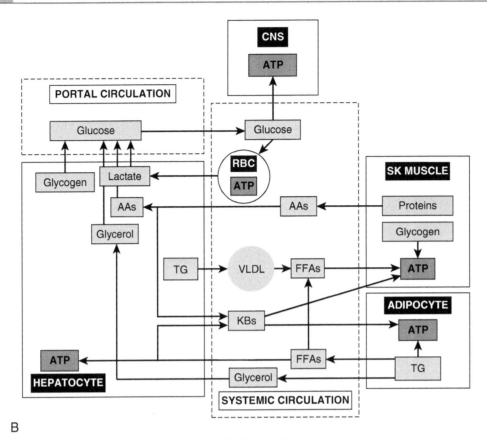

B

Fig. 3.1, cont'd

phase hormone that promotes the movement of fuels out of the circulation and into cells, and their subsequent oxidation for energy or polymerization for storage or, in the case of AAs, for the synthesis of functional proteins. Insulin also promotes anabolic pathways that consume carbons from glucose, FFAs, and AAs, as well as consuming ATP, to build macromolecules to maintain cellular integrity and viability, or to promote cell growth and proliferation.

Nutrient Partitioning: The Fasting Phase

During the interdigestive phase between meals, the fasting phase during sleep and daytime fasting, and during prolonged physical work or exercise, the levels of circulating fuels begin to decline. In a normal, nonprotracted fasting phase (i.e., 8 to 12 hours), the brain is absolutely dependent on blood glucose for normal function. *Thus a major challenge associated with the fasting phase is the maintenance of blood glucose levels above a critical threshold (60 to 70 mg/dL).* This is required to avoid autonomic responses

(e.g., nausea, heart racing), neuroglycopenic symptoms (e.g., confusion, lethargy), and even coma and death, due to increasingly severe degrees of hypoglycemia. Blood glucose levels are maintained by two processes (see Fig. 3.1B):

1. **Hepatic glucose production.** During the initial period of a fast, the liver breaks down stored glycogen via glycogenolysis to glucose-6-phosphate (G6P), converts G6P to glucose by the liver-specific enzyme, glucose-6-phosphatase, and exports glucose through the bidirectional GLUT2 transporter. As a fasting phase progresses, hepatic glucose production switches from primarily glycogenolysis to primarily gluconeogenesis, or the production of glucose from 3-carbon metabolites, including lactate, pyruvate, glycerol, and several "glucogenic" AAs that are released from proteolysis.

2. **Glucose sparing.** Most cell types can utilize fuels other than glucose, thereby sparing glucose for use by the central nervous system (CNS). First, low levels of insulin during the fasting phase minimize the

flow of glucose into skeletal muscle and adipocytes. TGs within adipocytes are mobilized so that FFAs are released into the circulation as FFAs, and preferentially used by skeletal and cardiac muscle, adipocytes, and other cell types for ATP production. Also, during the fasting phase, the liver converts FFAs and some "ketogenic" AAs into ketone bodies, and exports these fuels into the circulation for use by extrahepatic tissues. During a prolonged fast (i.e., 1 to 2 weeks), the CNS itself switches to the utilization of ketone bodies. Finally, skeletal muscle stores glycogen, which is mobilized especially during exercise/work for use within the muscle fiber.

The hormones **glucagon** and **epinephrine**, along with the sympathetic neurotransmitter, **norepinephrine**, represent the primary signals that induce the mobilization of energy stores and new synthesis of glucose and ketone bodies during the fasting phase, thereby preventing blood glucose from declining to dangerously low levels (see later). Several other hormones, including **cortisol** and **growth hormone**, also play important roles in the mobilization of energy stores, the control of circulating glucose and lipids, and the balance between protein synthesis and degradation; these are discussed in Chapters 5 and 7.

KEY HORMONES INVOLVED IN METABOLIC HOMEOSTASIS

Endocrine Pancreas

The **islets of Langerhans** constitute the endocrine portion of the pancreas (also called the **endocrine pancreas**; Fig. 3.2). About 1 million islets, making up about 1% to 2% of total pancreatic mass, are spread throughout the pancreas. The islets are composed of several cell types, each producing a different hormone. In islets situated in the body, tail, and anterior portion of the head of the pancreas (all of which have a common embryologic origin), the most abundant cell type is the β cell. The β cells make up about three-fourths of islet cells and produce the hormone **insulin**. The α cells comprise about 10% of these islets and secrete the hormone **glucagon**. The third major cell type of the islets within these regions is the Δ **cells**, which make up about 5% of the cells and produce the peptide **somatostatin** (gastric somatostatin was discussed in Chapter 2, as an inhibitor of gastrin secretion). A fourth cell type, the F cell, represents about 80% of the cells in the islets situated within the posterior portion of the head of the pancreas (including the uncinate process) and secretes the peptide, **pancreatic polypeptide**.

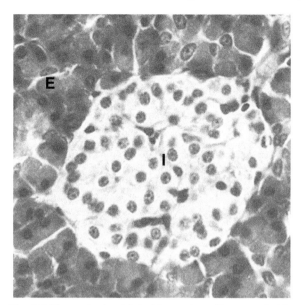

Fig. 3.2 The endocrine Islet of Langerhans (*I*) surrounded by exocrine pancreatic tissue (*E*).

Because the physiologic function of pancreatic polypeptide in humans remains obscure, it is not further discussed here. Blood flow through the islets is somewhat autonomous from the blood flow to the surrounding exocrine tissue. Insulin secreted from the inner β cells reaches the outer α cells. Consequently, the first cells affected by circulating insulin are the α cells, in which insulin inhibits glucagon secretion.

Insulin

Insulin is the primary anabolic hormone that is responsible for maintaining the upper limit of blood glucose and FFA levels. Insulin achieves this by the following mechanisms:
1. Increasing glucose uptake by skeletal muscle and adipocytes.
2. Increasing metabolism of glucose in liver, skeletal muscle, and adipocytes.
3. Increasing glycogen storage in liver and skeletal muscle.
4. Increasing the clearance of chylomicrons from the blood.
5. Increasing TG synthesis and storage in the liver and adipose tissue.
6. Suppressing glucose output by the liver.
7. Suppressing lipolysis of adipose TG stores.
8. Suppressing very-low-density lipoprotein (VLDL) production by the liver.

Insulin also promotes protein synthesis from AAs and inhibits protein degradation in peripheral tissues. Finally, insulin regulates metabolic homeostasis through effects on satiety.

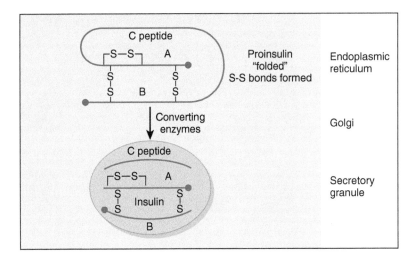

Fig. 3.3 Structure of insulin. (Modified from Koeppen BM, Stanton BA, editors: *Berne & Levy Physiology*, 6th ed., Philadelphia, 2010, Mosby.)

Insulin Structure, Synthesis, and Secretion

Insulin is a protein hormone that belongs to a gene family that also includes **insulin-like growth factors I and II (IGF-I, IGF-II), relaxin,** and several insulin-like peptides. Organized, functional islets appear in the human pancreas at the beginning of the third trimester of gestation. Insulin gene expression and islet cell biogenesis are dependent on several transcription factors (e.g., hepatocyte nuclear factor-4 [HNF-4α], HNF-1α, or HNF-1β; pancreatic and intestinal homeobox-1 [PDX1]; neuroD1) (Clinical Box 3.1).

The insulin gene encodes **preproinsulin.** Preproinsulin is converted to **proinsulin** by microsomal enzymes as the peptide enters the endoplasmic reticulum. Proinsulin is packaged in the Golgi apparatus into membrane-bound secretory granules. Proinsulin contains the AA sequence of insulin plus the 31-amino acid C (**connecting**) **peptide.** The proteases that leave proinsulin, prohormone (or proprotein) convertase-2 and -3, are packaged with proinsulin within the secretory vesicle. The mature hormone consists of two chains, an α chain and a β chain, connected by two disulfide bridges (Fig. 3.3). Insulin is stored in secretory vesicles in zinc-bound crystals. Because the entire contents of the granule are released, equimolar amounts of insulin and C peptide are secreted, as are small amounts of proinsulin. C peptide has no known biologic activity, and proinsulin has about 7% to 8% of the biologic activity of insulin.

Measurements of C peptide in the blood are used to quantify endogenous insulin production in patients receiving exogenous insulin, which has been purified from C peptide. Insulin has about a 5-minute half-life and is cleared rapidly from the circulation by receptor-mediated endocytosis. It is degraded by lysosomal **insulin degrading enzyme (IDE)** in the liver, kidneys, and other tissues. Because insulin is secreted into the hepatic portal vein, almost one half of the insulin is degraded before leaving the liver. Recombinant human insulin and insulin analogs are now available, with different characteristics of onset and duration of action and peak activity.

Serum insulin levels normally begin to rise within 10 minutes after food ingestion and reach a peak in 30 to 45 minutes. The higher serum insulin level rapidly lowers blood glucose to baseline values. When insulin secretion is stimulated, insulin is released rapidly (within minutes), and this is called the early phase of insulin secretion. If the stimulus is maintained, insulin secretion falls within 10 minutes and then slowly rises over a period of about 1 hour. The second phase is referred to as the *late phase* of insulin release.

Glucose is the primary stimulus of insulin secretion (Fig. 3.4). Glucose entry into β cells is facilitated by the **GLUT2 transporter.** Once glucose enters the β cell, it is phosphorylated to **G6P** by the low-affinity **hexokinase, glucokinase (GK).** GK is referred to as the **glucose sensor** of the β cell because the rate of glucose entry is correlated to the rate of glucose phosphorylation, which, in turn, is directly related to insulin secretion. Heterozygous mutations in GK are one defect that leads to inadequate insulin release in patients with **mature-onset diabetes of the young (MODY).** G6P is metabolized by β cells, increasing the intracellular **ATP levels** and closing an **ATP-sensitive K⁺ channel** (see Fig. 3.4). This results in depolarization of the β-cell membrane, which opens **voltage-gated Ca²⁺ channels.** Increased intracellular Ca²⁺ levels activate exocytosis of secretory vesicles.

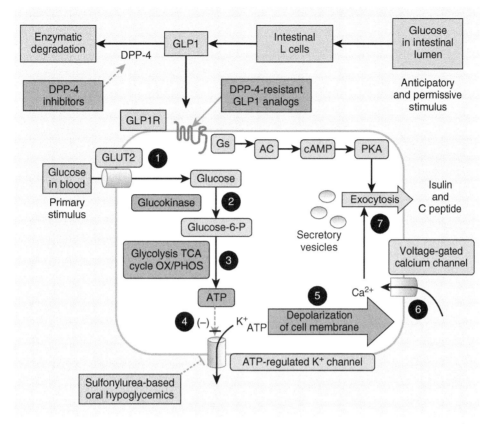

Fig. 3.4 Regulation of insulin secretion from β cells by nutrients (glucose, amino acids, FFAs) and the hormones/neurotransmitters, glucagon-like peptide-1 (GLP1), epinephrine, norepinephrine, and acetylcholine. (Modified from Koeppen BM, Stanton BA, editors: *Berne & Levy Physiology*, 7th ed., Philadelphia, 2018, Mosby.)

CLINICAL BOX 3.1

Heterozygous mutations in any one of the islet transcription factors, as well as glucokinase (see later), result in progressively inadequate production of insulin. This leads to MODY, which typically manifests in patients younger than 25 years of age.

- TYPE gene mutated (requires insulin or oral hypoglycemic)
- MODY 1 HNF-4α (yes)
- MODY 2 Glucokinase (no)
- MODY 3 HNF-1α (yes)
- MODY 4 IPF-1 (yes)
- MODY 5 HNF-1β (yes)
- MODY 6 Neuro D1 (yes)

In addition to glucose, certain AAs (leucine) and vagal (parasympathetic) cholinergic innervation (i.e., in response to a meal) also stimulate insulin through increasing intracellular Ca^{2+} levels. Long-chain FFAs also increase insulin secretion, although to a lesser extent than glucose and AAs.

As discussed in Chapter 2, nutrient-dependent stimulation of insulin release is enhanced **by the incretin hormones, glucagon-like peptide-1 (GLP-1) and gastric inhibitory peptide** (GIP) and possibly other gastrointestinal (GI) hormones (e.g., cholecystokinin [CCK]). These act primarily by raising intracellular cyclic AMP (cAMP) within the β cell, which amplifies the intracellular effects of glucose on Ca^{2+} (see Fig. 3.4). Intracellular cAMP acts both through phosphokinase A (PKA)-dependent and EPAC (exchange protein activated by cAMP)–dependent pathways (see Chapter 1) in β cells. Incretin hormones minimally increase insulin secretion in the absence of glucose.

Insulin secretion is inhibited by α_2-**adrenergic receptors**, which are activated by epinephrine (from the adrenal medulla) and norepinephrine (from postganglionic sympathetic fibers). The α_2-adrenergic receptors are coupled to a Gi-containing trimeric G-protein complex that inhibits adenylyl cyclase and decreases cAMP levels. Adrenergic inhibition of insulin serves to protect against hypoglycemia, especially during exercise. Although somatostatin from D cells inhibits both insulin and glucagon, its physiologic role in pancreatic islet function is unclear. Nevertheless, somatostatinomas are malignant tumors of the islets that produce high levels of somatostatin, which can lead to mild glucose intolerance.

CLINICAL BOX 3.2

The ATP-sensitive K⁺ channel is a protein complex that contains an ATP-binding subunit called **SUR1**. This subunit is also activated by **sulfonylurea** and **meglitinide drugs**, which are used as ingested drugs (**oral hypoglycemics**) to treat hyperglycemia in patients with partially impaired β-cell function (see Fig. 3.4). As these drugs act within the direct pathway for **glucose-stimulated insulin secretion (GSIS)**, they are associated with **hypoglycemic episodes** as a side effect. Rare mutations in the ATP-sensitive K⁺ channel that keep it in the open conformation, thereby blocking glucose-induced insulin secretion, result in early-onset diabetes.

Analogs of **GLP-1** (so-called "glutide" drugs) are also used to enhance GSIS (see Fig. 3.4).

GLP-1 is rapidly degraded by the enzyme **dipeptidyl dipeptidase-4 (DPP-4)**. Inhibitors of DPP-4 (so-called "gliptin" drugs) are also effective at enhancing GSIS. Both glutides and gliptins confer a significantly lower risk of hypoglycemia, as they only act in the presence of elevated glucose.

Insulin Receptor

The insulin receptor is a member of the receptor tyrosine kinase (RTK) family (see Chapter 1), which includes receptors for several other growth factors, such as IGFs, platelet-derived growth factor (PDGF), and epidermal growth factor (EGF). The insulin receptor is expressed on the cell membrane as a homodimer composed of α/β monomers (Fig. 3.5). The α/β monomer is synthesized as one protein, which is then proteolytically cleaved, with the two fragments connected by a disulfide bond. The two α/β monomers are also held together by a disulfide bond between the α subunits. The α subunits are external to the cell membrane and contain the hormone-binding site. The β subunits span the membrane and contain tyrosine kinase on the cytosolic surface.

Insulin binding to the insulin receptor induces the β subunits to cross-phosphorylate each other on three tyrosine residues. These phosphotyrosine residues recruit two major classes of adaptor proteins: insulin-receptor substrate isoforms 1 to 4 (IRS1-4) and Shc

protein (see Fig. 3.5). The IRS proteins are phosphorylated by the tyrosine kinase activity of the insulin receptor. The phosphotyrosine residues on IRS recruit PI3 kinase to the membrane, where it is phosphorylated and activated by the insulin receptor. PI3 kinase converts phosphoinositide-4,5-bisphosphate (PIP2) to phosphoinositide-3,4,5-triphosphate (PIP3). PIP3 recruits to the membrane and leads to the activation of a pleiotropic protein kinase, called Akt (see Fig. 3.5).

Akt regulates numerous enzymes and transcription factors that mediate the metabolic actions of insulin. Akt acts in five general ways that largely account for the metabolic effects of insulin (Fig. 3.6):

1. Phosphorylation of exocytosis components that induce the insertion of GLUT4 glucose transporters into the cell membranes of muscle and adipose tissue (see later). This action requires combined IRS/PI3K-dependent signaling and an additional adaptor protein-dependent pathway that activates a small G-protein pathway (not shown).
2. Activation of protein phosphatases that, in turn, regulate metabolic enzymes through dephosphorylation. For example, dephosphorylation of liver pyruvate kinase activates the enzyme, whereas phosphorylation by cAMP/PKA signaling inactivates it.
3. Activation of mammalian target of rapamycin complex-1 (mTORC1) (see later). mTORC1 is a kinase complex that promotes ribosomal RNA synthesis, ribosome assembly, and protein synthesis. mTORC1 also increases sterol-regulatory element–binding protein-1c (SREBP1c) activity.
4. Direct induction of synthesis and activation of the lipogenic transcription factor, the SREBP1c. SREBP1c coordinately stimulates the expression of enzymes involved in glycolysis, lipogenesis, and the pentose phosphate pathway.
5. Phosphorylation and inactivation of the hepatic transcription factor, FOXO1.
6. FOXO1 stimulates the expression of some gluconeogenic enzymes, as well as VLDL-related apoprotein B100.

The Shc protein is linked to the mitogen-activated protein kinase (MAPK) pathway (see Fig. 3.5), which mediates the growth and mitogenic actions of insulin (in conjunction with the activation of mTORC1).

The termination of insulin receptor signaling is a topic of high interest because these mechanisms potentially play a role in insulin resistance. Insulin induces the downregulation of its own receptor by receptor-mediated endocytosis. Additionally, several serine and threonine protein kinases are indirectly activated by insulin and by other molecules (such as inflammatory cytokines) and subsequently inactivate the insulin receptor or IRS proteins. These include mTORC1, which negatively feeds back on IRS proteins

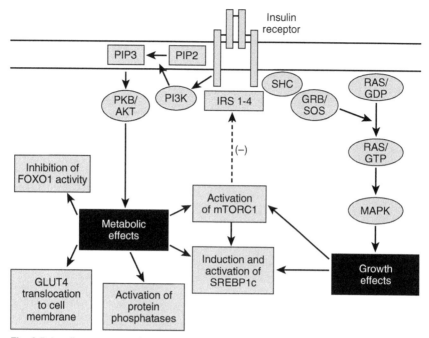

Fig. 3.5 Insulin receptor and postreceptor signaling pathways. See text for abbreviations.

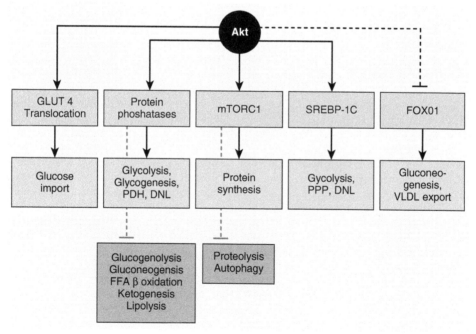

Fig. 3.6 Summarized actions of insulin/insulin receptor-activated Akt kinase. *DNL*, de novo lipogenesis. (Modified from Koeppen BM, Stanton BA, editors: *Berne & Levy Physiology*, 7th ed., Philadelphia, 2018, Mosby.)

(see Fig. 3.5). Another serine threonine kinase that reduces activity or levels of the insulin receptor and IRS proteins is the suppressor of cytokine signaling (SOCS) family of proteins. In the presence of inflammation, proinflammatory cytokines activate SOCS kinase, which negatively feeds back on both the cytokine receptors and the insulin receptor. Thus inflammation can lead to insulin resistance. Finally, intracellular accumulation of TGs and other lipids increase cytosolic levels of lipid intermediates such as diacylglycerol (DAG) and ceramide. These intermediates lead to the activation of serine/threonine kinases such as protein kinase C (PKC) isoforms that phosphorylate and inhibit the insulin receptor and IRS proteins.

Glucagon

Glucagon is an important counterregulatory hormone that opposes insulin actions, and increases blood glucose levels through its effects on liver glucose output. Glucagon promotes the production of glucose through elevated hepatic glycogenolysis and gluconeogenesis and through decreased glycolysis and glycogen synthesis. Glucagon inhibits hepatic FFA synthesis (de novo lipogenesis) from glucose. Glucagon also maintains blood glucose indirectly through stimulation of ketogenesis, which provides an alternative energy source that leads to glucose sparing in many tissues.

Glucagon Structure, Synthesis, and Secretion

As discussed in Chapter 2, glucagon is a member of the secretin gene family. Preproglucagon is proteolytically cleaved in the pancreatic islet α cell in a cell-specific manner to produce the 29-AA glucagon (see Fig. 2.9). Glucagon is highly conserved among mammals.

Like insulin, glucagon circulates in an unbound form and has a short half-life (about 6 minutes). The predominant site of glucagon degradation is the liver, which degrades as much as 80% of the circulating glucagon in one pass. Because glucagon (either from the pancreas or the gut) enters the hepatic portal vein and is carried to the liver before reaching the systemic circulation, a large portion of the hormone never reaches the systemic circulation. The liver is the primary target organ of glucagon, with lesser effects on adipose tissue. As discussed later, glucagon opposes the actions of insulin. Thus several factors that stimulate insulin inhibit glucagon. Indeed, it is the insulin-to-glucagon ratio that determines the net flow of hepatic metabolic pathways. A major stimulus for glucagon secretion is a drop in blood glucose, which is primarily an indirect effect via the removal of inhibition of glucagon secretion by insulin (Fig. 3.7). Circulating catecholamines, which inhibit insulin secretion through

α_2-adrenergic receptors, stimulate glucagon secretion through β_2-adrenergic receptors (see Fig. 3.7). Serum AAs also stimulate glucagon secretion. This means that a protein meal will increase postprandial levels of glucagon along with insulin, thereby protecting against hypoglycemia. In contrast, a carbohydrate-only meal stimulates insulin secretion and inhibits glucagon secretion.

Glucagon Receptor

The glucagon receptor is a 7-transmembrane receptor primarily linked to Gs-containing heterotrimeric G-protein complex (see Chapter 1). Consequently, glucagon increases intracellular cAMP levels in the liver. The increase leads to activation of protein kinase A (PKA). Glucagon stimulated PKA opposes the effects of insulin/Akt-activated protein phosphatases at several steps within hepatic and adipocyte metabolic pathways. The glucagon receptor is expressed by hepatocytes and adipocytes, but not by skeletal muscle.

Epinephrine and Norepinephrine

The other major counterregulatory factors are the catecholamines, epinephrine and norepinephrine. Epinephrine, and to a much lesser extent norepinephrine, are secreted by the adrenal medulla (see Chapter 7), whereas only norepinephrine is released from postganglionic sympathetic nerve endings. The direct metabolic actions of catecholamines are mediated primarily by β_2- and β_3-adrenergic receptors located on muscle, adipose, and liver. Like the glucagon receptor, β-adrenergic receptors are linked to a Gs signaling pathway that increases intracellular cAMP. Epinephrine also promotes glycogenolysis and gluconeogenesis through the α_1-adrenergic receptor, which is coupled to the Gq/IP3/DAG signaling pathway.

Catecholamines are released from sympathetic nerve endings and the adrenal medulla in response to decreased glucose concentrations, stress or alarm, and exercise. Decreased glucose levels (i.e., hypoglycemia) are primarily sensed by hypothalamic neurons, which initiate a sympathetic response to release catecholamines.

Catecholamines circulate in the blood as free hormones, and both circulating and tissue catecholamines are rapidly enzymatically inactivated (see Chapter 7).

Intracellular Sensors and Regulators

Importantly, all cells must balance energy needs associated with their differentiated function with other uses of carbon, especially the synthesis of macromolecules (lipids, nucleic acids, proteins) and the assembly of organelles that is associated with maintenance of cellular viability. There are several master regulatory nutrient and energy sensors

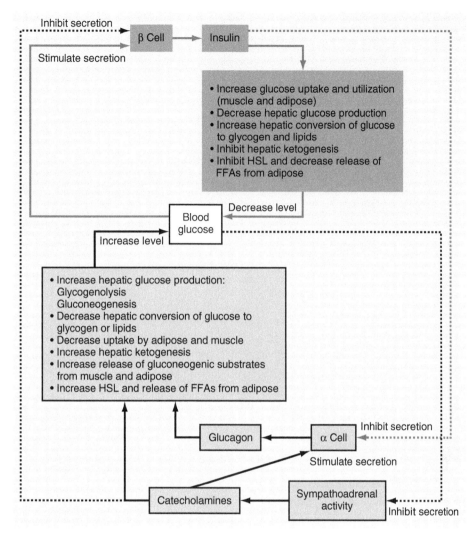

Fig. 3.7 Interaction of insulin, glucagon, and catecholamines in the regulation of each other and of blood glucose (the primary secretogogue for insulin). (Modified from Koeppen BM, Stanton BA, editors: *Berne & Levy Physiology*, 6th ed., Philadelphia, 2010, Mosby.)

that monitor intracellular nutrient levels and the relative amount of ATP to balance anabolic pathways with catabolic ones.

Two of these regulatory factors are **mTORC1** and **AMP-activated kinase (AMPK**; also a multimeric complex). In the presence of insulin and high levels of intracellular nutrients (AAs, glucose) that signal an abundance of carbons, mTORC1 promotes energy-consuming anabolic pathways, such as ribosomal RNA production and ribosome assembly, protein synthesis, and lipogenesis (Fig. 3.8). Also, activation of mTORC1 inhibits the breakdown of

intracellular macromolecules and organelles for energy and survival, a process termed **autophagy**. In contrast, a drain on energy supply associated with an elevation of AMP levels, or an indication of high energy use such as elevated intramuscular Ca^{2+} levels and or reduced O_2, activates AMPK (see Fig. 3.8). Hormones associated with a fasting state (ghrelin, adiponectin; discussed later) also activate AMPK. Active AMPK inhibits anabolic pathways (in part by inhibiting mTORC1 activity) and promotes energy-generating catabolic pathways, including glycolysis and β-oxidation of FFAs (see later). Although other

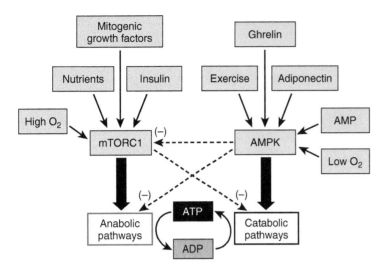

Fig. 3.8 mTORC1 and AMPK act as nutrient and energy sensors and regulate metabolism in conjunction with hormones.

important energy-sensing factors exist in cells, mTORC1 and AMPK have emerged as two centrally important factors involved in cellular energy balance, and the interaction of these two complexes with hormonal signaling is discussed later.

METABOLIC HOMEOSTASIS: THE INTEGRATED OUTCOME OF HORMONAL AND SUBSTRATE/PRODUCT REGULATION OF METABOLIC PATHWAYS

The hormonal regulation of the major metabolic pathways, with emphasis on key regulated enzymes and transporters, during the digestive phase compared with the fasting phase is presented in this section.

Energy Metabolism During the Digestive Phase

During the digestive phase, circulating nutrient levels increase. Following are some basic facts concerning the metabolism of glucose, FFAs and AAs during the digestive phase, with emphasis on hepatocytes, skeletal muscle and adipocytes.

Overview of Glucose Metabolism During the Digestive Phase

Glucose Transport Across the Cell Membrane

Glucose is a universal and normally abundant fuel. Glucose enters most cell types via facilitative, bidirectional transporters called GLUTs.

1. **GLUT1** is expressed in most cell types, including erythrocytes. GLUT1 deficiency is accompanied by severe neurologic disorders (e.g., epilepsy), emphasizing the importance of GLUT1 in the function of the blood-brain barrier and CNS.
2. **GLUT2** is a low affinity, high capacity transporter that is expressed in **hepatocytes** and **pancreatic β cells**. GLUT2 is paired with a low affinity, high V_{max} hexokinase, GK, which can both act as a **sensor** of glucose levels, and allow for a high flux of glucose import.
3. **GLUT3** is expressed primarily in the CNS.
4. **GLUT4** is expressed primarily in skeletal muscle and adipocytes. During the fasting phase, GLUT4 is inactive because it resides within cytoplasmic "**glut storage vesicles**." In response to insulin signaling during the digestive phase, GLUT4-containing vesicles are inserted into and fuse with the cell membrane, thereby targeting the GLUT4 transporters to the cell membrane where they can actively import glucose. Because skeletal muscle (and in some individuals, adipocytes) represent an abundant cell type, insulin-dependent GLUT4 translocation and activation plays a central role in the removal of glucose from the circulation after a meal. Insulin resistance leads to deficient GLUT4 insertion into the cell membrane of skeletal myocytes and adipocytes, which contributes significantly to excessive blood glucose levels associated with **glucose intolerance** and type 2 diabetes mellitus (T2DM).

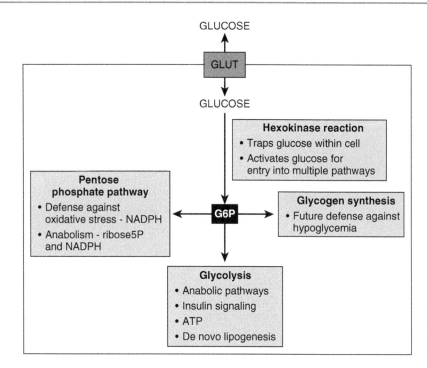

Fig. 3.9 Overview of the hexokinase reaction, and the metabolic pathways that glucose-6-phosphate *(G6P)* can potentially enter.

CLINICAL BOX 3.3

In addition to GLUT transporters, there also exist sodium/glucose-linked transporters, **SGLT1** and **SGLT2**, primarily found in the brush borders of the **small intestine** and **proximal convoluted tubule**, respectively. **Sodium** is actively transported out of the cell through the basolateral membrane by an **Na⁺/K⁺-ATPase**. This allows sodium to be transported through SGLTs into the cell down a concentration gradient. SGLTs are symporters, in that glucose is transported into cells along with sodium. Glucose is then exported through the basolateral membrane through GLUT2 transporters, and then enters capillary beds through GLUT1 transporters in endothelial cells. SGLT2 is highly expressed in the proximal (S1) segment of the proximal convoluted tubule, and plays a major role in the recapture of sodium and glucose that exit the blood at the glomerulus. Normally, 100% of filtered glucose is recaptured by the proximal convoluted tubule and returned to the circulation. **"Gliflozin" drugs** inhibit SGLT2 and thus renal reabsorption of glucose, and are currently being used to treat **T2DM**.

Utilization of Glucose

Glucose is rapidly phosphorylated to G6P by the family of hexokinases (Fig. 3.9). This reaction traps glucose within the cell, in that G6P cannot exit through bidirectional GLUT transporters. The hexokinase reaction also "activates" glucose, so that as G6P, the carbons within glucose can potentially enter several pathways (see Fig. 3.9):

1. Glycogen synthesis in hepatocytes and skeletal muscle. Glycogen is a storage form that can be accessed during fasting and exercise.
2. Pentose phosphate pathway (PPP). The PPP generates riboses that are used for nucleotide and nucleic acid synthesis, as well as NADPH, which is a cofactor for antioxidant defense pathways and anabolic pathways.
3. Glycolysis:
   a. Glycolysis converts G6P to pyruvate and generates a net of two molecules of ATP/G6P. Glycolysis occurs in the cytoplasm and does not require O_2, so that erythrocytes can use glucose to generate ATP, and convert pyruvate to lactate, which is exported.
   b. Side reactions of glycolysis contribute to several pathways, including those involved in protein glycosylation, AA synthesis, single carbon metabolism that contributes to folate-dependent synthesis of nucleic acids, and glycerol-3-phosphate that is used for TG synthesis.

4. **Mitochondrial utilization of pyruvate.** Most normal cells further metabolize pyruvate through **mitochondrial respiration**, which requires O_2. This involves conversion of pyruvate to **acetyl CoA** by **pyruvate dehydrogenase (PDH) complex**, complete oxidation of acetyl CoA to CO_2 through the **TCA cycle**, and oxidation of the TCA cycle-generated **NADH** and **FADH$_2$** through the **electron transport system** and **ATP synthase** to generate ATP.
5. **De novo lipogenesis**—this is discussed later in the context of hepatocyte metabolism during the digestive phase.

Glucose is produced and exported by the liver through **glycogenolysis** and **gluconeogenesis**, collectively referred to as **hepatic glucose production.** Insulin has *direct inhibitory actions* on hepatic glucose production during the digestive phase. It must be stressed that glucose is a reactive molecule and prolonged, inappropriately elevated levels of circulating and, consequently, intracellular glucose leads to the nonenzymatic **glycation** of proteins and lipids. Glycation of these molecules leads to aberrant processing, folding, secretion (e.g., of extracellular matrix proteins), and function. Glucose also contributes to the **osmolarity** of fluids, so that as excessive glucose is cleared by the kidney, it drags water with it, causing potentially dangerous **dehydration.** Therefore it is important that blood glucose levels remain below a critical threshold (e.g., fasting blood glucose should be below 100 mg/dL). Chronic elevation of glucose, due to the inability of certain tissues/organs to import and metabolize glucose, and/or due to inappropriate hepatic glucose production, is defined as **glucose intolerance** (fasting blood glucose between 100 to 125 mg/100 dL); or **diabetes mellitus (DM)** (fasting blood glucose higher than 125 mg/100 dL). As discussed later, DM imposes a broad range of stresses on cells that ultimately are manifested by the compromised function or failure of specific organs. Thus it is important to understand that insulin imposes important negative actions on metabolism that contribute to the maintenance of blood glucose levels below the upper normal limit (i.e., below 100 mg/dL for an overnight fasting glucose).

Overview of Metabolism of Selected Amino Acids During the Digestive Phase

The flow of AAs into hepatocytes during the digestive period is coupled to deamination and entry of ammonia into the urea cycle, and the conversion of deaminated carbon skeletons of AAs into pyruvate, acetyl CoA, or intermediates of the TCA cycle (Fig. 3.10). AAs are also used in several anabolic pathways, including of course protein synthesis, but also including glutathione synthesis, nucleotide synthesis, and glucosamine synthesis during the digestive phase. Insulin both promotes the synthesis of many macromolecules (e.g., protein synthesis), as well as inhibiting their degradation (e.g., proteosomal degradation of proteins).

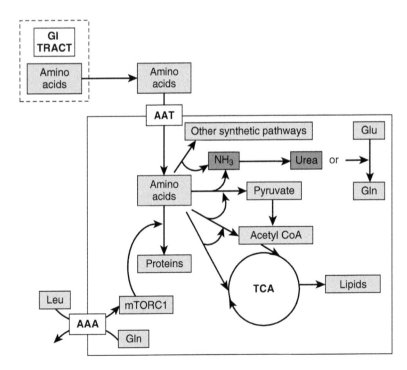

Fig. **3.10** Overview of use of amino acids within energy metabolism. *AAA,* Amino acid antiporter; *AAT,* amino acid transporter. In hepatocytes, most ammonia is converted to urea. In other cell types, amino groups are transferred to glutamate *(Glu)* to form glutamine *(Gln).*

AAs that are not metabolized by the liver enter the general circulation for use by other cells. The most abundant circulating AA is glutamine (Gln), due to its abundance in the diet and to its generation from the transfer of amino groups to glutamate (Glu) in most cells. Gln is required for the hexosamine pathway that is involved in protein glycosylation, nucleotide biosynthesis, and can be exchanged for leucine (Leu) through several cell membrane antiporters. Leu, in turn, is a strong activator of mTORC1, which promotes RNA, protein and lipid synthesis (see Fig. 3.10). Leu also stimulates insulin secretion in β cells. Gln can also be converted to Glu, which can be used to synthesize several other AAs, protein, as well as the antioxidant molecule, glutathione. Glu can also be converted to the TCA cycle intermediate, α-ketoglutarate (also designated 2-oxoglutarate). This is especially important in the hepatocyte during de novo lipogenesis, in that α-ketoglutarate replaces carbons ("anaplerosis") that exit the TCA cycle as citrate ("cataplerosis"). Thus Gln and Glu contribute to de novo lipogenesis, as well as ATP generation. Other AAs can be converted to pyruvate or TCA cycle intermediates and also contribute to de novo lipogenesis and ATP production.

Overview of Long-Chain Free Fatty Acid Metabolism During the Digestive Phase

Long chain FFAs (designated herein simply as FFAs), with 13 to 21 carbons, are common in the diet. These lipids are absorbed by the intestinal enterocytes as either FFAs or as 2-monoglyceride. Within the enterocytes, FFAs are re-esterified to the 2-monoglyceride to form TG. TG, in turn, is assembled with the apoprotein B48 and other lipids to form nascent chylomicrons. Chylomicrons are too large to enter capillaries, and instead enter lymphatics that convey them to the thoracic duct that empties directly into the circulation near the left venous angle. Thus unlike glucose and AAs, chylomicrons are not directly conveyed to hepatocytes via the hepatic portal vein, but enter the systemic circulation close to the heart (see Fig. 3.1A).

Within the circulation, chylomicrons mature by having other apoproteins transferred to them from high-density lipoprotein (HDL) particles. As chylomicrons enter the capillary beds within adipose tissue, they undergo lipolysis that is catalyzed by lipoprotein lipase (LPL). In response to high insulin during the digestive phase, LPL is synthesized within adipocytes, secreted, and ultimately becomes noncovalently attached to the luminal membrane of the endothelial cells that line the capillary beds. LPL-mediated digestion releases FFAs from chylomicron-associated TGs (discussed later). The FFAs are transported across the endothelial cells and into the adipocytes. As stated previously, adipocytes convert a significant fraction of glucose to glycerol-3-phosphate, which is used as the backbone for reesterification of the imported FFAs for storage as TG within the adipocyte.

Several intracellular lipases can reverse this process, potentially releasing FFAs into the blood through an inappropriate futile cycle during the digestive phase. FFAs would compete for glucose utilization, thereby promoting glucose intolerance. A key hormone-regulated intracellular lipase is called hormone-sensitive lipase (HSL). During the digestive phase, high insulin levels directly inhibit HSL activity and prevent the lipolysis of newly synthesized TG.

TG is stored as cytoplasmic lipid droplets (CLDs) within adipocytes. These CLDs are coated primarily by the perilipin isoform, PLIN1. Perilipins interact with lipases and lipase-activating proteins that stabilize CLDs during the digestive phase, but reconfigure CLDs in the presence of PKA signaling from catecholamines and glucagon to allow for lipolysis and release of FFAs and glycerol.

The partially digested chylomicrons become chylomicron remnants as they move through adipose capillary beds. Chylomicron remnants eventually bind to apoprotein E–related receptors on hepatocytes and undergo receptor-mediated endocytosis and digestion within lysosomes. The residual FFAs that are released from the remnants are reesterified to TGs, and thus contribute to the total intrahepatic TG.

Hepatic Metabolism During The Digestive Phase
Anatomic Considerations

The liver is anatomically and functionally situated between the GI tract and the heart. The main veins that drain the GI tract of its ingested nutrients all converge to form the hepatic portal vein. A "portal vein" is defined as a vein that conveys the contents of a capillary bed (or many convergent capillary beds) to a second set of capillary beds before reaching the heart. In the case of the hepatic portal vein, it receives the venous drainage of the GI tract and then ends at the hepatic sinusoids (a sinusoid is a discontinuous capillary). This means that the liver is the first organ to receive the ingested carbohydrates and AAs before they reach the general circulation (as stated previously, FFAs and TGs initially bypass the liver because they enter lymphatics as chylomicron particles). The liver is also the first organ to respond to hormones and cytokines from the pancreas and intraabdominal adipose tissue.

Hormonal Regulation of Key Reactions in the Liver During the Digestive Phase
Intracellular Transport and Trapping of Monosaccharides

Ingested monosaccharides (glucose, fructose, and galactose) reach the liver sinusoids and flow down their concentration gradient into hepatocytes through the bidirectional,

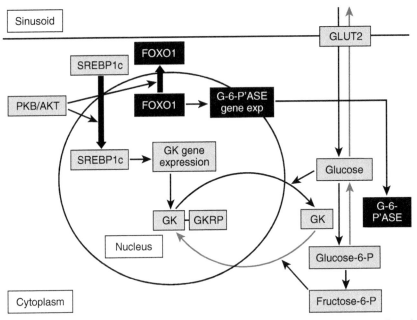

Fig. 3.11 Regulation of glucokinase *(GK)* and glucose-6-phosphatase *(G-6-P'ASE)* during digestive phase *(black arrows)* and fasting phase *(orange arrows)* stages.

facilitative transporter, GLUT2 (Fig. 3.11). GLUT2 is a low-affinity, high-capacity facilitative transporter well-suited to moving high amounts of absorbed glucose during and soon after a meal. GLUT2 expression or localization at the hepatocyte cell membrane is largely not regulated.

Intrahepatic glucose is trapped by phosphorylation to G6P by the enzyme, GK (see Fig. 3.11). GK has a low affinity and high Vmax. Thus GK, which is a member of the hexokinase family of enzymes, is paired with GLUT2 in the β cell and hepatocyte. GK can only catalyze the phosphorylation of glucose, not its dephosphorylation (i.e., the reaction is irreversible). Normally, dephosphorylation of G6P to glucose is catalyzed by the liver-specific enzyme, glucose-6-phosphatase (G-6-P'ASE) during the fasting phase (see Fig. 3.11).

Hepatic GK is tightly regulated by metabolites and by insulin (see Fig. 3.11). In the absence of glucose, GK is sequestered in the nucleus by binding to GK regulatory protein (GKRP). Increased glucose promotes the dissociation of GK from its GKRP and translocation into the cytoplasm, where it converts glucose to G6P. The downstream product, fructose-6-phosphate, inhibits GK by promoting its sequestration.

Insulin, acting through the AKT signaling pathway, stimulates the new synthesis of GK through activation of SREBP1c (see Fig. 3.11; Table 3.1). Insulin/Akt promotes the nuclear localization of SREBP1c, which in turn stimulates GK gene expression (see Fig. 3.11). Insulin/Akt

also inhibits expression of G-6-P'ASE (reverse reaction) through the inactivation of FOXO1. Nuclear FOXO1 stimulates G-6-P'ASE gene transcription. AKT phosphorylates FOXO1, thereby sequestering FOXO1 in the cytoplasm (see Fig. 3.11).

As stated previously (see Fig. 3.9), the conversion of glucose to G6P essentially "activates" glucose so that it can now enter several metabolic pathways.

Storage of Glucose as Glycogen

Insulin/Akt signaling increases the activity of glycogen synthase in several ways (Fig. 3.12). Insulin/Akt indirectly increases glycogen synthase through increased expression of GK because high levels of G6P allosterically increase glycogen synthase activity. Insulin/Akt increases the activity of protein phosphatase-1 (see Fig. 3.12), which dephosphorylates and thereby activates glycogen synthase. Insulin/Akt also inactivates glycogen synthase kinase-3 (GSK3β), which, in turn, promotes the accumulation of dephosphorylated (active) glycogen synthase. Insulin/Akt prevents the futile cycle of glycogen synthesis and glycogenolysis through inhibition of glycogen phosphorylase (see Fig. 3.12). Insulin/Akt-activated protein phosphatase-1 dephosphorylates and inactivates glycogen phosphorylase as well as phosphorylase kinase. Glycogen phosphorylase is also inactivated by glucose, G6P, and ATP.

TABLE 3.1 Hepatic Genes Stimulated by SREBP1c

Gene	Enzyme	Pathway
GCKR	Glucokinase (hexokinase-4)	Glycolysis
PKLR	Pyruvate kinase (liver and red blood cells)	Glycolysis
ACLY	Adenosine triphosphate and citrate lyase	De novo lipogenesis
ACACA	Acetyl coenzyme A (CoA) carboxylase-1(acetyl CoA carboxylase-α)	De novo lipogenesis
ACACB	Acetyl CoA carboxylase-2 (acetyl CoA carboxylase-β)	De novo lipogenesis
FASN	Fatty acid synthase	De novo lipogenesis
G6PD	Glucose-6-phosphate dehydrogenase	Pentose phosphate pathway (hexose monophosphate shunt)

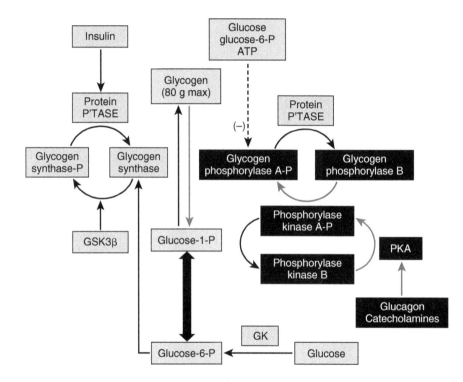

Fig. 3.12 Regulation of glycogen synthesis (*black arrows*, digestive) and glycogenolysis (*orange arrows*, fasting). protein P'TASE, protein phosphatase. *GK*, Glucokinase; *GSK*, glycogen synthase kinase.

Glycolysis

G6P is also metabolized through the glycolytic pathway. Once glycogen stores are filled, glycogen synthesis ceases, further increasing the flux of G6Pe through glycolysis. There are two hormonally regulated cytoplasmic enzymes within glycolysis (after GK): **phosphofructokinase-1 (PFK1)** and **liver-specific pyruvate kinase (PK-L)**.

Phosphofructokinase-1. The **PFK1 reaction** converts fructose-6-phosphate (F6P) to fructose-1,6-bisphosphate (F1,6bisP) (Fig. 3.13). This reaction is irreversible, requiring a separate enzyme, **fructose-1,6-bisphosphatase**, to

catalyze the reverse reaction. The PFK1 reaction is one of the most tightly regulated reactions in metabolism, and it is also one of the few reactions in hepatocytes that does not involve the transcription factor, SREBP1c. The PFK1 reaction is altered by allosteric regulators on a minute-to-minute basis. During the digestive phase, PFK1 activity is moderated by high levels of ATP and cytoplasmic citrate (as discussed earlier, citrate moves from the mitochondria to the cytoplasm at times when the TCA cycle is slowed down by abundant ATP and NADH during the digestive phase). In contrast, AMP allosterically activates PFK1.

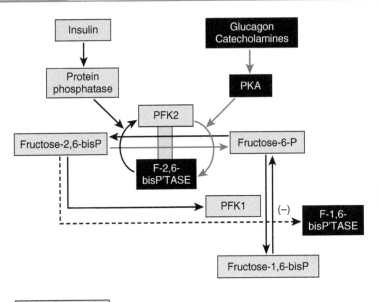

Fig. 3.13 Hormonal regulation of phosphofructose kinase-1 *(PFK1)* and fructose-1,6-bisphosphatase *(F-1,6-bisP'TASE)* by levels of fructose-2,6-bisphosphate. The dual activity enzyme, PFK2/F-2,6-bisP'TASE, acts as the kinase when dephosphorylated and as a phosphatase when phosphorylated. *Dashed lines* indicate allosteric inhibition.

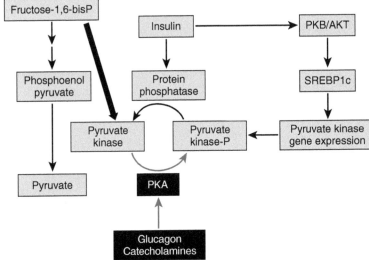

Fig. 3.14 Regulation of pyruvate kinase during the digestive phase *(black arrows)* and fasting phase *(orange arrows)* states. Fructose-1,6-bisphosphate is an allosteric activator of pyruvate kinase.

Another major allosteric activator of PFK1 is the glycolytic side product, **fructose-2,6-bisphosphate (F2,6bisP**; see Fig. 3.13). F2,6bisP is produced from F6P by the **phosphofructose kinase-2 (PFK2)** function of the **bifunctional enzyme, PFK2/fructose-2,6-bisphosphatase**. The PFK2 function of the enzyme is active when the enzyme is dephosphorylated by an insulin/Akt-activated protein phosphatase-1 (see Fig. 3.13). The fructose-2,6-bisphosphatase function is active when the enzyme is phosphorylated by a glucagon- and catecholamine-activated PKA (see Fig. 3.13). Through the generation of F2,6bisP, insulin/Akt commits G6P to glycolysis during the digestive phase.

The opposing reaction that converts F1,6bisP to F6P is catalyzed by the gluconeogenic enzyme, **fructose-**1,6-bisphosphatase. F2,6bisP is an allosteric inhibitor offructose-1,6-bisphosphatase (see Fig. 3.13), thereby inhibiting inappropriate hepatic glucose production during the digestive phase.

Pyruvate kinase. The **pyruvate kinase** reaction is also irreversible and converts phosphoenolpyruvate (PEP) to pyruvate (Fig. 3.14). This reaction is coupled to ATP synthesis and accounts for the next two ATPs/molecule of glucose produced by glycolysis. Pyruvate kinase is allosterically activated by the upstream intermediate, **F1,6bisP** (see previous section). In this way, insulin/Akt activates pyruvate kinase indirectly through a feed-forward mechanism that is initiated by the insulin/Akt-induced production of F2,6bisP (see Fig. 3.14). Pyruvate kinase is also regulated by phosphorylation. Insulin/

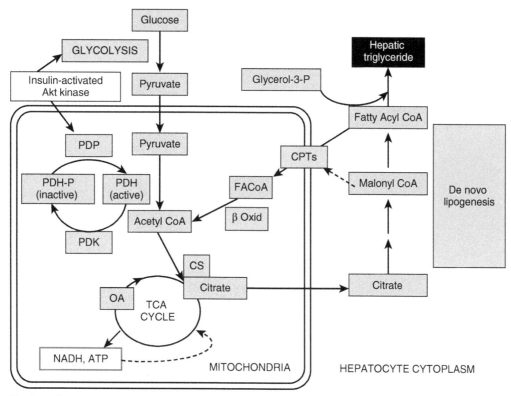

Fig. 3.15 Regulation of pyruvate dehydrogenase *(PDH)* by pyruvate dehydrogenase kinase *(PDK)* and pyruvate dehydrogenase phosphatase *(PDP)*. Also, de novo lipogenesis from the movement of citrate into the cytoplasm. *CS*, Citrate synthase.

Akt activates pyruvate kinase through dephosphorylation by protein phosphatases. Insulin also has a longer-term effect on pyruvate kinase gene transcription through the AKT-activated SREBP1c pathway (see Fig. 3.14).

Entry of Pyruvate into the Tricarboxylic Acid Cycle

Glycolysis generates pyruvate, which can be converted to lactate by lactate dehydrogenase. This replenishes NAD+ levels required for glycolysis to continue. In hepatocytes with active mitochondria, NAD+ is continually regenerated from NADH through the electron transport chain. This promotes the entry of pyruvate into the mitochondria (Fig. 3.15), where it enters the TCA cycle. This first requires the conversion of pyruvate into acetyl CoA (AcCoA), as catalyzed by the PDH complex. PDH kinase is associated with the PDH complex, and phosphorylation of the PDH complex inhibits its activity (see Fig. 3.15). PDH kinase is activated by ATP, acetyl CoA, and NADH. However, in the face of high glycolytic flux during the digestive phase, abundant pyruvate acts as a potent allosteric inhibitor of PDH kinase, thereby activating PDH and promoting the conversion of pyruvate to acetyl CoA (see Fig. 3.15). In addition, insulin/Akt stimulates PDH

phosphatase, which dephosphorylates and activates PDH. The conversion of pyruvate to AcCoA generates 1 molecule of NADH, as well as 1 molecule of CO_2. Oxidation of NADH back to NAD+ will generate 3 ATPs through the processes of the electron transport chain and oxidative phosphorylation.

Tricarboxylic Acid Cycle

Acetyl CoA (2 carbons) is condensed with oxaloacetate (4 carbons) to form citrate (6 carbons), as catalyzed by citrate synthase. In the absence of abundant energy, citrate is cycled through seven reactions back to oxaloacetate, generating 3 NADH and 1 FADH2, which will generate 11 ATPs through processing by the electron transport chain and oxidative phosphorylation. Another reaction within the TCA cycle generates GTP, which is converted to ATP. As the digestive phase progresses, intramitochondrial NADH and ATP become increasingly abundant and allosterically inhibit the progression of the TCA cycle after citrate. The slowing of the TCA cycle allows citrate to accumulate andultimately flow through citrate transporters into the cytoplasm. Cytoplasmic citrate is the first intermediate in de novo lipogenesis (see Fig. 3.15).

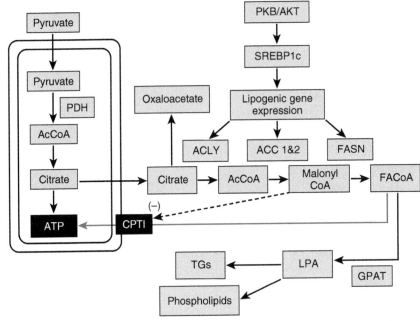

Fig. 3.16 Regulation of de novo lipogenesis. *ACC,* Acetyl CoA carboxylase; *AcCoA,* acetyl CoA; *ACLY,* ATP-citrate lyase; *CPTI,* carnitine palmitoyl transferase; *FACoA,* fatty acyl CoA; *FASN,* fatty acid synthase; *GPAT,* glycerol phosphate acyltransferase; *LPA,* lysophosphatidic acid; *TG,* triglyceride.

De Novo Lipogenesis

De novo lipogenesis normally occurs only in the liver, adipose tissue, and lactating mammary glands. New synthesis of fatty acyl CoAs involves three hormonally regulated enzymes: ATP-citrate lyase (ACLY), acetyl CoA carboxylase (ACC1 and ACC2), and fatty acid synthase (FASN). Cytoplasmic citrate is converted to acetyl CoA, and acetyl CoA can be used for fatty acyl CoA synthesis (Fig. 3.16) or cholesterol synthesis (not shown). ACC converts acetyl CoA to malonyl CoA, which is the key substrate for production of fatty acyl CoAs by FASN (see Fig. 3.14). FASN requires NADPH, which is obtained by the PPP (see the following text), and the conversion of cytoplasmic oxaloacetate (from the ACLY reaction on citrate) to malate, followed by conversion to pyruvate by malic enzyme (NAD$^+$-dependent malate dehydrogenase).

The expression of ACLY, ACC1, ACC2, FASN, as well as **glycerol-3-phosphate acyltransferase (GPAT;** generates lysophosphatidic acid [LPA]) is coordinately stimulated by insulin-activated SREBP1c (see Fig. 3.16). LPA is then converted to TG. In addition, ACC1 activity is increased by insulin/Akt-activated dephosphorylation (Fig. 3.17). Conversely, ACC1 and ACC2 are phosphorylated and inactivated by AMPK during the fasted state. The production of malonyl CoA by ACC1 is also antagonized by AMPK-activated **malonyl CoA decarboxylase (MDC;** see Fig. 3.17). Whereas ACC1 is in the cytoplasm (cyto), ACC2 is localized to the

outer mitochondrial membrane. The malonyl CoA generated by ACC2 directly inhibits **carnitine-palmitoyl transferase-I (CPTI)** on the outer mitochondrial membrane. Thus ACC1 promotes lipogenesis, whereas ACC2 inhibits fatty acyl oxidation and ketogenesis during the digestive phase (see Fig. 3.17).

NADPH PRODUCTION THROUGH THE PENTOSE PHOSPHATE PATHWAY

As stated previously, de novo lipogenesis is dependent on abundant NADPH as a cofactor. NADPH is derived primarily from the PPP and from malic enzyme. Insulin promotes the flux of G6P into the PPP (see Fig. 3.9) through the stimulation of **glucose-6-phosphate dehydrogenase** gene transcription by SREBP1c.

In summary, in the liver, insulin promotes the following:
- Glycogen synthesis
- Glycolysis
- De novo lipogenesis, leading to production of cholesterol, phospholipids, and TG
- NADPH production through the PPP
- Protein and organelle synthesis, in part through mTORC1 (not discussed)

In the liver, insulin inhibits the following:
- Hepatic glucose production by inhibiting glycogenolysis and gluconeogenesis

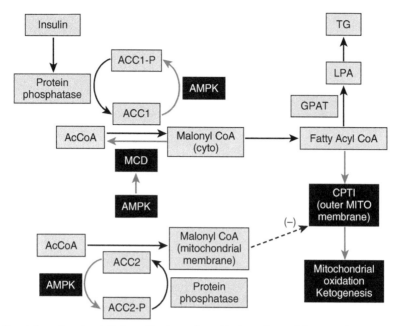

Fig. 3.17 Regulation of malonyl CoA synthesis as the critical regulator of lipogenesis versus oxidation of lipid. *AcCoA*, Cytoplasmic acetyl CoA; *ACC*, acetyl CoA carboxylase; *AMPK*, AMP-activated kinase; *CPTI*, carnitine-palmitoyl transferase-I; *GPAT*, glycerol phosphate acyltransferase; *LPA*, lysophosphatidic acid; *MCD*, malonyl CoA decarboxylase.

- Fatty acid oxidation and ketogenesis
- Proteolysis

In terms of the intracellular nutrient and energy sensors:

1. mTORC1 is activated in the digestive phase by a combination of increased AAs and insulin-PKB/AKT signaling. mTORC1 stimulates protein synthesis. mTORC1 also stimulates de novo lipogenesis through stimulating SREBP1c activity.
2. In the digestive phase, with a surfeit of ATP, AMPK is inactive.

Skeletal Muscle Metabolism During The Digestive Phase

The glucose that is not metabolized by the liver contributes to the postprandial rise in glucose levels in the peripheral circulation. **Glucose intolerance** refers to the inability to minimize the degree and duration of excursions of blood glucose concentrations. A primary way in which insulin prevents glucose intolerance is through promoting the uptake of glucose into skeletal muscle (Fig. 3.18). Insulin stimulates the translocation of preexisting **GLUT4 transporters** within to the cell membrane. In the absence of insulin, GLUT transporters reside in **GLUT storage vesicles**, which are largely retained in the cytoplasm. Insulin signaling, both through PKB/AKT and a small G-protein pathway, significantly increasing insertion of GLUT storage vesicles into the cell membrane.

As in the liver, insulin also promotes the storage of intramyocellular glucose by stimulating **glycogen synthesis** in muscle, and the use of glucose for ATP synthesis through glycolysis and the TCA cycle. Insulin stimulates muscle-associated isoforms of hexokinases (converting glucose to G6P) and glycolytic enzymes. Importantly, in the presence of excessive carbohydrate intake, insulin increases TG synthesis from glucose in skeletal muscle (through activation of SREBP1c), which can lead to ectopic intramyocellular TG and associated lipids. The intramyocellular lipid load may lead to lipotoxicity and insulin resistance (see later). Note that **exercise** increases intracellular Ca^{2+} and the **AMP/ATP ratio**, both of which stimulate **AMPK**, which inhibits lipogenesis and stimulates oxidation of FFAs.

Skeletal muscle contains a large amount of protein. During the digestive phase, insulin and AAs stimulate mTORC1, which in turn stimulates protein synthesis.

Adipocyte Metabolism During the Digestive Phase

Insulin stimulates GLUT4-dependent uptake of glucose and subsequent glycolysis in **adipocytes** as it does in skeletal muscle (Fig. 3.19). Adipocytes use glycolysis for energy needs, but also for the generation of **glycerol-3-phosphate**, which is required for the reesterification of FFAs into TGs. As discussed previously, most dietary FFAs reach the adipocytes in the form of TGs within

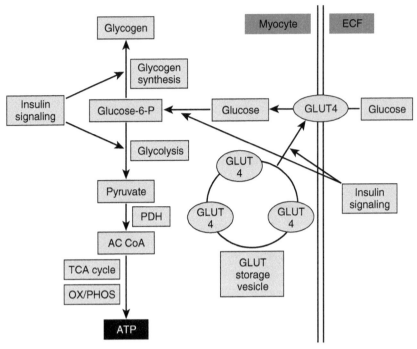

Fig. 3.18 Regulation of glucose uptake and use in skeletal muscle during the digestive phase.

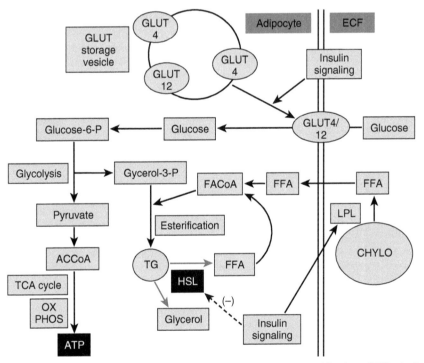

Fig. 3.19 Regulation of glucose uptake, lipolysis of chylomicrons, and reesterification of FFAs in the adipocyte during the digestive phase. *HSL*, Hormone-sensitive lipase; *LPL*, lipoprotein lipase.

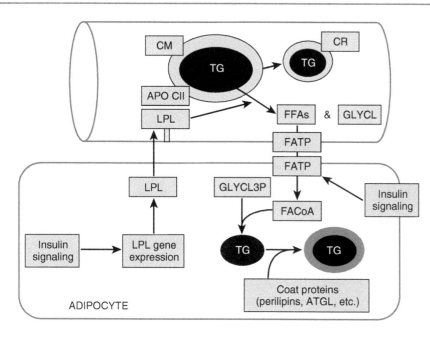

Fig. 3.20 Regulation of lipoprotein lipase *(LPL)* synthesis secretion and transcellular transport to the apical membrane of endothelial cells. *CM,* Chylomicron; *CR,* chylomicron remnant; *GLYCL3P,* glycerol-3-phosphate.

chylomicrons. The TGs within the chylomicrons are digested by the extracellular lipase, LPL. Insulin stimulates the expression of LPL within adipocytes and its exocytosis and migration to the apical side of endothelia of adipose capillary beds (Fig. 3.20). This action of insulin thereby promotes the release of FFAs from chylomicrons within the capillary beds of adipose tissue. Insulin also stimulates the expression of fatty acid transport proteins (e.g., CD36) into the cell membrane. Fatty acid transport proteins facilitate the movement of FFAs into the adipocyte and the activation of FFAs by their conversion to fatty acyl CoAs. Insulin/Akt stimulates glycolysis in adipocytes, which generates the glycerol-3-phosphate required for reesterification of FFAs into TGs (see Figs. 3.19 and 3.20). Insulin/Akt stimulates protein phosphatases, which, in turn, dephosphorylate and inactivate HSL and dephosphorylate and stabilize TG droplet coat proteins (e.g., perilipin 1) (see Fig. 3.20).

Insulin/Akt signaling also activates a nuclear receptor, called peroxisome proliferator activated receptor-γ (PPARγ). PPARγ promotes the differentiation of preadipocytes into adipocytes. As in liver and skeletal muscle, insulin and AAs promote the protein synthesis through activation of mTORC1.

In considering glucose and lipid metabolism during the digestive phase as stated previously, it becomes apparent that two major sources of TG in hepatocytes are de novo lipogenesis from glucose, fructose (and AAs), and from the endocytosis of chylomicron remnants (Fig. 3.21). A

third source comes from the expression of hepatic lipase (HL), which is expressed on the cell membrane of hepatocytes, and drives lipolysis of TGs associated with smaller lipoprotein particles, including intermediate-density lipoprotein (IDL) particles, HDL particles, and low-density lipoprotein (LDL) particles (discussed further in the following text). The liver is not able to store large amounts of TG safely, and extensive intrahepatic lipids is referred to as hepatic steatosis or fatty liver. Further, turnover of TGs to metabolites such as DAG leads to the activation of signaling pathways (e.g., DAG activates isoforms of PKC) that inhibit the insulin receptor signaling pathway, causing insulin resistance. Normally, hepatocytes do not become too engorged with intrahepatic lipid, because they package TGs and other lipids with apoprotein B100 (apoB100) to form VLDL particles, and export the VLDL particles to the blood so that they can be used for fuel by several tissues, including skeletal and cardiac muscle. In general, chylomicrons are the dominant large, TG-rich lipoproteins during the digestive phase, whereas VLDL are the same for the fasting phase. Secretion of VLDL during the digestive phase would dangerously increase blood TG levels. Accordingly, insulin inhibits apoB100 expression and stability during the digestive phase. But in the face of hepatic steatosis and insulin resistance, excessive TG-rich VLDL is secreted continuously (see Fig. 3.21). This results in abnormally high blood TG levels. VLDL particles are first converted to IDL particles by muscle LPL, and then to cholesterol-rich LDLs by hepatic lipase. High TG-rich

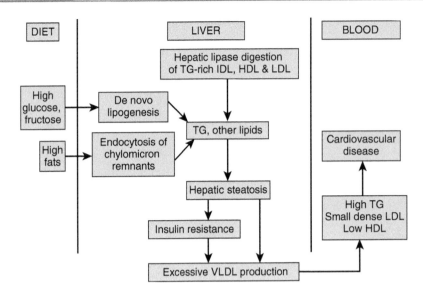

Fig. 3.21 Sources of hepatic lipids that, in excess, lead to hepatic steatosis, insulin resistance, and excessive TG-rich VLDL production, ultimately leading to small dense LDL, low levels of HDL, and high blood TG, all of which potentially lead to cardiovascular disease.

VLDL results in the transfer of TG to LDL and HDL particles, making them good substrates for HL. Digestion by HL of TG-rich LDL lead to small dense LDL particles, which are atherogenic. Digestion of TG-rich HDL leads to lipid-poor apoprotein A1, which is then excreted at the kidney. This results in low HDL levels, and thus poor transfer of cholesterol away from sites of cholesterol accumulation (e.g., atherogenic cholesterol-laden macrophages).

OVERVIEW OF ENERGY METABOLISM DURING THE FASTING PHASE

The Big Picture

The liver, skeletal muscle, and adipose tissue largely act independently during the digestive phase. In contrast, there is considerable interaction among these organs during the fasting phase in an effort to (1) provide the fuels and energy to all cells for the continuation of bodily functions and (2) preventing blood glucose from falling too low and causing acute CNS stress and dysfunction. Key processes/adaptations to fasting include:

- breakdown of liver glycogen (glycogenolysis) for release of glucose into the blood, followed by the synthesis of glucose from 3-carbon metabolites (lactate, pyruvate, glycerol, glucogenic AAs) through gluconeogenesis (hepatic glucose production);
- minimal glucose uptake by skeletal muscle and adipocytes due to retention of GLUT4 within cytoplasmic vesicles (glucose sparing);

- the release of FFAs from adipocytes for use by adipocytes and other cells (e.g., skeletal muscle) (glucose sparing);
- the release of TG-rich VLDL lipoproteins for delivery of FFAs and other lipids to skeletal and cardiac muscle (glucose sparing);
- the conversion of a fraction of FFAs (released by adipocytes) and ketogenic AAs (released primarily from skeletal muscle) into ketone bodies within hepatocytes for use by other nonhepatic cell types. The CNS is able to utilize ketone bodies for ATP production during an extended fast (glucose sparing).

Several hours after a meal, especially during sleep, nutrient levels fall, leading to lower levels of insulin secretion. Consequently, the actions of insulin on hepatic, muscle, and adipose tissue are attenuated. The decrease in insulin also relieves inhibition of glucagon secretion. During the fasting phase, glucagon and catecholamines promote hepatic glucose production, VLDL assembly and export, FFA oxidation, and ketone body synthesis and release (Fig. 3.22). Another major consequence of low insulin is the release of Akt-induced inhibition of the transcription factor FOXO1. FOXO1 promotes gluconeogenesis and VLDL assembly in the liver.

During the fasting phase, with low insulin levels, muscle fibers import minimal amounts of glucose because of basal levels of GLUT4 in their plasma membrane. Muscle fibers switch from using glucose to using abundant FFAs, as well as ketone bodies in a longer fast, for ATP synthesis (Fig. 3.23). Skeletal muscle also releases lactate and AAs. During exercise or in response to a fight-or-flight situation, muscle mobilizes its glycogen stores for ATP production (see Fig. 3.23).

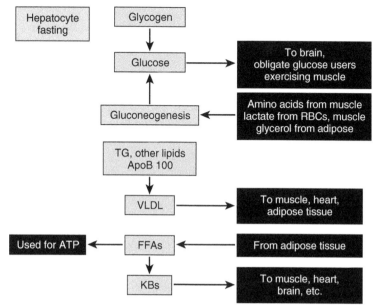

Fig. 3.22 Overview of hepatocyte function during the fasting phase.

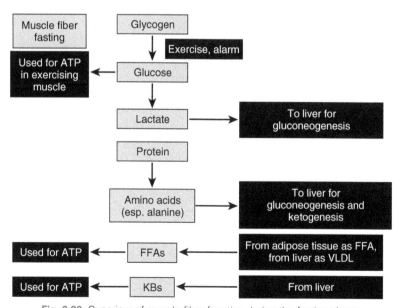

Fig. 3.23 Overview of muscle fiber function during the fasting phase.

The adipocytes also have low GLUT4 levels at their cell membrane during the fasting phase and consequently cannot generate glycerol-3-phosphate for TG synthesis. The low insulin and high catecholamine levels promote lipolysis of TG and the release of FFAs into the blood (Fig. 3.24). Adipocytes will also switch to FFAs and ketone bodies for ATP synthesis.

Adipocyte Metabolism During the Fasting Phase

In adipose tissue, catecholamines (and to a lesser extent, glucagon) stimulate phosphorylation of HSL and perilipin proteins that surround and stabilize fat droplets (Fig. 3.25). Phosphorylated perilipins reconfigure the triglyceride-cytoplasm interface and allow access to adipocyte triglyceride lipase (ATGL) and HSL (a DAG lipase),

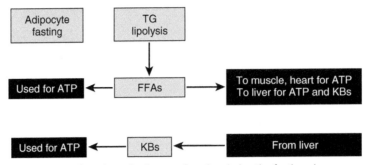

Fig. 3.24 Overview of adipocyte function during the fasting phase.

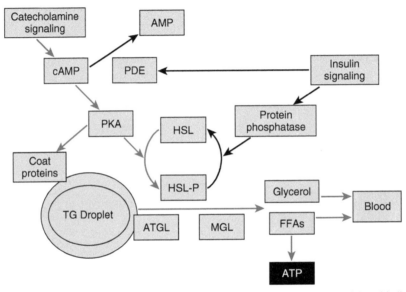

Fig. 3.25 Regulation of lipolysis in the adipocyte during the fasting. *ATGL,* Adipocyte triglyceride lipase; *HSL,* hormone-sensitive lipase; *MGL,* monoglyceride lipase; *PDE,* cyclic AMP phosphodiesterase; *PKA,* protein kinase A.

which is activated by phosphorylation. After the final monoglycerol lipase (MGL) reaction, FFAs and glycerol are released. FFAs circulate in the blood as FFA-albumin complexes, and, as discussed previously, become a very important source of energy substrate in muscle and liver. This use of FFAs, especially by skeletal muscle, plays an essential glucose-sparing role.

The adipocyte uses FFAs (and ketone bodies) for ATP synthesis because it has very little access to carbohydrates in the fasting phase. The ability of adipocytes to import glucose is very low because only basal levels of insulin-dependent GLUT4 transporters are localized at the cell membrane, and the adipocyte does not store glycogen. The low abundance of glucose also results in very low levels of glycerol-3-phosphate. This results in minimal reesterification

of released FFAs back to acylglycerides, avoiding a futile cycle.

Skeletal Muscle Metabolism During the Fasting Phase

During the fasting phase, with low insulin levels, muscle fibers import minimal amounts of glucose because of basal levels of GLUT4 in their plasma membrane. Muscle fibers switch from using glucose to using abundant FFAs, as well as ketone bodies in a longer fast, for ATP synthesis (see Fig. 3.23). FFAs enter myocytes through transporters and generate high levels of intramitochondrial acetyl CoA by β-oxidation (Fig. 3.26). FFAs and FFA derivatives act as ligands and activate a member of the nuclear receptor family (see Chapter 1), called PPARα. Activated PPARα stimulates the expression of CPTI and the enzymes involved in β-oxidation, thereby promoting fatty acid oxidation. PPARα is also activated by glucagon- and catecholamine-PKA signaling and by AMPK.

Pyruvate dehydrogenase complex is inhibited by the relatively abundant acetyl CoA. Thus more pyruvate is converted to lactate (there is no gluconeogenesis in muscle), and the released lactate is used by the liver for gluconeogenesis. Skeletal muscle also expresses LPL in an insulin-independent manner, and skeletal muscle LPL increases during the fasting phase and exercise. This allows skeletal muscle to import FFAs from two sources: circulating FFA-albumin complexes and VLDL from liver.

Catecholamine/PKA and fatty acids activate the transcription factor, PPARα, which drives the process of mitochondrial lipid β-oxidation. The switch from glucose to FFAs as a source of energy, along with low levels of GLUT4 in the cell membrane (due to low insulin), allows the skeletal muscle to spare glucose for the brain and obligate glucose users (e.g., erythrocytes, lens cells of the eye).

During exercise, muscle glycogen is mobilized for ATP production (see Fig. 3.26). Glycogenolysis in muscle is largely driven by intracellular Ca^{2+}, which activates phosphorylase kinase as a Ca^{2+}-calmodulin complex.

In response to acute stress or alarm, norepinephrine is released as a fight-or-flight reaction. Norepinephrine signals through the α1-adrenergic receptor that is coupled to a Gq/phospholipase C signaling pathway. This ultimately causes a rapid release of intracellular Ca^{2+} (see Chapter 1). AMP is also an allosteric activator of muscle-specific glycogen phosphorylase. During exercise in a fasted individual, the depletion of ATP also leads to activation of AMPK, which also activates PPARα and promotes β-oxidation of FFAs. However, AMPK also increases GLUT4 transporters at the cell membrane, thereby increasing glucose uptake, and activates the glycolytic pathway. Thus exercise has the potential of causing hypoglycemia.

In the skeletal muscle, a high catecholamine-to-insulin ratio promotes increased proteolysis and decreased protein synthesis. This results in the release of gluconeogenic and ketogenic AAs for use by the liver. In summary, both skeletal muscle and adipose tissue contribute to circulating blood glucose through the release of gluconeogenic substrates (lactate, AAs, glycerol) and indirectly through the release of FFAs by adipocytes, which allow skeletal muscle and other tissues to consume less glucose (glucose-sparing). Finally, release of FFAs and ketogenic amino acids supports ketogenesis by the liver.

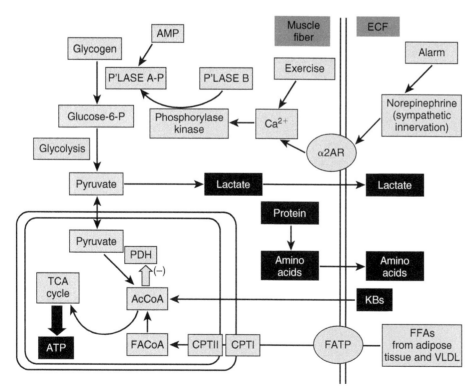

Fig. 3.26 Regulation of muscle metabolism during fasting phase and during exercise of a fight-or-flight alarm response. *α2AR*, $α_2$-adrenergic receptor.

LIVER METABOLISM DURING THE FASTING PHASE

Hormonal Regulation of Key Reactions in the Liver During the Fasting Phase

(See Fig. 3.22 for an overview).

Hepatic Glucose Production

Glycogenolysis. Glucagon and catecholamines, acting through Gs-coupled receptors (glucagon receptor and β₂-adrenergic receptor, respectively) stimulate PKA, leading to the phosphorylation and activation of phosphorylase kinase and glycogen phosphorylase (see Fig. 3.12). Additionally, the loss of insulin/Akt signaling prevents the dephosphorylation and activation of glycogen synthase. Collectively, these actions lead to the increase in hepatic G6P levels. For G6P to leave the liver through the GLUT2 transporter (and contribute to hepatic glucose production), it needs to be dephosphorylated to glucose. This reaction is catalyzed by G-6-P'ASE within the smooth endoplasmic reticulum (see Fig. 3.11). In the absence of insulin/AKT signaling, the transcription factor, FOXO1, remains in the nucleus and stimulates G-6-P'ASE gene expression. Glycogenolysis supports hepatic glucose production for about 12 to 16 hours at the beginning of a fast.

Gluconeogenesis. Gluconeogenic enzymes include pyruvate carboxylase (PC), PEP carboxykinase (PEPCK), and fructose-1,6-bisphosphatase, as well as glucose-6-phosphatase (in the previous text). All of these reactions are irreversible (i.e., opposed by a separate glycolytic enzyme). Gluconeogenesis can continue for days and weeks, as long as glucogenic substrates (lactate, glucogenic AAs, glycerol) are delivered to the liver.

Pyruvate Carboxylase. During the fasting phase, hepatic pyruvate is primarily generated from lactate and alanine, as opposed to glucose (Fig. 3.27). Furthermore, little pyruvate is decarboxylated to acetyl CoA by the PDH

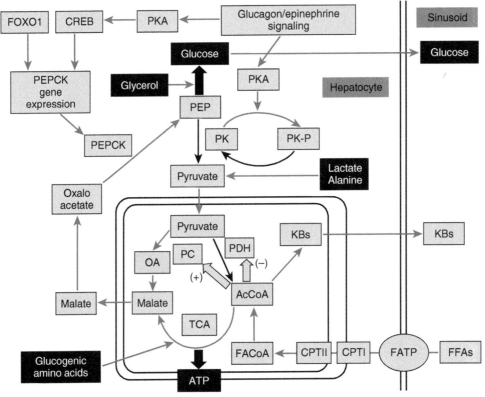

Fig. 3.27 Regulation in hepatocyte of the gluconeogenic enzymes, pyruvate carboxylase *(PC)* and phosphoenolpyruvate carboxykinase *(PEPCK)* during the fast stage. *CPT,* carnitine-palmitoyl transferase (CPTI is in outer mitochondrial membrane; CPTII is in inner mitochondrial membrane; *CREB,* cyclic AMP response element binding protein; *FATP,* fatty acid transport protein; *KBs,* ketone bodies (acetoacetate and hydroxybutyrate); *OA,* oxaloacetate; *PDH,* pyruvate dehydrogenase; *PK,* pyruvate kinase; *PKA,* protein kinase A.

complex. Rather, pyruvate is converted to the 4-carbon oxaloacetate by PC. This switch occurs primarily in response to an increase in FFA oxidation. FFAs from adipocytes are readily oxidized in the liver. Loss of insulin/Akt signaling decreases malonyl CoA levels, removing the inhibition on CPTI and allowing FFAs to enter the mitochondria (see Figs. 3.15, 3.16, and 3.17). As FFAs undergo β-oxidation, the massive amounts of acetyl CoA released activate PDH kinase and inhibit the PDH complex. In contrast, high acetyl CoA levels allosterically activate PC. The oxaloacetate produced by PC is converted to malate and then exits the mitochondria through the malate shuttle to be used for gluconeogenesis (see Fig. 3.27).

PEPCK. Cytoplasmic oxaloacetate is converted to PEP by PEPCK (see Fig. 3.27). PEPCK gene expression is increased by glucagon- and epinephrine-PKA-CREB signaling (see Chapter 1) and by FOXO1, which remains active in the nucleus in the absence of insulin.

Importantly, PEP is not efficiently converted back to pyruvate (i.e., thereby causing a futile cycle) because glucagon and epinephrine phosphorylate and inactivate pyruvate kinase (see Fig. 3.27).

Fructose-1,6-Bisphosphatase. The absence of insulin/Akt signaling and increased glucagon/PKA signaling selectively increases the fructose-2,6-bisphosphatase activity of the bifunctional enzyme, phosphofructose kinase 2/ fructose-2,6-bisphosphatase. This causes the levels of the allosteric regulatory metabolite, F2,6bisP, to decrease. This reduces PFK1 activity, but releases inhibition of fructose-1,6-bisphosphatase (see Fig. 3.13). As this enzyme becomes activated, its substrate, F1,6bisP, reaches an equilibrium at a lower level. This further inhibits pyruvate kinase, which is allosterically activated by fructose-1,6-bisphosphate (see Fig. 3.14).

Once F1,6bisP is converted to F6P, it is converted to G6P, which, in turn, is converted to glucose that can exit the GLUT2 transporter.

Switch to Use of FFAs for ATP and Ketogenesis. As discussed earlier, adipose tissue releases FFAs during the fasting phase. FFAs are used by the hepatocytes for ATP production through β-oxidation (see Fig. 3.27). In the face of low insulin, malonyl CoA is not produced by acetyl CoA carboxylase-2, thereby allowing fatty acyl CoAs to enter the mitochondria through the CPT transporters. As discussed previously for muscle, intrahepatic FFAs and their derivatives, as well as glucagon- and catecholamine-PKA signaling activate PPARα. Activated PPARα stimulates the expression of CPTI and the enzymes involved in β-oxidation, thereby promoting fatty acid oxidation.

The oxidation of fatty acyl CoAs requires their conversion to acetyl CoA, and the continuation of fatty acyl oxidation requires the regeneration of free CoA. This

is accomplished in the liver by the formation of ketone bodies, acetoacetate (which degrades spontaneously to acetone), and β-hydroxybutyrate. The liver does not possess the enzymes for ketone body catabolism. Consequently, ketone bodies are released into the blood (see Fig. 3.27) and, because of their hydrophilic nature, easily circulate unbound to carrier proteins or particles. Ketone bodies can be used by all cells with mitochondria for ATP production and are used by the brain during an extended fast or starvation.

ADIPOSE TISSUE–DERIVED HORMONES AND ADIPOKINES

White adipose tissue (WAT) contributes to the regulation of energy metabolism in the adult through the production of hormones and adipokines. Adipose tissue is composed of several cell types. The TG-storing cell is called the adipocyte. These cells develop during gestation in humans from preadipocytes. This process of adipocyte differentiation, which may continue throughout life, is promoted by several transcription factors. One of these factors is SREBP1c, which regulates genes involved in FFA and TG synthesis. SREBP1c is activated by lipids as well as insulin and several growth factors and cytokines. Another important transcription factor in adipose tissue is PPARγ. PPARγ is a member of the nuclear receptor superfamily and the natural ligands for PPARγ are FFAs and their derivatives. Activated PPARγ promotes expression of genes involved in TG storage. Thus an increase in food consumption leads to SREBP1c and PPARγ activation, which increases preadipocyte differentiation into small adipocytes, and an upregulation of enzymes within these cells to allow storage of the excess fat.

In addition to adipocytes, about 50% of WAT is composed of nonadipocyte cells including resident connective tissue cells (e.g., fibroblasts, macrophages) and a connective tissue matrix, cells associated with blood vessels, and cells associated with inflammatory and immune responses. WAT also receives a rich autonomic innervation. Several cell types contribute to the integrated endocrine function of WAT.

WAT is divided into subcutaneous and intraabdominal (visceral) depots. Intraabdominal WAT refers primarily to omental and mesenteric fat and is the smaller of the two depots. These depots receive different blood supplies that are drained in a fundamentally different way, in that the venous return from the intraabdominal fat leads into the hepatic portal system. Thus intraabdominally derived FFAs are mostly cleared by the liver, whereas subcutaneous fat is the primary site for providing FFAs to muscle during exercise or fasting. The regulation of intraabdominal and subcutaneous adipose tissue also differs. These depots are innervated by distinct sets of neurons within autonomic

TABLE 3.2   Adipose Tissue- and Stomach-Derived Hormones Involved in Metabolism, Appetite, and Insulin Resistance and Sensitivity

Hormone/ Cytokine	Cell of Origin	SC vs. IA	Stimulus for Secretion	Primary Target	Actions
Leptin	Adipocyte	SC > IA	Increased adiposity	Hypothalamus	Decreases appetite Increases energy expenditure in adipose and nonadipose tissue Improves insulin sensitivity Allows for reproductive maturity
Adiponectin	Adipocyte	SC > IA	Weight loss (including surgical)	Muscle Liver Blood vessels and heart Macrophages	Activates oxidation of free fatty acids Antiinflammatory/antioxidant Improves insulin sensitivity Improves health of cardiovascular tissues and protects against cell death
Tumor necrosis factor-α	Adipocyte White adipose tissue Macrophage	IA > SC	Engorgement of adipocytes	Liver Muscle Adipocytes Other organs	Reduces adipocyte mass Proinflammatory Opposes insulin signaling Increases insulin resistance Atherogenic
Interleukin-6	White adipose tissue Macrophage	IA > SC	Other inflammatory cytokines	Liver Muscle Adipocytes Other organs	Opposes insulin signaling Increases insulin resistance Increases acute-phase protein production by liver Proinflammatory systemically
Ghrelin	P/D1 cells of stomach ε cells of islets	Not applicable	Empty stomach	Pituitary gland Hypothalamus	Increases growth hormone secretion (Opposes glucoregulatory and liporegulatory actions of insulin) Increases insulin resistance Increases appetite

SC, subcutaneous adipose; *IA,* intra-abdominal adipose

nuclei in the spinal cord and brainstem and are influenced differently by sex steroids. Men tend to gain fat in the intraabdominal depot (**android [apple-shaped] adiposity**), whereas women tend to gain fat in the subcutaneous depot, particularly in the thighs and buttocks (**gynecoid [pear-shaped] adiposity**). Finally, these two depots display differences in hormone production and enzyme activities (Table 3.2).

Visceral adipose tissue secretes less **adiponectin**, which normally has beneficial effects on insulin resistance through activation of PPARα and AMPK. Adiponectin also has a strong beneficial action on cardiovascular tissue, including exerting antiinflammatory effects, opposing oxidative stress, and increasing cell survival in response to disease or stress (see Table 3.2).

Visceral adipose tissue also secretes less **leptin**. Leptin has an important role in liporegulation in peripheral tissues. Leptin protects peripheral tissues (i.e., the liver, skeletal muscle, cardiac muscle, β cells) from the accumulation of too much lipid, directing storage of excess caloric intake into adipose tissue. This action of leptin, although opposing the lipogenic actions of insulin, contributes significantly to the maintenance of insulin sensitivity (as defined by insulin-dependent glucose uptake) in peripheral tissues. Leptin also acts as a signal that the body has sufficient energy stores to allow for reproduction and to enhance erythropoiesis, lymphopoiesis, and myelopoiesis. For example, in women suffering from **anorexia nervosa**, leptin levels are extremely low, resulting in low ovarian steroids, amenorrhea (lack of menstrual bleeding), anemia due to low red blood cell production, and immune dysfunction, which promotes lipid oxidation and glucose uptake and use in nonadipose tissue.

Visceral adipose tissue secretes more inflammatory cytokines than subcutaneous adipose tissue, including tumor necrosis factor-α (TNF-α) and interleukin-6 (IL-6). These cytokines oppose insulin signaling at the receptor and postreceptor levels.

APPETITE CONTROL AND OBESITY

The amount of energy stored by an individual is determined by calorie intake and calories expended as energy/day. In many individuals, input and output are in balance, so the weight of that individual remains relatively constant. However, the abundance of inexpensive high-fat, high-carbohydrate food, along with more sedentary lifestyles, is contributing to a pandemic of obesity and the pathologic sequelae of obesity, including T2DM and cardiovascular disease. The preponderance of stored energy consists of fat, and individuals vary greatly in the amounts and percentages of body weight that are accounted for by adipose tissue. About 25% of the variance in total body fat appears to be accounted for by genetic factors. A genetic influence on fat mass is supported by the following:

- Tendency to correlate better with that of their biologic parents than with that of their adoptive parents
- Greater similarity of adipose stores in identical (monozygotic) twins, whether reared together or apart, than in fraternal (dizygotic) twins
- Greater correlation between the gains in body weight and in abdominal fat in identical twins than in fraternal twins when they are fed a caloric excess
- Discovery of several genes that cause obesity

In addition, the gestational environment has a profound effect on the body mass of the adult. The effect of maternal diet on the weight and body composition of offspring is called fetal programming. Low birthweight correlates with increased risk for obesity, cardiovascular disease, and diabetes. These findings suggest that the efficiency of fetal metabolism has plasticity and can be altered by the environment in utero. The development of a thrifty metabolism would be advantageous to an individual born to a mother who received poor nutrition and into a life that meant chronic undernourishment. However, a thrifty metabolism increases the risk for obesity in the face of the caloric excess often confronting today's individuals.

Body Mass Index

One measure of adiposity is the body mass index (BMI). The BMI of an individual is calculated as follows:

$$BMI = weight\ (in\ kilograms)/height\ (in\ meters^2)$$

The BMI of healthy lean individuals ranges from 20 to 25. A BMI greater than 25 indicates that the individual is overweight, whereas a BMI over 30 indicates obesity. The condition of being overweight or obese is a risk factor for multiple pathologies, including insulin resistance, dyslipidemia, diabetes, cardiovascular disease, and hypertension.

Clearly, an excess of abdominal fat poses a greater risk factor for the pathologies mentioned previously. Thus another indicator of body composition is circumference of the waist (measured in inches around the narrowest point between ribs and hips when viewed from the front after exhaling) divided by the circumference of the hips (measured at the point where the buttocks are largest when viewed from the side). This waist-to-hip ratio may be a better indicator than BMI of body fat, especially as it relates to the risk for developing diseases. A waist-to-hip ratio of greater than 0.95 in men, or 0.85 in women, is linked to a significantly higher risk for developing diabetes and cardiovascular disease.

Hypothalamic Neurons and Appetite Control

The arcuate (ARC) nucleus (a nucleus is a collection of neuronal cell bodies within the central nervous system) in the hypothalamus is the key regulator of fuel sensing and food intake (Fig. 3.28). One group of ARC neurons synthesizes proopiomelanocortin (POMC) and cocaine and amphetamine-regulated transcript (CART). As discussed more in Chapter 5, POMC is proteolytically processed in a cell specific manner: in the ARC POMC/CART neurons, POMC is processed to form α-melanocyte stimulating hormone (α-MSH). POMC/CART neurons project to second-order neurons located in several areas of the brain, including the ventromedial hypothalamus, the lateral hypothalamus, and the brainstem. α-MSH binds to the melanocortin receptors, MC3R and MC4R, on second-order neurons, which innervate other areas of the CNS and orchestrate the cessation of eating (anorexigenic effect) and an increase in energy output. These circuits also coordinate autonomic nervous system activity, with diverse endocrine actions on thyroid gland function, reproduction, and growth. CART has a similar anorexigenic action. A second group of neurons expresses the peptides, NPY and agouti-related peptide (AgRP). AgRP competes for α-MSH at MC4R receptors and inhibits their activation. NPY acts at NPY receptors and is a potent orexigen. Thus the NPY/AgRP neurons increase eating (orexigenic effect) and diminish energy use.

Leptin represses signaling from the NPY/AgRP and stimulates the production of POMC-derived α-MSH and the production of CART, both of which inhibit food

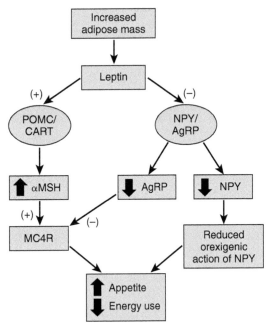

Fig. 3.28 Regulation of appetite by the action of leptin on two groups of neurons in the arcuate nucleus of the hypothalamus. See text for explanation. Thin arrows denote inhibited action.

intake. Thus leptin acts as a satiety signal that decreases food consumption and increases energy expenditure (see Fig. 3.28). To maintain overall energy homeostasis, the system must also balance specific nutrient intake and expenditure, for example, CHO intake with CHO oxidation. This may account for some specificity in neuropeptide and neurotransmitter responses to meals. Serotonin produces satiety after glucose ingestion. GI

hormones, such as CCK and GLP-1, produce satiety by humoral effects, but their local production in the brain may participate in nutrient and caloric regulation. Insulin is also an important regulator of appetite. The recently discovered hormone ghrelin (see Table 3.2) is an acylated peptide with potent orexigenic activity that arises in endocrine cells in the mucosa of the stomach. Plasma levels of ghrelin rise in humans in the 1 to 2 hours that precede their normal meals. The plasma levels of ghrelin fall drastically to minimal values about 1 hour after eating. Ghrelin appears to stimulate food intake by reacting with its receptor in hypothalamic neurons that express NPY.

Long-Term Sequelae of Diabetes Mellitus

Hyperglycemia leads to elevated intracellular glucose in specific cell types, especially endothelial cells in the retina, kidney, and capillaries associated with peripheral nerves. This glucotoxicity alters cell function in several ways that may contribute to pathologic changes. These include increased synthesis of polyols, hexosamines, and DAG (which activates PKC). Although the exact mechanisms by which intracellular accumulation of these molecules causes abnormal cell function remain unclear, current thinking indicates that these changes lead to increased oxidative stress within the cell. Additionally, intracellular nonenzymatic glycation of proteins gives rise to advanced glycation end products (AGEs). Intracellular AGEs have altered function, whereas secreted AGEs in the extracellular matrix interact abnormally with other matrix components and matrix receptors on cells. Finally, some secreted AGEs interact with receptors on macrophages and endothelial cells. Endothelial receptors for AGEs (RAGEs) lead to proinflammatory gene expression.

CLINICAL BOX 3.4

Diabetes Mellitus (DM)

DM is a disease in which insulin levels and/or the responsiveness of tissues to insulin are insufficient to maintain normal levels of plasma glucose. Although the diagnosis of DM is based primarily on plasma glucose, DM also causes dyslipidemia (high TG-rich lipoproteins, low HDL). Normal fasting (i.e., no caloric intake for at least 8 hours) plasma glucose levels should be below 100 mg/dL. A patient is considered to have impaired glucose control (glucose intolerance) if the fasting plasma glucose is between 110 and 126 mg/dL, and the diagnosis of DM is made if the fasting plasma glucose exceeds 126 mg/dL on two successive days. Another approach to the diagnosis of diabetes is the

oral glucose tolerance test. After overnight fasting, the patient is given a bolus amount of glucose (usually 75 g) orally, and blood glucose levels are measured at 2 hours. The glucose is administered orally rather than intravenously (IV) because the insulin response to an oral glucose load is faster and greater than the response to an IV load (i.e., the incretin effect; see previous text). A 2-hour plasma glucose greater than 200 mg/dL on 2 consecutive days is sufficient to make the diagnosis of DM. The diagnosis of diabetes is also indicated if the patient presents with symptoms associated with diabetes (see later) and has a nonfasting plasma glucose value of greater than 200 mg/dL.

Diabetes Mellitus (DM)

Type 1 DM (T1DM) and T2DM represent the two major forms of DM. T1DM accounts for about 10% of newly diagnosed cases. T1DM usually, but not always, occurs in the preteenage and early teenage years. T1DM involves an autoimmune-mediated destruction of the islet β cells. T1DM represents an absolute deficit in insulin. Untreated T1DM results in runaway catabolic and starvation-associated metabolism, in which FFAs released from adipose tissue flood the liver and are converted into ketone bodies, while hepatic glucose production is increased and glucose uptake by muscle is minimal. The rampant ketogenesis leads to diabetic ketoacidosis, which is a form of metabolic acidosis. Uncorrected ketoacidosis can lead to cardiovascular collapse and coma. Diabetic ketoacidosis also results in the loss of K^+ from the intracellular compartment and ultimately from the body through increased renal excretion. Thus K^+ replacement needs to be one component of the treatment of diabetic ketoacidosis. Hyperglycemia causes osmotic diuresis and dehydration but ultimately can lead to systemic hyperosmolality and neurologic dysfunction and coma. T1DM is usually not associated with obesity. Instead, muscle wasting and dehydration promote weight loss, muscle pain, and weakness. Patients experience frequent urination (polyuria) matched with excessive thirst and frequent drinking (polydipsia). Patients also experience hunger due to imbalances in the hypothalamic signaling, leading to frequent eating (polyphagia). Patients with T1DM require insulin replacement therapy. T2DM is by far the more common form, accounting for 90% of diagnosed cases. However, T2DM is often a progressive and insidious disease that remains undiagnosed in a significant percentage of patients for several years. T2DM is often associated with visceral obesity and lack of exercise; indeed, obesity-related T2DM is reaching epidemic proportions worldwide. Usually, there are multiple causes for the development of T2DM in a given individual that are associated with defects in the ability of target organs to respond to insulin (i.e., insulin resistance), along with an increasing degree of β-cell damage and deficiency as the disease progresses. Insulin sensitivity can be compromised at the level of the insulin receptor (IR) or, more commonly, at the level of postreceptor signaling. T2DM appears to be the consequence of insulin resistance, followed by reactive hyperinsulinemia. As β cells succumb to increased oxidative damage trying to compensate for hyperglycemia, relative hypoinsulinemia appears (i.e., inadequate release of insulin to compensate for the end

organ resistance). Although insulin resistance specifically refers to an inability of insulin to maintain blood glucose levels below normal upper limits, the underlying causes of insulin resistance differ among patients. Three major underlying causes of obesity-induced insulin resistance are as follows:

1. A decreased ability of insulin to increase GLUT4-mediated uptake of glucose, especially by skeletal muscle. This function, which is specifically a part of the glucometabolic regulation by insulin, may be due to the excessive accumulation of TG in the muscle of obese individuals. Excessive caloric intake induces hyperinsulinemia. Initially, this leads to excessive glucose uptake into skeletal muscle. Just as in the liver (see Fig. 3.13), excessive calories in the form of glucose promote lipogenesis and, through the generation of malonyl CoA, repression of fatty acyl CoA oxidation. Byproducts of fatty acid and TG synthesis, such as DAG and ceramide, may accumulate and stimulate signaling pathways (e.g., PKC-dependent pathways) that antagonize signaling from the insulin receptor or IRS proteins. Thus insulin resistance in the skeletal muscle of obese individuals may be due to lipotoxicity. High caloric intake is also associated with abundant circulating AAs, which stimulate mTORC1. mTORC1 negatively feeds back on the insulin receptor and IRS proteins.

2. A decreased ability of insulin to repress hepatic glucose production. The liver makes glucose by glycogenolysis in the short term and by gluconeogenesis in the long term. The ability of insulin to repress key hepatic enzymes in both of these pathways is attenuated in insulin-resistant individuals. Insulin resistance in the liver may also be due to lipotoxicity in obese individuals (e.g., fatty liver or hepatic steatosis). The degree of insulin resistance is correlated to degree of visceral (e.g., abdominal) obesity. Note that secreted products of visceral adipose tissue enter the hepatic portal system, conveying these products directly to hepatocytes.

Visceral adipose tissue is likely to affect insulin signaling at the liver in several ways, in addition to the effects of lipotoxicity. For example, visceral adipose tissue releases proinflammatory cytokines, such as TNF-α, which has been shown to antagonize insulin signaling pathways. Also, TG in visceral adipose tissue has a high rate of turnover (possibly due to a rich sympathetic innervation) so that the liver is exposed to high levels of FFAs, which further exacerbate hepatic lipotoxicity.

Continued

CLINICAL BOX 3.4—cont'd

Diabetes Mellitus (DM)

3. An inability of insulin to repress HSL or increase LPL in adipose tissue. High HSL and low LPL are major factors in the dyslipidemia associated with insulin resistance and diabetes. The dyslipidemia is characterized as hypertriglyceridemia and large TG-rich VLDL particles produced by the liver. Because of their high TG content, large VLDLs give rise to TG-rich intermediate-density-lipoprotein (IDL) particles. These IDL particles are excellent substrates for digestion by the ectoenzyme, hepatic lipase. Ultimately, small, dense LDL particles are generated, which are very atherogenic. In contrast, small HDL particles are inherently unstable and rapidly cleared. Thus HDL, which normally plays a protective role against vascular disease, drops to low levels. Insulin resistance in adipose tissue is likely due to the production of antiinsulin local factors, such as TNF-α and other inflammatory cytokines. Note that reduction of LPL in adipose tissue results in the import of more TG by the liver upon endocytosis of TG-rich chylomicron remnants, further exacerbating hepatic steatosis.

CLINICAL BOX 3.5

Exercise and weight loss are effective treatments for obesity-related insulin resistance and T2DM. The beneficial effects from exercise are due, in part, to the activation of AMPK. AMPK activates PPARγ and lipid oxidation and inhibits de novo lipogenesis. The oral hypoglycemic agent, metformin, is a front-line therapy for T2DM and appears to act, in part, through activation of AMPK. Metformin is readily transported by hepatocytes and inhibits hepatic glucose production and increases lipid oxidation. Metformin also uncouples oxidative phosphorylation, allowing more calories to be lost as heat. Fibrate drugs target PPARα, which stimulates FFA oxidation. Fibrates are used to lower circulating lipids in T2DM patients with dyslipidemia.

CLINICAL BOX 3.6

The ability of hepatocytes to export TG is critical to their viability and normal function. TGs are not normally stored in the liver to a large extent. However, a sedentary lifestyle and overeating can result in intrahepatocyte TG levels that are out of balance with VLDL synthesis and export as well as FFA oxidation. This leads to the development of hepatic steatosis (fatty liver) and insulin resistance at the liver. Hepatic steatosis predisposes the liver to more serious disease, such as hepatocellular carcinoma and fibrotic changes. Hepatic steatosis represents the inability of the liver to form and export VLDL at a pace that equals the influx of TG (via chylomicron remnants), FFAs, and carbohydrates and is closely associated with diet-induced obesity.

Numerous other factors promote insulin resistance and may act at skeletal muscle, liver, and adipose tissue. Hyperinsulinemia per se causes down regulation of the insulin receptor and components of the insulin receptor signaling pathway (especially IRS proteins) and activates intracellular negative feedback pathways such as the suppressor of cytokine signaling-3 (SOCS3) pathway and mTORC1. Inflammatory cytokines (e.g., IL-6) similarly increase SOCS3, thereby inducing a crossover negative feedback loop in which insulin signaling is inhibited. Glucocorticoids, which are released in response to stress and acute hypoglycemia, are diabetogenic. Sex steroids also antagonize insulin signaling. The growth hormone prolactin and its homolog human placental lactogen (which is also high during pregnancy) also induce insulin resistance. Finally, the ARC region of the hypothalamus, acting through the autonomic nervous system, can induce insulin resistance.

As insulin resistance worsens, reactive hyperinsulinemia progressively increases in an attempt to regulate glucose. This often leads to some degree of compromised β-cell function; patients with T2DM may require insulin therapy at some point in their life. Patients with T2DM can also benefit from agents that optimize β-cell function, such as sulfonylurea drugs or GLP-1 analogs.

An important circulating product of glycation is hemoglobin A1c (HbA1c), which is a useful marker for long-term glucose regulation. A red blood cell has a 120-day life span; once glycation occurs, the hemoglobin remains glycated for the remainder of the red blood cell's life span. The proportion of HbA1c present in a nondiabetic person is low. However, a diabetic patient who has had prolonged periods of hyperglycemia over the past 8 to 12 weeks will have elevated levels. HbA1c measurements are clinically useful for checking treatment compliance.

Retinopathies are various forms of retinal abnormalities that develop in diabetic patients. Retinopathies are the major cause of new-onset blindness in preretirement adults in the United States. Hyperglycemia results in high intracellular glucose concentrations in retinal endothelial cells and pericytes (capillary supportive cells). This is due to the inability of these cells specifically to adapt to hyperglycemia by decreasing GLUT expression. As discussed earlier, elevated intracellular glucose initiates multiple mechanisms that ultimately lead to endothelial cell dysfunction, leading to increased resistance, hypertensive-induced changes, and cell death. These microvascular changes lead to microaneurysms, increased capillary permeability, small retinal hemorrhages, and excessive microvascular proliferation. Proliferative retinopathy is caused by impaired blood flow to the retina and subsequent tissue hypoxia. Subsequent vascular degeneration can produce vitreal hemorrhage, retinal detachment, and neovascular glaucoma, all of which can lead to severe vision loss. As blood glucose and therefore blood osmolarity rise, the volume of the lens changes, distorting vision. Diabetic patients commonly have cataracts, and sorbitol and glycosylated protein accumulation have been proposed as mechanisms for inducing cataract formation. Peripheral nerve damage (neuropathy) can occur as a result of metabolic, oxidative, or immune-related damage to neurons or Schwann cells. Additionally, the microvasculature of peripheral nerves undergoes changes similar to those seen in retinopathies and may represent an event that is concurrent with, or causal to, peripheral neuropathy. Schwann cells (supportive cells involved in myelination) are among those shown to accumulate sorbitol as a result

of hyperglycemia. Diabetic patients can exhibit sensory loss, paresthesias, and even pain as a result of the neurologic damage. Neuropathies of the autonomic nerves also develop in diabetic patients, which can lead to numerous symptoms in multiple organ systems, including erectile dysfunction, postural hypotension, and heat intolerance. The sensory loss is more apparent in the extremities, particularly the lower portions of the legs and feet. This poses particular problems because, as diabetic patients lose cutaneous sensation in the feet, they become unaware of poorly fitting shoes and are more prone to injuries. Poor peripheral circulation aggravates this problem.

Because diabetic patients have impaired wound healing, foot ulcerations can become a serious threat. Diabetes is a common cause of impairment of renal function (nephropathy) and is the greatest cause of end-stage renal disease in North America. Clinical or overt diabetic nephropathy is characterized by the loss of greater than 300 mg of albumin in the urine over a 24-hour period (microalbuminuria) and progressive decline of renal function. Nephropathies develop from microvascular changes that occur in the glomerular capillaries. The glomerular capillary basement membrane thickens, resulting in thicker walls and narrower lumina (glomerulosclerosis) and expansion of the supportive mesangial cells. Podocytes detach and undergo apoptosis. Poor renal filtration also leads to activation of the renin-angiotensin system (see Chapter 7), inducing hypertension.

Atherosclerosis develops in diabetic patients at an accelerated rate (macroangiopathies). Diabetic patients are more likely to have coronary artery disease and myocardial infarction than are nondiabetic individuals. Macrovascular disease is also associated with necrosis of lower extremities and the need for amputation. Many diabetic patients with coronary artery disease have the additional risk factors of hypertension, abdominal obesity, insulin resistance, and dyslipidemia. This cluster of factors has been identified as the metabolic syndrome (also called syndrome X, insulin resistance syndrome, and cardiovascular dysmetabolic syndrome). Some of the consequences of visceral obesity, insulin resistance, and dyslipidemia were discussed earlier.

SUMMARY

1. Cells must continually make ATP to meet their energy needs. ATP is made by glycolysis and by the TCA cycle coupled to oxidative phosphorylation.
2. Cells can oxidize carbohydrate (primarily in the form of glucose), amino acids, and FFAs to make ATP. Additionally, the liver makes ketone bodies (as well as glucose) for other tissues to oxidize for energy in times of fasting.

3. Some cell types are limited in what energy substrates they can oxidize for energy. The brain is normally exclusively dependent on glucose for energy. Thus blood glucose must be maintained above 60 mg/dL for normal autonomic and central nervous system function.

4. Conversely, inappropriately high levels of glucose (i.e., fasting glucose above 100 mg/dL) promote glucotoxicity in specific cell types, leading to the long-term complications of diabetes.

5. The endocrine pancreas produces the hormones insulin, glucagon, somatostatin, gastrin, ghrelin, and pancreatic polypeptide.

6. Insulin is produced from the β cells and is an anabolic hormone that is secreted in times of excess nutrient availability. It allows the body to use carbohydrates as energy sources to store nutrients, and to use nutrients for anabolic pathways.

7. Major stimuli for insulin secretion include increased serum glucose and certain amino acids. Cholinergic (muscarinic) receptor activation also increases insulin secretion, whereas $α_2$-adrenergic receptors inhibit insulin secretion. The GI tract releases incretin hormones that stimulate pancreatic insulin secretion. GLP-1 and GIP are particularly potent in augmenting glucose-dependent stimulation of insulin secretion.

8. Insulin binds to the insulin receptor, which is linked to multiple pathways that mediate metabolic and growth effects of insulin.

9. During the digestive phase, insulin acts on the liver to promote conversion of glucose to glucose-6-phosphate. Insulin also increases glycogenesis, glycolysis, and fatty acid synthesis (de novo lipogenesis) in the liver. Insulin inhibits hepatic glucose production (glycogenolysis and gluconeogenesis) and ketogenesis. Insulin regulates hepatic metabolism by both regulating gene expression, especially through its effects on SREBP1c and FOXO1, and posttranslational dephosphorylation events.

10. Insulin increases GLUT4-mediated glucose uptake in muscle and adipose tissue.

11. Insulin increases glycogenesis, glycolysis, and, in the presence of caloric excess, lipogenesis in skeletal muscle. Insulin increases muscle amino acid uptake and protein synthesis.

12. In adipocytes, insulin increases glucose uptake, glycolysis, and the production of glycerol-3-phosphate. Insulin also increases the expression and export to capillary beds of lipoprotein lipase (LPL), import of FFAs and their reesterification into TG and cytoplasmic lipid droplets. Insulin dephosphorylates and thereby decreases activity of hormone sensitive lipase (HSL).

13. Glucagon is a catabolic hormone. Its secretion increases during periods of food deprivation, and it acts to mobilize nutrient reserves.

14. Glucagon is released in response to decreased serum glucose (and therefore decreased insulin), increased serum amino acid levels, and β-adrenergic signaling.

15. Glucagon binds to the glucagon receptor, which is linked to Gs/PKA-dependent pathway

16. The primary target organ for glucagon is the liver. Glucagon increases hepatic glucose output by increasing glycogenolysis and gluconeogenesis. It also increases oxidation of fatty acids and ketogenesis.

17. Glucagon regulates hepatic metabolism by both regulating gene expression and through posttranslational PKA-dependent phosphorylation events.

18. The major counterregulatory factors in muscle and adipose tissues are the adrenal hormone epinephrine, and the sympathetic neurotransmitter norepinephrine. These two factors act through β2- and β3-adrenergic receptors to increase cAMP levels. Epinephrine and norepinephrine increase glycogenolysis and fatty acyl oxidation in muscle and increase hormone-sensitive lipase in adipose tissue.

19. Cells express intracellular sensors of nutrients and energy. Two of these are: mTORC1, which senses amino acids and growth factor/insulin signaling and promotes anabolic pathways; and AMP-activated kinase (AMPK), which senses a low level of energy (AMP/ATP ratio) and inhibits anabolic pathways, while driving catabolic pathways (glycolysis).

20. It is increasingly well established that adipose tissue has an endocrine function, especially in terms of energy homeostasis. Hormones produced by adipose tissue include leptin and adiponectin. Adipose tissue also releases proinflammatory cytokines, including IL-6, and TNF-α, that can induce insulin resistance.

21. The ARC of the hypothalamus is the central regulator of appetite and energy use.

22. The POMC/CART neurons secrete α-MSH, which acts on second-order neurons to promote satiety and increase energy expenditure (i.e., anorexigenic). NPY/AgRP neurons act to promote eating and reduce energy expenditure (i.e., orexigenic). Several hormones act on these neurons to control nutrient and energy balance, including leptin, insulin, CCK, and ghrelin.

23. Two forms of DM are classified as type 1 (T1DM) and type 2 (T2DM). T1DM is characterized by the destruction of pancreatic β cells and requires exogenous insulin for treatment. T2DM accounts for as much as 90% of all diabetes. T2DM can be due to numerous factors but usually is characterized as insulin resistance coupled to some degree of β-cell deficiency. Patients with T2DM may require exogenous insulin at some point to maintain blood glucose levels. Obesity-associated T2DM is currently at epidemic proportions worldwide.

24. Obesity-associated T2DM is characterized by insulin resistance due to lipotoxicity, hyperinsulinemia, and inflammatory cytokines produced by adipose tissue.

T2DM is often associated with obesity, insulin resistance, hypertension, and coronary artery disease. This constellation of risk factors is referred to as metabolic syndrome.

25. Major symptoms of DM include hyperglycemia, polyuria, polydipsia, polyphagia, muscle wasting, electrolyte depletion, and ketoacidosis (in T1DM). Long-term complications of poorly controlled diabetes are due to excess intracellular glucose (glucotoxicity) in specific cells, especially in the retina, kidney, and peripheral nerves. This leads to retinopathies, nephropathies, and neuropathies. Diabetes also increases the risk for cardiovascular disease and loss of adequate blood flow in the lower extremities.

CLINICAL BOX 3.7

Statin drugs are used to treat individuals with hypercholesterolemia due to excessive LDL cholesterol. Statins target 3-hydroxy-3-methylglutaryl (HMG) CoA reductase, so one effect of these drugs is to simply lower cholesterol synthesis. Additionally, lowering cholesterol synthesis in the liver leads to an activation of SREBP2 and an increase in LDL receptor expression. This allows the liver to increase the clearance of LDL cholesterol form the blood. Why is LDL cholesterol a risk factor for cardiovascular disease? LDL particles are relatively small and make their way into the lamina propria of the tunica intima (the layer just below the endothelial lining) of blood vessels at regions of endothelial damage and death due to hypertension, cigarette smoke, or other factors. Oxidation of LDL components leads to engulfment by macrophages that ultimately become engorged with cholesterol. At this point, macrophages are called foam cells. Foam cells become participants in a series of events that lead to the development of an atherosclerotic plaque. Plaques are dangerous because they can become unstable and rupture. Once this happens, the blood is exposed to prothrombic molecules. This induces the formation of blood clots (thrombi) that can occlude the arterial lumen. In the coronary arteries, a thrombus potentially leads to myocardial infarction, and in arteries in the brain, a thrombus causes a stroke.

SELF-STUDY PROBLEMS

1. During the fed state, how does the role of glycolysis in the liver differ from the role of glycolysis in adipose tissue?

2. How does the function of glycogen differ in the liver versus the skeletal muscle?

3. Normally, the brain is dependent on glucose. What other energy substrate is used by the brain during a prolonged fast? What is the origin of this substrate?

4. What is the relation between mitochondrial citrate levels and lipogenesis?

5. What two enzymes in adipocytes are dysregulated in DM that contribute to high levels of circulating TGs?

6. Why does loss of the LDL receptor give rise to high blood cholesterol?

7. What futile cycle do high levels of malonyl CoA prevent?

8. How would a mutant glucokinase with decreased transport activity affect insulin secretion?

9. How does insulin regulate the following hepatic enzymes: (a) glucokinase, (b) fructose-1,6- bisphosphatase, (c) pyruvate kinase, (d) acetyl CoA carboxylase, (e) PEPCK? Be specific.

10. What is the basis for ketoacidosis in patients with poorly managed type 1 diabetes mellitus?

11. How is obesity related to insulin resistance?

KEYWORDS AND CONCEPTS

Digestive phase versus fasting phase

Glucose, amino acids, free fatty acids, ketone bodies as fuels

Glycogen, triglyceride, protein as storage forms of fuels

Pancreatic Islet Cells (especially β cells and α cells)

Insulin and C Peptide

GLUT transporters (especially GLUT2 and GLUT4)

Glucagon-like peptide 1 and the incretin effect

Sulfonylurea drugs and ATP-regulated K^+ channel

Insulin receptor, AKT kinase, insulin resistance

Type 1 and type 2 diabetes mellitus

SREBP1c and FOXO1

AMP-activated protein kinase (AMPK) & mTORC1

Hexokinase, glucokinase versus glucose-6-phosphatase

Pentose phosphate pathway and NADPH

Glycogen synthase versus glycogen phosphorylase

Glycolysis: phosphofructokinase-1 (PFK1), pyruvate kinase

Pyruvate dehydrogenase (PDH) and PDH kinase, PDH phosphatase

Gluconeogenesis: phosphoenolpyruvate carboxykinase (PEPCK) and fructose 1,6-bisphosphatase

Mitochondrial TCA cycle, NADH, $FADH_2$, electron transport system and ATP synthase

De novo lipogenesis: ATP-citrate lyase (ACLY), acetyl CoA carboxylase (ACC1, ACC2), fatty acid synthase (FASN), malonyl CoA

Mitochondrial oxidation of FFAs, carnitine palmitoyl transporter 1 (CPT1)

Lipoprotein lipase versus hormone-sensitive lipase

Chylomicron, chylomicron remnant, very-low-density lipoprotein (VLDL), low-density-lipoprotein (LDL), high-density-lipoprotein (HDL), hepatic lipase

Hepatic steatosis/fatty liver

POMC/CART neurons, NPY/AgRP neurons, satiety, orexigenic, anorexigenic, leptin, adiponectin

Body mass index, visceral versus subcutaneous adipose tissue

Calcium and Phosphate Homeostasis

OBJECTIVES

1. Describe the structure and synthesis of parathyroid hormone (PTH), the regulation of PTH secretion, and the nature of the PTH receptor.
2. Describe the structure and synthesis of 1,25-dihydroxyvitamin D, the regulation of 1,25-dihydroxyvitamin D production, and the receptor for 1,25-dihydroxyvitamin D.
3. Discuss the roles of the gastrointestinal (GI) tract, bone, and kidneys in calcium (Ca^{2+})/phosphate (Pi) homeostasis.
4. Discuss the actions of calcitonin, PTH–related peptide (PTHrP), fibroblast growth factor-23 (FGF23), and gonadal and steroid hormones on Ca^{2+}/Pi metabolism.
5. Discuss the pathophysiology associated with imbalances in PTH and 1,25-dihydroxyvitamin D.

Calcium (Ca^{2+}) and phosphate (Pi) are essential to human life, playing important structural roles in hard tissues (i.e., bones and teeth) and important regulatory roles in metabolic and signaling pathways. The two primary sources of circulating Ca^{2+} and Pi are the diet and the skeleton (Fig. 4.1).

Two hormones, **1,25-dihydroxyvitamin D** (also called **calcitriol**) and **parathyroid hormone (PTH)**, regulate intestinal absorption of Ca^{2+} and Pi and the release of Ca^{2+} and Pi into the circulation during bone resorption. The primary processes for removal of Ca^{2+} and Pi from the blood are renal excretion and bone formation (see Fig. 4.1), and 1,25-dihydroxyvitamin D and PTH regulate these processes as well. Other hormones and paracrine growth factors, including the rapidly emerging role of **fibroblast growth factor-23 (FGF23)**, also have clinical relevance to Ca^{2+} and Pi homeostasis.

CALCIUM AND PHOSPHORUS ARE IMPORTANT DIETARY ELEMENTS THAT PLAY MANY CRUCIAL ROLES IN CELLULAR PHYSIOLOGY

Calcium is an essential dietary element. In addition to getting calcium from the diet, humans contain a vast store (>1 kg) of calcium in their bones, which can be called on to maintain normal circulating levels of calcium in times of dietary restriction and during the increased demands of pregnancy and nursing. Circulating calcium exists in three forms (Table 4.1): free ionized calcium (Ca^{2+}), protein-bound calcium, and calcium complexed with anions (e.g., phosphates, bicarbonate, citrate). The ionized form represents about 50% of circulating calcium, and because this form is so critical to many cellular functions, Ca^{2+} levels in both extracellular and intracellular compartments are tightly controlled (see Chapter 1 for discussion of Ca^{2+}-dependent signaling pathways). Circulating Ca^{2+} is under direct hormonal control and is normally maintained in a relatively narrow range. Either too little Ca^{2+} (**hypocalcemia**; total serum Ca^{2+} < 8.5 mg/dL [2.1 mM]) or too much Ca^{2+} (**hypercalcemia**; total serum Ca^{2+} > 10.5 mg/dL [2.6 mM]) in the blood can lead to a broad range of pathophysiologic changes, including neuromuscular dysfunction, central nervous system dysfunction, renal insufficiency, calcification of soft tissue, and skeletal pathologies.

Phosphorus is also an essential dietary element and is stored in large quantities in bone complexed with calcium. In the blood at physiologic pH, **inorganic phosphate (Pi)** exists as hydrogen phosphate (HPO_4^{2-}) or dihydrogen phosphate ($H_2PO_4^-$). Most circulating Pi is in the ionized form, but some Pi (<20%) circulates as a protein-bound form or

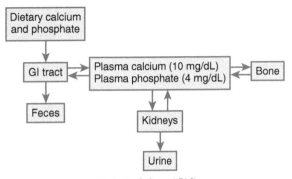

Fig. 4.1 Daily Ca^{2+} and Pi fluxes.

TABLE 4.1 Forms of Ca^{2+} and Pi in Plasma

Ion	Concentration (mg/dL)	Ionized (%)	Protein Bound (%)	Complexed (%)
Ca^{2+}*	10	50	45	5
Pi	4	84	10	6

*Ca^{2+} is bound (i.e., complexed) to various anions in the plasma, including HCO_3^-, citrate, Pi, and SO_4^-. Pi is complexed to various cations, including Na^+ and K^+.
From Koeppen BM, Stanton BA: *Renal Physiology*, 4th ed., Philadelphia, 2007, Mosby.

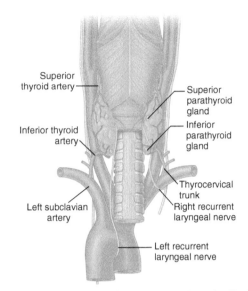

Fig. 4.2 Anatomic position of the parathyroid glands. (Redrawn from Drake RL, Vogl W, Mitchell AWM: *Gray's Anatomy for Students*, Philadelphia, 2005, Elsevier.)

complexed with cations (see Table 4.1). Phosphorus also exists as pyrophosphate (two Pi groups in a covalent linkage), an important inhibitor of mineralization. Unlike Ca^{2+}, phosphate is incorporated covalently as single or multiple phosphate groups into many molecules, and consequently, soft tissues contain about 10-fold more phosphate than Ca^{2+}. This means that significant tissue damage (e.g., crush injury with massive muscle cell death) can result in **hyperphosphatemia**, which can then complex with Ca^{2+} to cause acute hypocalcemia. Phosphate represents a key intracellular component. Indeed, it is the high-energy phosphate bonds of adenosine triphosphate (ATP) that maintain life. Phosphorylation and dephosphorylation of proteins, lipids, second messengers, and cofactors represent key regulatory steps in numerous metabolic and signaling pathways, and phosphate also serves as the backbone for nucleic acids.

PHYSIOLOGIC REGULATION OF CALCIUM AND PHOSPHATE: PARATHYROID HORMONE, 1,25-DIHYDROXYVITAMIN D, AND FGF23

PTH and 1,25-dihydroxyvitamin D have long been recognized as the physiologically important hormones that are dedicated to the maintenance of normal blood

Ca^{2+} and Pi levels in humans. As such, they are referred to as **calciotropic hormones**. The structure, synthesis, and secretion of these two hormones and their receptors will be discussed here. In the following section, the detailed actions of PTH and 1,25-dihydroxyvitamin D on the three key sites of Ca^{2+}/Pi homeostasis (i.e., gut, bone, and kidney) will be discussed. The emerging role of FGF23 in the regulation of Pi metabolism and its interaction with PTH and 1,25-dihydroxyvitamin D will then be addressed.

Parathyroid Hormone

PTH is a key hormone that maintains serum calcium levels and protects against a hypocalcemic challenge. The primary targets of PTH are bone and kidneys. PTH also functions in a positive feed-forward loop by stimulating 1,25-dihydroxyvitamin D production.

Parathyroid Glands

The **parathyroid glands** develop from the endodermal lining of the third and fourth branchial pouches. They usually develop into four glands, with the two superior glands derived from the fourth branchial pouch and the two inferior glands from the third. The embryonic anlage of the parathyroids is associated with the caudal migration of the thyroglossal duct, so the parathyroid glands usually become situated on the dorsal side of the right and left lobes of the thyroid gland (Fig. 4.2). The exact positions of the parathyroid glands are variable, and more than 10% of humans

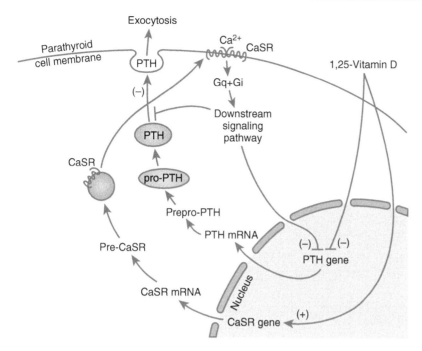

Fig. 4.3 Regulation of PTH gene expression and PTH secretion. The primary regulator of PTH is extracellular Ca²⁺, which is sensed by the Ca²⁺-sensing receptor (CaSR). The CaSR is a G-protein–coupled receptor (GPCR) linked to Gq and Gi that inhibits PTH secretion and PTH gene expression. 1,25-Dihydroxyvitamin D inhibits PTH gene expression directly and indirectly by stimulating CaSR gene expression.

harbor a fifth parathyroid gland. The predominant parenchymal cell type in the parathyroid gland is the **principal** (also called **chief**) **cell**. With age, a large mitochondria-rich, eosinophilic cell type, the **oxyphil cell**, appears. Although the oxyphil cell is not normally important in PTH secretion, PTH-overproducing tumors (i.e., primary hyperparathyroidism) can be derived from both principal and oxyphil cells.

Structure, synthesis, and secretion of parathyroid hormone. Secreted PTH is an 84-amino acid polypeptide. PTH is synthesized in principal cells as **prepro-PTH**, which is proteolytically processed to **pro-PTH** in the endoplasmic reticulum, then to mature PTH in the Golgi and secretory vesicles. The primary signal that stimulates PTH secretion is a decrease in circulating Ca^{2+} levels (Fig. 4.3). The extracellular Ca^{2+} concentration is sensed by the parathyroid principal cells through a Ca^{2+}**-sensing receptor (CaSR)**. The CaSR is a member of the seven-transmembrane G-protein–coupled receptor superfamily that forms disulfide-linked dimers in the plasma membrane. The CaSR is also expressed in calcitonin-producing C cells, renal tubules, and several other tissues. In the parathyroid gland, increasing amounts of extracellular Ca^{2+} bind to the CaSR and activate downstream signaling pathways that inhibit PTH secretion Conversely, decreasing amounts of Ca^{2+} reduces CaSR signaling, resulting in increased PTH secretion. The serum Ca^{2+} concentration that results in a half-maximal rate of PTH secretion has been referred to as the setpoint. Although the CaSR binds to extracellular Ca^{2+} with relatively low affinity, it is extremely sensitive to *changes* in extracellular Ca^{2+} above or below the setpoint. A 0.1 mM difference in serum Ca^{2+} spans the entire range of PTH secretion rates from basal (5% of maximum) to maximal levels (Fig. 4.4). Thus the CaSR regulates PTH output in response to subtle fluctuations in Ca^{2+} on a minute-to-minute basis. It should be noted that the CaSR is also stimulated by high levels of magnesium, so hypermagnesemia also inhibits PTH secretion.

In addition to inhibiting secretion, the CaSR also regulates degradation of newly synthesized PTH. Intracellular degradation of PTH is increased during hypercalcemia, thereby reducing the availability of intact PTH, while increasing the secretion of inactive fragments. This, coupled with rapid extracellular degradation of PTH, necessitates serum PTH assays that are specific for intact hormone. Consistent with its role in minute-to-minute regulation of serum Ca^{2+}, circulating intact PTH has a very short half-life (< 5 minutes). This allows intraoperative assessment of serum PTH levels during a surgical procedure to remove a PTH-secreting parathyroid adenoma.

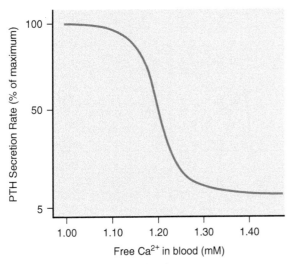

Fig. 4.4 Ca^{2+}/PTH secretion dose-response curve.

CLINICAL BOX 4.1

Patients with **familial hypocalciuric hypercalcemia (FHH)** are heterozygous for inactivating mutations of the CaSR. In these patients, reduced expression of the CaSR requires higher levels of Ca^{2+} to inhibit PTH, resulting in an elevated setpoint. The CaSR also plays a direct role in Ca^{2+} reabsorption in the kidney (specifically the thick ascending limb of the loop of Henle) to protect against hypercalcemia. The **hypocalciuria** (i.e., the inappropriately low Ca^{2+} excretion in the face of high circulating Ca^{2+} levels) in patients with FHH is due to the reduced ability of the CaSR to respond to hypercalcemia by increasing urinary Ca^{2+} excretion. FHH is a benign condition that must be distinguished from primary hyperparathyroidism in a hypercalcemic patient by clinical criteria, including normal to only slightly elevated serum PTH levels and low urinary calcium.

PTH production is also regulated at the level of gene transcription (see Fig. 4.3). Chronic activation of the CaSR signaling pathway causes repression of PTH gene expression. The PTH gene is also repressed by 1,25-dihydroxyvitamin D (acting through vitamin D–responsive elements, discussed later). The ability of 1,25-dihydroxyvitamin D to hold PTH gene expression in check is reinforced by the coordinated upregulation of CaSR gene expression by positive vitamin D–responsive elements in the promoter of the CaSR gene (see Fig. 4.3).

Parathyroid Hormone Receptor

The classic PTH receptor (PTH1R) is a seven-transmembrane, G-protein–coupled membrane receptor that is activated by both PTH and PTH–related peptide (PTHrP). PTH1R is primarily coupled to a Gαs signaling pathway that leads to increased cyclic adenosine monophosphate (cAMP), although it also is coupled to Gαq/11-phospholipase C–dependent pathways. PTH1R is expressed on osteoblasts in bone, and in the proximal and distal tubules of the kidney, as the receptor for the systemic actions of PTH. However, PTH1R is also expressed in many developing structures (e.g., the growth plate) in which PTHrP has an important paracrine function.

Vitamin D

Vitamin D is actually a prohormone that must undergo two successive hydroxylations to become the active hormone, **1,25-dihydroxyvitamin D** (Fig. 4.5). Vitamin D plays a critical role in Ca^{2+} absorption, and to a lesser extent Pi absorption, by the small intestine. Vitamin D also regulates aspects of bone remodeling and facilitates renal reabsorption of Ca^{2+}.

Structure, Synthesis, and Transport of Active Vitamin D Metabolites

Vitamin D_3 (D_3; also called **cholecalciferol**) is synthesized by ultraviolet (UV) light–mediated conversion of 7-dehydrocholesterol in the more basal layers of the skin (Fig. 4.6). UV radiation (specifically UVB) opens up the B ring of cholesterol, generating previtamin D_3, which then undergoes a temperature-dependent isomerization to D_3. Vitamin D_3 is therefore referred to as a **secosteroid**, a class of steroids in which one of the cholesterol rings is opened. Vitamin D_2 (D_2, also called **ergocalciferol**) is the form produced in plants. Vitamin D_3, and to a lesser extent D_2, are absorbed from the diet and are both effective after conversion into active hydroxylated forms.

CLINICAL BOX 4.2

The balance between UV-dependent, endogenously synthesized vitamin D_3 and the absorption of dietary forms of vitamin D becomes important in certain situations. Individuals with higher epidermal melanin content and those who live at higher latitudes convert less 7-dehydrocholesterol into vitamin D_3 and thus are more dependent on dietary sources of vitamin D, especially in winter. Some dairy products, including milk, are enriched in vitamin D_3, but not all individuals tolerate or consume dairy products. Institutionalized, sedentary elderly patients who stay indoors and avoid dairy products are particularly at risk for developing **vitamin D deficiency**.

D_3 is transported in the blood from the skin to the liver. Dietary D_3 and D_2 reach the liver directly via the portal circulation and indirectly through chylomicrons (see Fig. 4.6).

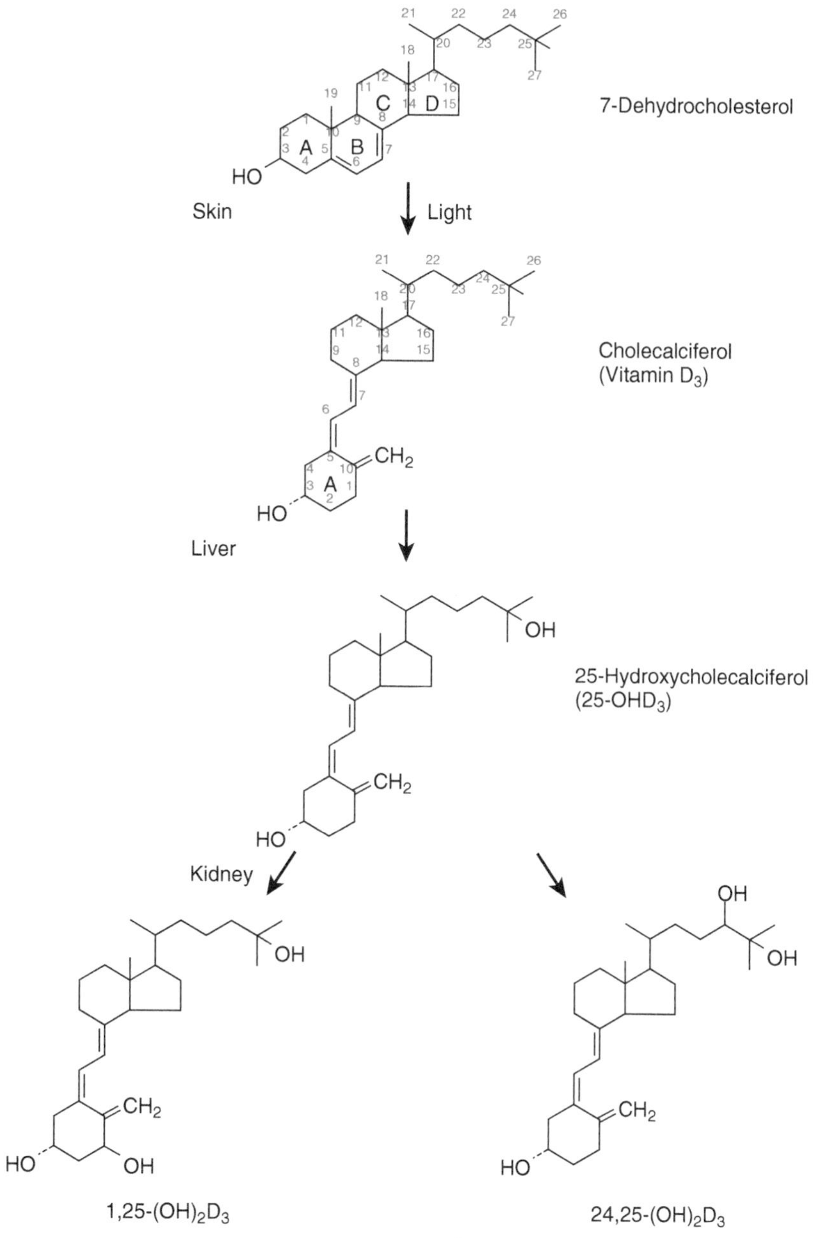

Fig. 4.5 Biosynthesis of 1,25-dihydroxyvitamin D (dihydroxycholecalciferol).

In the liver, D_2 and D_3 are hydroxylated at the 25-carbon position to yield **25-hydroxyvitamin D** (no further distinction will be made between D_3 and D_2 metabolites). Hepatic 25-hydroxylase is constitutively expressed, so circulating levels of 25-hydroxyvitamin D reflect the amount of precursor available for 25-hydroxylation. For this reason, assay of serum 25-hydroxyvitamin D levels is used to assess a patient's vitamin D status. Because the hydroxyl group at the

25-carbon position represents the second hydroxyl group on the molecule, 25-hydroxyvitamin D is also referred to as **calcifediol** (see Fig. 4.6).

25-Hydroxyvitamin D is further hydroxylated in the mitochondria of the proximal tubules of the kidney at either the 1α-carbon or 24-carbon position (see Figs. 4.5 and 4.6). The 1α-hydroxylase (gene symbol CYP27B1) generates **1,25-dihydroxyvitamin D** (also called **calcitriol**),

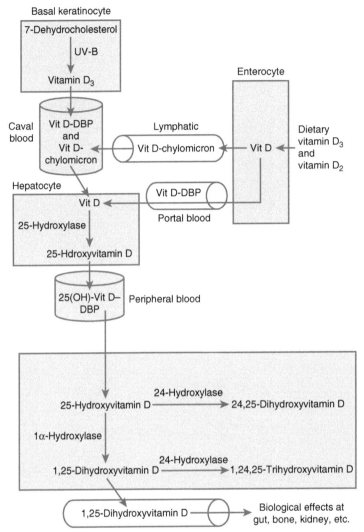

Fig. 4.6 Vitamin D metabolism. Vitamin D can be synthesized by skin keratinocyte or absorbed from the gastrointestinal tract enterocyte. Vitamin D is transported to the liver hepatocyte, where it undergoes constitutive hydroxylation at the 25-carbon position. 25-Hydroxyvitamin D is carried in the blood by vitamin D–binding protein (DBP) to the renal proximal tubules, where it is hydroxylated at either the 1α position (activating) or the 24 position (inactivating). This represents the key regulated step in the production of 1,25-dihydroxyvitamin D.

which is the most active form of vitamin D. Hydroxylation at the 24 position, generating **24,25-dihydroxyvitamin D** and **1,24,25-trihydroxyvitamin D**, represents an inactivation pathway.

Vitamin D and its metabolites circulate in the blood primarily bound to **vitamin D–binding protein (DBP)**. DBP is a serum glycoprotein of about 60 kDa that is related to the albumin gene family and is synthesized by the liver. DBP binds more than 85% of 25-hydroxyvitamin D and 1,25-dihydroxyvitamin D. As a result

of binding to other proteins, only 0.4% of the active metabolite, 1,25-dihydroxyvitamin D, circulates as free steroid. DBP allows for the movement of the highly lipophilic molecules within the aqueous environment of the blood and provides a reservoir of vitamin D metabolites that protects against vitamin D deficiency. The bound fractions of vitamin D metabolites have a circulating half-life of several hours.

There are several factors that regulate renal 1α-hydroxylase activities (see Fig. 4.6). Low serum Ca^{2+} is associated with increased 1α-hydroxylase activity, an effect that is primarily mediated by elevated levels of PTH. Similarly, it has long been known that hypophosphatemia is associated with increased production of 1,25-dihydroxyvitamin D. Recent elucidation of the role of FGF23 on Pi metabolism has shed light on the mechanism. FGF23 acts on the FGFR1/Klotho receptor complex in the proximal tubule to inhibit Pi reabsorption and 1α-hydroxylase activity. Conversely, low serum Pi inhibits the production of FGF23 in bone, leading to enhanced Pi reabsorption and stimulation of 1α-hydroxylase activity in the kidney. Lastly, there is evidence for a short feedback loop in which 1,25-dihydroxyvitamin D inhibits 1α-hydroxylase expression. Regulation and activity of the 24-hydroxylase inactivation pathway generally exhibits reciprocity to that of the 1α-hydroxylase.

Vitamin D Receptor

1,25-Dihydroxyvitamin D exerts its actions primarily through binding to the nuclear vitamin D receptor (VDR). The VDR is a 50-kDa protein and is a member of the nuclear hormone receptor superfamily, which also includes steroid and thyroid hormone receptors and metabolic receptors such as the peroxisome proliferator–activated receptors (see Chapter 1). The VDR is a transcription factor that binds to DNA sequences (vitamin D–response elements) as a heterodimer with the retinoid X receptor (RXR). Thus a primary action of 1,25-dihydroxyvitamin D is to regulate gene expression in its target tissues, including the small intestine, bone, kidneys, and parathyroid gland.

SMALL INTESTINE, BONE, AND KIDNEY DETERMINE CA²⁺ AND PI LEVELS

The general effects of PTH and 1,25-dihydroxyvitamin D on Ca^{2+} and Pi levels on the small intestine, bone, kidneys, and parathyroid glands are summarized in Table 4.2.

Handling of Ca²⁺ and Pi by the Small Intestine

Dietary levels of calcium can vary, but in general, North Americans consume about 1.5 g of calcium per day. Of this, about 200 mg is absorbed by the proximal small intestine. Importantly, fractional absorption of calcium is stimulated by 1,25-dihydroxyvitamin D, so absorption can be made more efficient in the face of declining dietary calcium.

Ca^{2+} is absorbed from the duodenum and jejunum both by a passive paracellular route and by a transcellular active transport process that is hormonally regulated. In the transcellular route, Ca^{2+} enters the intestinal enterocyte down a concentration and electrical gradient primarily through an apical epithelial calcium channel called TRPV6 (Fig. 4.7). Once inside, Ca^{2+} binds to a 9-kd cytoplasmic transport protein called calbindin-D_{9K}. Calbindin-D_{9K} serves to maintain the low cytoplasmic free Ca^{2+} concentration, preserving the favorable lumen-to-enterocyte concentration gradient, and shuttles Ca^{2+} across the cell. Ca^{2+} is actively transported across the basolateral membrane, against an electrochemical and concentration gradient, by the plasma membrane calcium ATPase (PMCA). The sodium-calcium exchanger (NCX) may also contribute to the active transport of Ca^{2+} across the basolateral membrane. 1,25-Dihydroxyvitamin D stimulates the expression of all of the components (i.e., TRPV6, calbindin-D_{9K}, and PMCA) involved in Ca^{2+} uptake by the small intestine. PTH affects Ca^{2+} absorption at the gut indirectly by stimulating renal 1α-hydroxylase activity to increase circulating 1,25-dihydroxyvitamin D.

The fraction of phosphate absorbed by the jejunum remains relatively constant at about 70% and is under minor hormonal control by 1,25-dihydroxyvitamin D. The limiting process in transcellular Pi absorption is transport across the apical brush border, which is carried out by an isoform of the sodium-Pi cotransporter, NPT2.

Handling of Ca²⁺ and Pi by Bone

In addition to its structural role, bone represents a massive and dynamic extracellular depot of Ca^{2+} and Pi. Even after growth is completed, the adult skeleton is constantly remodeled through the concerted activities of the resident bone cell types. The processes of bone formation and bone resorption are in balance in an active, healthy, well-nourished adult. Of approximately 1 kg of calcium contained in bone, about 500 mg (i.e., 0.05% of skeletal calcium) is mobilized from and deposited into bone each day. However, the process of bone remodeling can be modulated to provide a net gain or loss of Ca^{2+} and Pi to the blood and is responsive to physical activity, diet, age, and hormonal regulation. Because the integrity of bone is absolutely dependent on Ca^{2+} and Pi, chronic dysregulation of Ca^{2+} and Pi levels, or of the hormones that regulate Ca^{2+} and Pi, leads to pathologic changes in bone.

Histophysiology of Adult Bone

The biogenesis, growth, and remodeling of bone is a complex process that will not be fully explained here. The key features required to understand the role of adult bone in the hormonal regulation of calcium-phosphate metabolism are discussed.

TABLE 4.2   Actions of Parathyroid Hormone and 1,25-Dihydroxyvitamin D on Ca²⁺/Pi Homeostasis

	Small Intestine	Bone	Kidney	Parathyroid Gland
PTH	No direct action	Regulates osteoclast differentiation and function via RANKL/OPG expression by osteoblasts Chronic high levels promote bone resorption Intermittent PTH administration increases bone formation by osteoblasts Possible stimulation of FGF23 by osteocytes?	Stimulates 1α-hydroxylase activity and 1,25-dihydroxyvitamin D production Stimulates Ca^{2+} reabsorption in distal nephron Inhibits Pi reabsorption by proximal tubule (inhibits NPT2a)	No direct action
1,25-Dihydroxy-vitamin D	Increases Ca^{2+} absorption by increasing TRPV channels, calbind-inD_{9K}, and PMCA expression Marginally increases Pi absorption	Regulates osteoclast differentiation and function via RANKL/OPG expression by osteoblasts Promotes bone mineralization by maintenance of serum Ca^{2+} and Pi levels Feedback inhibition of FGF23 expression by osteocytes	Permissive action on Ca^{2+} reabsorption by upregulating calbindinD$_{28k}$ in the distal tubule Promotes Pi reabsorption by proximal nephron (stimulates NPT2a expression)	Feedback inhibition of PTH gene transcription Directly stimulates CaSR gene expression
FGF23	No direct action	FGF23 is produced by osteocytes	Inhibits Pi reabsorption by proximal tubule (inhibits NPT2a) Inhibits 1α-hydroxylase activity and 1,25-dihydroxyvitamin D production	Possible feedback inhibition of PTH?

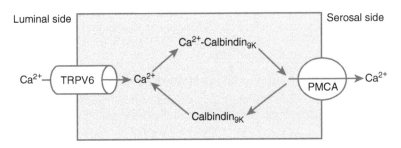

Fig. 4.7 Intestinal absorption of Ca²⁺ through the transcellular route. Ca²⁺ enters through the TRPV6 Ca²⁺ channel in the luminal membrane of the enterocyte. Ca²⁺ is then shuttled from the apical side of the cell to the basal side by the carrier protein, calbindin-D$_{9K}$. Ca²⁺ is then actively transported across the basolateral membrane by the plasma membrane Ca²⁺ ATPase (PMCA, and calbindin-D$_{9K}$ recycles). 1,25-Dihydroxyvitamin D increases the expression of all these proteins in the gastrointestinal tract.

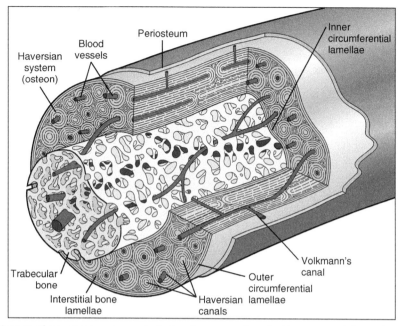

Fig. 4.8 Diagram of a typical long bone shaft showing compact cortical bone around the perimeter and trabecular (cancellous) bone in the center. (From Stevens A, Lowe J: *Human Histology*, 3rd ed., Philadelphia, 2005, Mosby.)

Most of the skeleton (about 75%) consists of **compact, cortical bone** that makes up the outer surfaces of long and flat bones (Fig. 4.8). The inner skeletal component is composed of an interconnecting network of plates and spicules located toward the end of the bone in the metaphyseal region. The prevalent orientation of this so-called **trabecular** or **cancellous** bone becomes organized by stress forces. Although it makes up only 25% of total bone mass, its surface area is several-fold greater than that of cortical bone. The greater surface area means that trabecular bone is much more accessible to bone cells and thus more dynamic in its turnover. This is an important concept, because bone loss in regions that are structurally dependent on trabecular bone (e.g., vertebrae, hip) renders them susceptible to osteoporotic fracture.

In the adult, bone remodeling involves the resorption of existing bone, with the commensurate release of Ca^{2+} and Pi into the blood. This is followed by the synthesis of new bone matrix (osteoid) at the site of resorption that will subsequently undergo mineralization to form mature bone. These processes are closely coupled so that under normal circumstances old bone is replaced without losing bone mass. Bone remodeling is therefore accomplished by teams of osteoclasts and osteoblasts (see later in the text), collectively referred to as the **basic multicellular unit.** At any one time, there are about 2 million basic multicellular units remodeling bone at discreet sites throughout the skeleton.

The cells involved in bone remodeling fall into two major classes: cells that promote the formation of bone (**osteoblasts**) and cells that promote the resorption of bone (**osteoclasts**). However, it should be emphasized that bone remodeling is a highly integrated process, and osteoblasts also play a primary role in the initiation and regulation of bone resorption (Fig. 4.9). Osteoblasts develop from mesodermally derived stromal cells that have the potential to differentiate into muscle, adipose, cartilage, and bone (i.e., osteoblasts) cells. Several paracrine and endocrine factors modulate the osteoblast differentiation program, which is dependent on the expression of bone-specific transcription factors. For example, the transcription factor Runx2 is essential for osteoblast differentiation and is mutated in patients with **cleidocranial dysplasia**, a congenital syndrome characterized by multiple defects in bone formation.

Osteoblasts express factors that induce osteoclast differentiation from cells of the monocyte-macrophage lineage and activate osteoclast function (see Fig. 4.9). Osteoblasts release **monocyte colony-stimulating factor (M-CSF)**, a secreted cytokine that binds to its receptor, **c-Fms**, on osteoclast precursor cells. M-CSF induces processes that lead to the production of osteoclast progenitor cells expressing the receptor activator of NF-κB (RANK) on their surface. RANK is structurally related to the receptor for **tumor necrosis factor-α (TNF-α)** and signals through

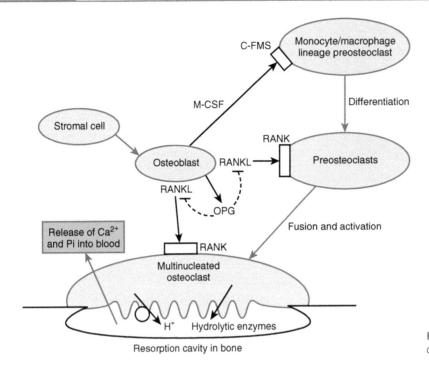

Fig. 4.9 Osteoblast regulation of osteoclast differentiation and function.

NF-κB–related pathways to induce osteoclastogenesis. RANK ligand (RANKL) is a 40- to 45-kDa protein on the cell membrane of osteoblasts. RANKL binds to RANK on osteoclast precursor membranes, which ultimately promotes the fusion of several osteoclast precursors, giving rise to a fused, multinucleated osteoclast. The perimeter of the osteoclast membrane facing a mineralized bone surface adheres tightly to it, essentially sealing off the area of osteoclast-bone contact (see Fig. 4.9). Within this region of the cell, a specialized structure called the ruffled border is formed, from which enzymes (e.g., cathepsin K) and HCl are secreted. The acid dissolves the mineral phase and the secreted lysosomal enzymes hydrolyze type I collagen and other matrix components. Osteoclast differentiation and function is also under negative control by osteoblasts. Osteoprotegerin (OPG) is a soluble decoy receptor for RANKL (see Fig. 4.9) that blocks its interaction with RANK. Consequently, increased OPG expression relative to RANKL results in decreased osteoclast differentiation and bone resorption.

In trabecular bone, osteoclasts excavate a resorption cavity called a Howship's lacuna, which is subsequently filled in by osteoblasts. In cortical bone, on the other hand, osteoclasts form a *cutting cone* and tunnel through bone along its longitudinal axis. After a reversal phase in which macrophages remove debris, osteoblasts migrate into the resorbed area and begin to lay down osteoid. Some of the proteins in osteoid promote mineralization in conjunction with alkaline phosphatase, an enzyme expressed by osteoblasts that promotes mineralization by cleaving pyrophosphate. This process removes Ca^{2+} and Pi from the blood and deposits them first as calcium phosphate crystals that eventually grow into hydroxyapatite. The bone is laid down in successive organized layers, called *lamellae,* starting from the perimeter of the resorption cavity and progressing inward. In the fully repaired region, multiple concentric lamellae surround a central haversian canal that contains a nutritive blood vessel (see Fig. 4.8). As osteoblasts become surrounded by and entrapped within bone matrix, they become osteocytes that sit within small spaces in mineralized bone called lacunae. Osteocytes remain interconnected by long cell processes that run within minute canaliculi and form communicating junctions with adjacent cell processes. The new concentric layers of bone, along with the interconnected osteocytes and the central canal, are referred to collectively as a Haversian system or osteon.

Osteocytes are the mechanoreceptor cells of bone. They detect increased strain in response to a mechanical stress that causes deformation of bone. This results in reduced expression of a secreted protein called sclerostin (SOST). SOST is an inhibitor of bone formation that suppresses osteoblast differentiation by inhibiting Wnt signaling in osteoblast progenitor cells. Thus the repression of SOST promotes increased osteoblast differentiation and bone formation in response to mechanical loading. Homozygous loss-of-function mutations of the SOST gene in humans cause **sclerosteosis**, a disease caused by excessive bone mass, while heterozygous individuals have high bone mass that does not cause disease.

CLINICAL BOX 4.3

The importance of the RANK/RANKL/OPG system is made evident by rare mutations in the human genes for RANK, RANKL, and OPG. Loss of either RANK or RANKL causes autosomal recessive osteopetrosis due to dramatically reduced bone resorption, whereas OPG mutations cause excessive resorption and formation and consequent bone deformities. Development of Denosumab, a humanized monoclonal antibody directed against RANKL, has provided a new biological approach as an antiresorptive therapy to prevent bone loss.

Intermittent administration of PTH is the only currently approved anabolic therapy for treatment of osteoporosis (see later in the text). However, the development of a biologic strategy using monoclonal antibodies against SOST is currently in clinical trials, and holds promise for a targeted therapy to increase osteoblast differentiation and bone formation.

As a calciotropic hormone, PTH is the primary endocrine regulator of serum calcium. The PTH1R receptor is expressed on osteoblasts, but not on osteoclasts. PTH indirectly stimulates osteoclastic bone resorption through osteoblast-derived paracrine factors (i.e., M-CSF, RANKL). Elevated levels of PTH in response to hypocalcemia shift the balance to a relative increase in osteoclast activity in order to restore serum calcium levels. If this continues, it can eventually result in increased bone turnover and reduced bone mass. In contrast, intermittent administration of low dose PTH (one injection/day) promotes osteoblast survival and bone anabolic functions, increases bone density, and reduces the risk for fracture in humans. This effect of PTH involves multiple mechanisms, including increased production of IGF-I, reduced osteoblast apoptosis, and decreased SOST production.

CLINICAL BOX 4.4

Regulation of bone remodeling by PTH requires normal levels of 1,25-dihydroxyvitamin D. In vitamin D–deficient individuals, reduced efficiency of intestinal Ca^{2+} absorption causes a secondary increase in PTH and subsequent bone resorption in an attempt to maintain normocalcemia. However, PTH also inhibits Pi reabsorption in the kidney, potentially causing hypophosphatemia. The resulting reduction in the Ca^{2+} x Pi product, in turn, can lead to defective bone mineralization. In children, this causes **rickets**, in which growth of long bones is abnormal, with weakened bones leading to bowing of extremities and deformities of the rib cage (see later). In adults, vitamin D deficiency causes **osteomalacia**, which is characterized by poorly mineralized osteoid, bone pain, and increased fracture risk.

Handling of Ca^{2+} and Pi by the Kidneys

(Mosby Physiology Monograph Series cross reference: Chapter 9 in *Renal Physiology*, 6th Ed., BM Koeppen and BA Stanton)

The kidneys filter a large amount of Ca^{2+} (about 10 g) each day, but most of the filtered Ca^{2+} is reabsorbed by the nephron. Renal excretion typically accounts for the loss of about 200 mg of Ca^{2+} per day, which is counterbalanced by net intestinal absorption of about 200 mg/day. In the proximal tubule, most of the Ca^{2+} is reabsorbed by a passive, paracellular pathway. In the **thick ascending limb (TAL) of the loop of Henle, paracellular transport** is driven by a lumen-positive electrical gradient established by the Na-K-2Cl transporter in the luminal membrane following K^+ leakage back into the lumen. The CaSR is located in the basolateral membrane of TAL cells, and its activation by high serum calcium inhibits the Na-K-2Cl symporter and reduces paracellular Ca^{2+} transport (Fig. 4.10). Clinically, inhibition of this transporter by **loop diuretics** such as furosemide has been used to treat hypercalcemia. Transcellular Ca^{2+} transport in the **cortical portion of the TAL** and the **distal convoluted tubule** occurs by an active transport process that is stimulated by PTH (see Fig. 4.10). Inhibition of the thiazide-sensitive Na^+-Cl^- symporter in the luminal membrane of distal tubule cells enhances Ca^{2+} reabsorption. **Thiazide diuretics** are therefore used to prevent renal calcium wasting in idiopathic hypercalciuria.

As discussed earlier, intestinal absorption of phosphate is largely proportional to the amount of phosphate in the diet and is only slightly regulated by 1,25-dihydroxyvitamin D. This leaves the kidney with an important role in the

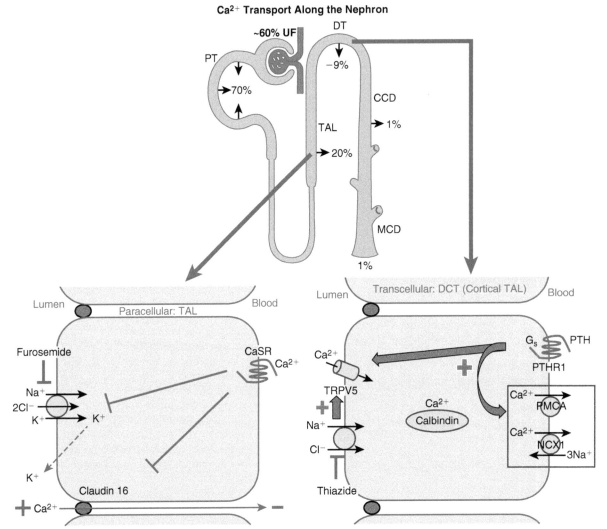

Fig. 4.10 Handling of Ca²⁺ by the distal nephron and proximal nephron (see text). Diagram of the nephron and the mechanisms and regulation of Ca²⁺ transport in the thick ascending limb (TAL) of the loop of Henle and the distal convoluted tubule (DCT). (Modified Koeppen BM, Stanton BA: *Renal Physiology*, 3rd ed., St. Louis, 2001, Mosby.)

regulation of circulating phosphate levels. Phosphate is mostly reabsorbed by the proximal convoluted tubule through a hormonally regulated transcellular route. Phosphate enters the apical surface of the proximal tubules in a rate-limiting manner through a **sodium-phosphate cotransporter (NPT)**. PTH downregulates NPT2 expression on the apical membrane of renal proximal tubule cells, thereby increasing phosphate excretion.

It is becoming clear that FGF23 is another key regulator of Pi metabolism (see Clinical Box 4.5). Osteocytes produce FGF23, and the levels of this hormone rise in response to a sustained elevation of serum Pi levels. Like PTH, FGF23 inhibits Pi reabsorption in the proximal tubule, but by a different mechanism—activation of the FGFR1/Klotho receptor complex (Fig. 4.11). In the same cells, FGF23 inhibits expression of the 1α-hydroxylase, thereby appropriately reducing circulating levels of 1,25-dihydroxyvitamin D. Conversely, reduced levels of FGF23 in response to low phosphate will allow increases in both Pi reabsorption and 1,25-dihydroxyvitamin D, helping to

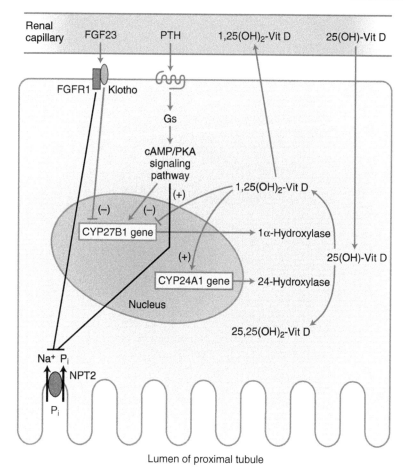

Fig. 4.11 Regulation of renal 1α-hydroxylase activity and Pi transport by PTH and FGF23 in proximal tubule cells. PTH stimulates and FGF23 inhibits 1α-hydroxylase activity and 1,25-dihydroxyvitamin D production. Both hormones reduce reabsorption of Pi by inhibition of NPT2 transporters located in the luminal membrane.

restore blood Pi levels. There is emerging evidence for a negative feedback loop in which 1,25-dihydroxyvitamin D inhibits FGF23 expression. Similarly, some new evidence suggests a possible feedback relationship between PTH and FGF23. However, many basic unanswered questions remain, including how and where circulating Pi levels are sensed.

Integrated Physiologic Regulation of Ca^{2+}/Pi Metabolism: Response of PTH and 1,25-Dihydroxyvitamin D to a Hypocalcemic Challenge

The integrated response of PTH and 1,25-dihydroxyvitamin D to a hypocalcemic challenge is shown in Fig. 4.12. Low blood Ca^{2+}, as detected by the CaSR on the parathyroid principal cells, stimulates PTH secretion. In bone, PTH stimulates osteoblasts to express RANKL, which increases osteoclast activity, leading to increased bone resorption and the release of Ca^{2+} and Pi into the blood. In the kidney, PTH rapidly increases Ca^{2+} levels by increasing reabsorption of Ca^{2+} in the distal renal tubule. PTH also inhibits the activity of the sodium-dependent phosphate transporter (NPT2) in the proximal tubule, thereby increasing Pi excretion. The relative loss of phosphate maintains normophosphatemia and serves to increase free, ionized Ca^{2+} in the blood. In a slower phase of the response to hypocalcemia, PTH stimulates 1α-hydroxylase expression in the proximal tubule, thereby increasing 1,25-dihydroxyvitamin D levels. In the small intestine, 1,25-dihydroxyvitamin D supports adequate Ca^{2+} levels in the long term by stimulating Ca^{2+} absorption. These effects occur over hours and days and involve increasing the expression of TRPV6 calcium channels, calbindin-D_{9K}, and PMCA. 1,25-dihydroxyvitamin D also stimulates osteoblast expression of RANKL, thereby amplifying the effect of PTH on bone.

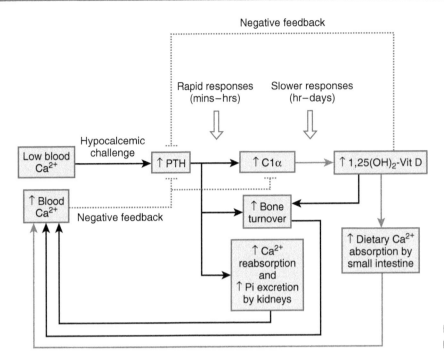

Fig. 4.12 Integrated response to a hypocalcemic challenge.

1,25-Dihydroxyvitamin D and the CaSR play key roles in negative feedback. Thus, elevated PTH stimulates 1,25-dihydroxyvitamin D production, which then inhibits PTH gene expression directly, and indirectly by upregulating the CaSR. 1,25-Dihydroxyvitamin D also represses renal 1α-hydroxylase activity while increasing 24-hydroxylase activity. While blood Ca^{2+} levels rise back to normal levels, PTH secretion and 1α-hydroxylase activity returns to normal as well.

Hormonal Regulation of Calcium and Phosphate: Pharmacologic Regulators

Calcitonin

The cells that produce calcitonin are called the parafollicular C cells. These cells are derived from the ultimobranchial bodies and become incorporated and interspersed among the thyroid follicles as the thyroglossal duct migrates caudally. Calcitonin is a 32-amino acid polypeptide. Calcitonins from other species are biologically active in humans. In fact, salmon calcitonin is about 20 times more potent in humans than human calcitonin, which has been used to clinical advantage. Alternative splicing of the calcitonin gene in other tissues can produce calcitonin gene–related peptide (CGRP), which is a potent vasodilator and positive cardiac inotrope. The secretion of calcitonin is primarily regulated by the same CaSR that regulates PTH secretion. However, in contrast to PTH, elevated extracellular Ca^{2+} levels stimulate the synthesis and secretion of calcitonin.

The primary action of calcitonin is a direct effect on osteoclasts to inhibit bone resorption. The calcitonin receptor, which is closely related to the secretin and PTH1R receptors, is a seven-transmembrane G protein–coupled receptor that acts primarily through cAMP-dependent signaling pathways. Calcitonin acts rapidly and directly on osteoclasts to suppress bone resorption.

In many species, calcitonin lowers serum calcium and phosphate levels, primarily by inhibiting bone resorption. In humans, however, calcitonin does not play a physiologic role in regulating serum Ca^{2+} levels. Consistent with this idea, total thyroidectomy does not result in hypercalcemia, nor does excess production of calcitonin in medullary thyroid carcinoma cause hypocalcemia. Medical interest in calcitonin stems from the fact that more potent forms of calcitonin (e.g., salmon calcitonin) have been used therapeutically as an anti-resorptive agent in the treatment of metabolic bone disease.

Hormonal Regulation of Calcium and Phosphate: Regulators Overexpressed by Cancers

PTH–Related Peptide

PTH–related peptide (PTHrP) is a peptide paracrine factor that shows limited structural similarity to PTH but nevertheless binds to and signals through the PTH1R. PTHrP is expressed in several developing tissues, including the growth plate of bones and the mammary glands. PTHrP is not regulated by circulating calcium and normally does not play a role in Ca^{2+}/Pi homeostasis in the adult. However, certain neoplasms such as lung carcinoma can secrete high levels of PTHrP, producing a paraneoplastic syndrome similar to hyperparathyroidism—the so-called hypercalcemia of malignancy.

CLINICAL BOX 4.5

Fibroblast growth factor-23 (FGF23) is an approximately 30-kDa peptide that is normally expressed by osteocytes. It acts on proximal tubule cells of the kidney to inhibit Pi reabsorption and promote phosphate excretion. FGF23 is inactivated by a protease that cleaves FGF23 into N-terminal and C-terminal peptides. One protease involved in FGF23 processing and inactivation, although not a direct substrate, is **PHEX** (**p**hosphate-regulating gene with **h**omologies to **e**ndopeptidases on the **X** chromosome). PHEX is mutated in **X-linked hypophosphatemic rickets**, which is caused by renal phosphate wasting and inappropriately low levels of 1,25-dihydroxyvitamin D relative to the degree of hypophosphatemia. Current evidence indicates that when PHEX is mutated, FGF23 levels increase and inhibit both phosphate reabsorption and 1α-hydroxylase in the proximal renal tubules. Increased activity of FGF23 has also been linked to **autosomal recessive hypophosphatemic rickets and tumor-induced osteomalacia**.

Regulation of Ca^{2+}/Pi Metabolism by Immune and Inflammatory Cells

It is interesting to note that the RANKL/RANK/osteoprotegerin signaling system is similar to the TNF receptor/NF-κB signaling pathways used in cells involved in the immune system and in inflammation. This link is further stressed by the fact that activated T cells express high levels of RANKL in response to stimulation by the cytokines, TNF-α, and several interleukins. Thus inflammatory bone diseases (e.g., rheumatoid arthritis) are associated with increased RANKL-to-osteoprotegerin ratios in the vicinity of the inflammatory site, with subsequent erosions of bone and osteoporosis.

RANKL is also overproduced by cells associated with several malignant bone diseases (e.g., multiple myeloma, skeletal metastatic breast cancer). As noted earlier, some malignant cells also overexpress PTHrP, which induces RANKL expression in neighboring osteoblasts. Thus several malignancies are associated with bone damage and hypercalcemia.

The 1α-hydroxylase enzyme is expressed by monocytes and peripheral macrophages. In the autoimmune disease of sarcoidosis, overactive macrophages produce high levels of 1,25-dihydroxyvitamin D, resulting in hypercalcemia.

Regulation of Ca^{2+}/Pi Metabolism by Gonadal and Adrenal Steroid Hormones

Gonadal and adrenal steroid hormones have profound effects on calcium and phosphate metabolism and skeletal health. Estradiol-17β (E_2; see Chapter 10) has a bone anabolic and calciotropic effect at several sites. E_2 stimulates intestinal calcium absorption and renal tubular calcium reabsorption. E_2 is also one of the most potent regulators of osteoblast and osteoclast function. Estrogen promotes survival of osteoblasts and apoptosis of osteoclasts, thereby favoring bone formation over resorption. In postmenopausal women, estrogen deficiency results in an initial phase of rapid bone loss that lasts about 5 years, followed by a second phase of slower bone loss. Exercise and high levels of dietary calcium with supplemental vitamin D can help to prevent postmenopausal osteoporosis. Androgens also have bone anabolic and calciotropic effects, although some of these effects are due to the peripheral conversion of testosterone to E_2 (see Chapter 9).

In contrast to gonadal steroids, high-dose glucocorticoids, either due to overproduction (i.e., Cushing's disease) or therapeutic administration of a chronic inflammatory disease, can cause glucocorticoid-induced osteoporosis. This involves multiple mechanisms, including inhibition of osteoblast differentiation and function, enhanced bone resorption, inhibition of intestinal calcium absorption, and renal calcium wasting.

PATHOLOGIC DISORDERS OF CALCIUM AND PHOSPHATE BALANCE

Primary Hyperparathyroidism

Primary hyperparathyroidism is caused by excessive production of PTH by the parathyroid glands. It is frequently caused by a single adenoma confined to one of the glands. A common cause of parathyroid adenoma is a gene

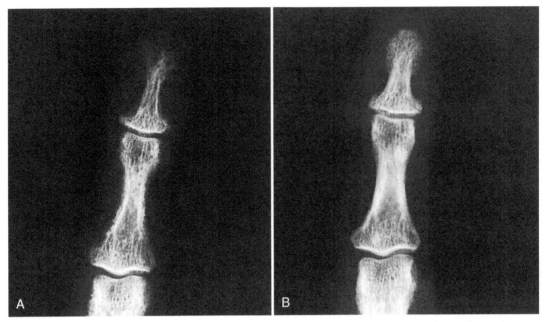

Fig. 4.13 Primary hyperparathyroidism. (A) Radiographs of middle and distal phalanges of index finger show subperiosteal bone resorption of shafts and tip of distal phalanx. (B) Second radiograph taken after bone had healed after treatment by removal of parathyroid hematoma. (From Besser GM, Thorner MO: *Clinical Endocrinology,* London, 1994, Mosby-Wolfe.)

rearrangement that drives overexpression of the *PRAD1* gene (parathyroid adenomatosis gene) encoding the cell cycle regulator cyclin D1.

Patients with primary hyperparathyroidism have high serum calcium levels and, in most cases, low serum phosphate levels. Hypercalcemia is a result of bone resorption, increased gastrointestinal (GI) calcium absorption (mediated by 1,25-dihydroxyvitamin D), and increased renal calcium reabsorption. Mild hyperparathyroidism may be asymptomatic but symptoms of the disorder that develop are directly related to increased bone resorption, hypercalcemia, and hypercalciuria (Fig. 4.13). The diagnosis is confirmed by the presence of elevated intact serum PTH.

High serum calcium levels decrease neuromuscular excitability. Patients with hyperparathyroidism often show psychological disorders, particularly depression, mental confusion, and fatigue, that are associated with hypercalcemia (Box 4.1). Hypercalcemia can also cause a number of cardiovascular symptoms including palpitations, arrhythmias, and hypertension. Along with other nonspecific GI symptoms (e.g. abdominal pain, nausea, constipation), hypercalcemia can result in peptic ulcer formation because calcium increases gastrin secretion (see Chapter 2). Kidney

> **BOX 4.1   Symptoms of Hyperparathyroidism**
>
> - Kidney stones
> - Osteoporosis
> - Gastrointestinal disturbances, peptic ulcers, nausea, constipation
> - Muscle weakness, decreased muscle tone
> - Depression, lethargy, fatigue, mental confusion
> - Polyuria
> - High serum phosphate concentration; low serum calcium concentration

stones (nephrolithiasis) are common because hypercalcemia leads to hypercalciuria and increased phosphate clearance in response to elevated PTH leads to phosphaturia. The high urinary calcium and phosphate concentrations increase the tendency for precipitation of calcium-phosphate salts in the soft tissues of the kidney. Calcium oxalate stones may also occur.

Patients with hyperparathyroidism have evidence of high bone turnover, such as elevated markers of bone formation (e.g., serum alkaline phosphatase and osteocalcin),

BOX 4.2   Symptoms of Hypoparathyroidism

- Tetany, convulsions, paresthesias, muscle cramps
- Decreased myocardial contractility
- First-degree heart block
- Central nervous system problems, including irritability and psychosis
- Intestinal malabsorption
- Low serum calcium concentration; high serum phosphate concentration

and increased markers of bone resorption (breakdown products of collagen). This high turnover state is frequently associated with bone loss and reduced bone mineral density. Some patients with hyperparathyroidism have the bone disorder osteitis fibrosa cystica, which is characterized by bone pain, cystic fibrous lesions (sometimes called "brown tumors"), a tendency for pathologic fractures of long bones, and histologic abnormalities of the bone.

Pseudohypoparathyroidism

Pseudohypoparathyroidism is a rare familial disorder characterized by tissue resistance to PTH. In many instances, the problem is thought to originate with the PTH receptor. Often there is a decrease in levels of the guanine nucleotide–binding protein, Gs. Individuals with pseudohypoparathyroidism demonstrate increased PTH secretion and low serum calcium levels, sometimes associated with congenital defects of the skeleton, including shortened metacarpal and metatarsal bones.

Hypoparathyroidism

Acquired hypoparathyroidism usually results from postsurgical or autoimmune loss of the parathyroid glands. It is associated with low serum calcium and high serum phosphate levels. Hypocalcemia results from reduced PTH and decreased production of 1,25-dihydroxyvitamin D by the kidney. Consequently, there is a decrease in bone calcium mobilization by osteoclastic bone resorption. Because 1,25-dihydroxyvitamin D is low, GI absorption of calcium is impaired. Although the filtered load of calcium is low, urinary calcium level is relatively high due to the loss of PTH-sensitive calcium reabsorption in the distal tubule. Bone mineral density in hypoparathyroid patients may be high relative to normal subjects.

Hypocalcemia alters cardiovascular function and may cause hypotension, a prolonged QT interval and cardiac arrhythmia. The most prominent symptom of hypoparathyroidism is increased neuromuscular excitability (Box 4.2). Low serum calcium concentrations decrease the neuromuscular threshold. This can be manifested as repetitive responses to a single stimulus and as spontaneous neuromuscular discharge. The increased neuromuscular excitability can result in tingling in the fingers or toes (paresthesia), muscle cramps, or even tetany. Laryngeal spasms can be life-threatening. Sometimes the serum calcium level is not low enough to produce overt tetany, but latent tetany can be demonstrated by inflating a blood pressure cuff on the arm to a pressure greater than systolic pressure for 2 min. The resultant oxygen deficiency precipitates overt tetany as demonstrated by carpal-pedal spasms. This is called Trousseau sign (Fig. 4.14A). Another test for latent tetany is to tap the facial nerve, which evokes facial muscle spasms (Chvostek sign).

Treatment of mild to moderate hypoparathyroidism is typically with calcium and vitamin D supplementation, and occasionally thiazide diuretics, which increase calcium reabsorption in the thick ascending limb of the loop of Henle. Administration of recombinant PTH may be required in more severe cases, in which supplementation alone is insufficient to maintain normocalcemia.

Hypomagnesemia resulting from either severe malabsorption or chronic alcoholism can cause hypoparathyroidism. Hypomagnesemia impairs the secretion of PTH and decreases the biologic response to PTH.

Vitamin D Deficiency

Vitamin D deficiency decreases GI absorption of calcium and phosphate. The drop in the serum calcium level secondarily stimulates PTH secretion, which in turn inhibits phosphate reabsorption. The resulting hypophosphatemia causes impaired bone mineralization because the calcium x phosphate product in serum is low. This leads to osteomalacia in adults or rickets in children. Rickets and osteomalacia are disorders in which bone mineralization is defective. Osteoid is formed, but it does not mineralize adequately. Rickets is caused by a vitamin D deficiency before skeletal maturation; it involves problems in not only the bone but also the cartilage of the growth plate (Fig. 4.14B and C). Osteomalacia is the term used when inadequate bone mineralization occurs after skeletal growth is complete and the epiphyses have closed.

Paget Disease

Paget disease results in bone deformities. It is characterized by an increase in bone resorption followed by an increase in bone formation. The new bone is generally abnormal and often irregular. Serum alkaline phosphatase and osteocalcin levels are dramatically increased, as are markers of bone resorption. Pain, bone deformity, and bone weakness can occur (Fig. 4.14D).

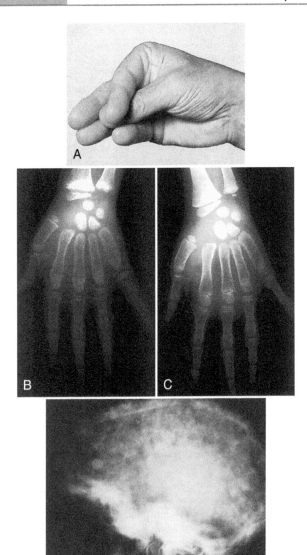

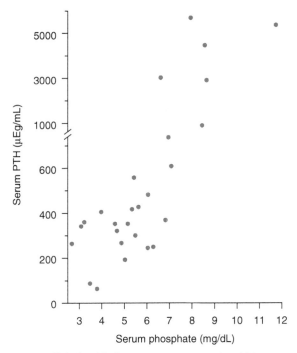

Fig. 4.15 Relationship between serum parathyroid hormone (PTH) level and serum phosphate level in patients with renal failure. (Redrawn from Bordier PF, Marie PF, Arnaud CD: Evolution of renal osteodystrophy: Correlation of bone histomorphometry and serum mineral and immunoreactive parathyroid hormone values before and after treatment with calcium carbonate or 25-hydroxycholecalciferol. *Kidney Int* 7[Suppl 2]:102, 1975.)

Bone Problems of Renal Failure (Renal Osteodystrophy)

Approximately 0.9 g, or more than 50% of dietary phosphate, is normally lost in the urine in a day. Consequently, the kidney serves as the major excretory route for phosphate. As renal function and phosphate clearance decreases, the serum phosphate concentration rises. The increase in serum phosphate concentration lowers serum calcium levels, which prompts an increase in PTH secretion (Fig. 4.15). Hyperphosphatemia also stimulates the production of FGF23 by osteocytes. The combination of kidney damage and high levels of FGF23 impairs production of 1,25-dihydroxyvitamin D, which decreases GI absorption of calcium. This further drop in the serum calcium level exacerbates the secondary hyperparathyroidism, potentially leading to osteitis fibrosa cystica. Fig. 4.16 shows the effect of renal impairment on phosphate, calcium, vitamin D, and PTH.

Fig. 4.14 (A) Position of hand in hypocalcemic tetany. (B) Radiograph of left hand of 9-year-old boy with rickets caused by malnutrition. In the distal radius there is poor mineralization of osteoid in the zone of provisional calcification. The growth plate therefore appears widened with evidence of metaphyseal cupping and fraying. (C) After 2 months of improved nutrition, note enhanced bone mineralization, decreased width of the growth plate and normalization of the metaphysis. (D) Radiograph of the skull in a patient with Paget disease. Thickness of the skull is increased, and sclerotic changes are seen scattered throughout, consistent with healing phase of Paget disease. (**A** from Hall R, Evered DC: *Color Atlas of Endocrinology,* 2nd ed., London, 1990, Mosby-Wolfe. **B** to **D,** Courtesy of Dr. C. Joe.)

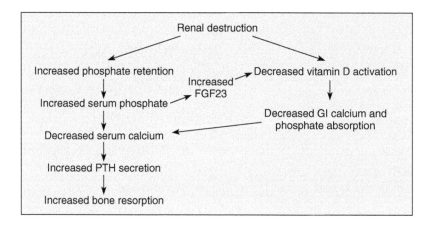

Fig. 4.16 The physiologic basis of bone loss in renal failure. *GI*, Gastrointestinal; *PTH*, parathyroid hormone.

SUMMARY

1. Serum calcium levels are a function of the rate at which calcium enters from GI absorption and bone demineralization and leaves through bone mineralization, GI excretion, and renal excretion. Serum calcium levels are normally maintained within a narrow range.

2. Serum phosphate levels are determined by the rate at which phosphate enters from GI absorption, soft tissue efflux, and bone resorption and leaves through GI excretion, soft tissue influx, bone mineralization, and renal excretion. Serum phosphate levels normally fluctuate over a relatively wide range.

3. The major physiologic hormones regulating serum calcium and phosphate levels are parathyroid hormone (PTH) and 1,25-dihydroxyvitamin D (calcitriol) and FGF23.

4. PTH is an 84-amino acid peptide, whose secretion is regulated by serum Ca^{2+} through the Ca^{2+}-sensing receptor (CaSR). PTH is made by the principal cells of the parathyroid glands. PTH binds to the PTH/PTHrP receptor, which is primarily coupled to a Gs/cAMP/PKA pathway.

5. Vitamin D can be acquired in the diet or synthesized from 7-dehydrocholesterol in skin in the presence of ultraviolet light. It is hydroxylated to 25-hydroxycholecalciferol (calcifediol) in the liver, then activated by renal 1α-hydroxylase to 1,25-dihydroxycholecalciferol (calcitriol) in the kidney. PTH and low phosphate (via FGF23), are the primary stimulators of renal 1α-hydroxylase activity. 1,25-Dihydroxyvitamin D binds to a nuclear vitamin D receptor (VDR), which regulates specific gene expression.

6. 1,25-Dihydroxyvitamin D strongly promotes intestinal Ca^{2+} absorption and weakly increases Pi absorption.

7. Osteoblasts are bone-forming cells of mesenchymal origin. They synthesize bone matrix and regulate its subsequent mineralization. Osteocytes are terminally differentiated cells of the osteoblast lineage that have become entrapped in bone. Osteoclasts are large, multinucleate cells derived from hematopoietic stem cells. Mature activated osteoclasts attach to mineralized bone, then secrete acid and hydrolytic enzymes to dissolve the mineral phase and digest the organic matrix, a process known as bone resorption.

8. The flux of Ca^{2+} and Pi into and out of bone is determined by the relative activities of osteoblasts versus osteoclasts, which exist as basic multicellular units at about 2 million sites within bone. Bone resorption is initiated by osteoblasts, which recruit and activate monocyte-macrophage-lineage cells to become mature polykaryonic osteoclasts. This occurs through the expression of M-CSF and RANKL by osteoblasts, which bind to their receptors, c-Fms and RANK, respectively, on osteoclast precursors to promote osteoclast differentiation and bone resorption. Osteoprotegerin (OPG) is a soluble decoy receptor produced by osteoblasts that can bind RANKL to inhibit osteoclast differentiation and function. Remodeling is completed by osteoblasts, which secrete osteoid that undergoes subsequent mineralization to form mature bone.

9. The PTH1R receptor is expressed on the osteoblast, not the osteoclast. PTH promotes osteoblast differentiation, proliferation, and survival. Intermittent administration of PTH promotes bone formation, whereas a chronic increase in PTH promotes M-CSF

and RANKL expression, shifting the balance in favor of bone resorption.

10. PTH inhibits phosphate reabsorption in the proximal tubule and increases the fractional reabsorption of calcium in the distal nephron.

11. Calcitonin can act on osteoclasts to inhibit bone resorption. Salmon calcitonin has been used therapeutically as an antiresorptive agent. However, endogenous human calcitonin does not play an important role in Ca^{2+}/Pi homeostasis.

12. Other factors that regulate Ca^{2+} and/or Pi levels, either physiologically or pathophysiologically, include PTHrP, FGF23, gonadal steroids, and adrenal steroids.

13. Patients with hyperparathyroidism typically have hypercalcemia, hypophosphatemia. They are prone to kidney stones because of hypercalciuria and hyperphosphaturia.

14. Patients with hypoparathyroidism typically have hypocalcemia and hyperphosphatemia. They may show symptoms of increased neuromuscular excitability such as paresthesias, muscle cramps, and tetany.

15. Children with a vitamin D deficiency are prone to develop rickets, whereas adults with a vitamin D deficiency develop osteomalacia. The vitamin D deficiency results in decreased GI absorption of calcium, phosphate, and magnesium.

SELF-STUDY PROBLEMS

1. How would vitamin D deficiency directly and indirectly alter PTH secretion?
2. What effect does vitamin D deficiency have on serum Pi, and what effect does that have, in turn, on bone?
3. What is the relationship between osteoblasts and bone resorption?
4. Why does unregulated overproduction of PTHrP (e.g., produced by a tumor) cause hypercalcemia?
5. What would be the effect of an elevated ratio of RANKL/OPG expression on bone density?
6. What is the role of FGF23 in the regulation of serum Pi, and what is its major target?

7. How can primary hyperparathyroidism and familial hypocalciuric hypercalcemia be distinguished clinically? Explain.
8. Draw schematic diagrams mapping the integrated hormonal responses to the following challenges:
   a. Vitamin D deficiency
   b. Hyperparathyroidism
   c. Hypocalcemia
   d. Hypophosphatemia

KEYWORDS AND CONCEPTS

1,25-Dihydroxyvitamin D
Adrenal corticoids (cortisol)
Autosomal-recessive hypophosphatemic rickets
Basic multicellular unit
Ca^{2+}-sensing receptor (CaSR)
Calbindin
Calcitriol
Cholecalciferol
Cortical (compact) bone
Estradiol-17β
Familial hypocalciuric hypercalcemia (FHH)
Fibroblast growth factor-23 (FGF23)
Hypercalcemia
Hyperphosphatemia
Hypocalcemia
Inorganic phosphate (Pi)

Monocyte colony–stimulating factor (M-CSF)
Osteoblasts
Osteoclasts
Osteoid
Osteoporosis
Parafollicular C cells
Parathyroid glands
Parathyroid hormone (PTH)
Parathyroid hormone–related peptide (PTHrP)
Principal (chief) cell
PTH/PTHrP receptor
RANKL/RANK
Trabecular (cancellous) bone
Vitamin D receptor (VDR)
Vitamin D–binding protein (DBP)
X-linked hypophosphatemia

Hypothalamus-Pituitary Complex

OBJECTIVES

1. Discuss the embryology and anatomy of the pituitary gland.
2. Review the function of the neurohypophysis (posterior pituitary), including the synthesis, regulation, and function of two neurohormones: antidiuretic hormone (ADH; also called *vasopressin*) and oxytocin.
3. Describe the neurovascular connection between the hypothalamus and the adenohypophysis (anterior pituitary).

4. Develop the concept of an endocrine axis.
5. Describe the cytology of the adenohypophysis, along with the structure and function of the six hormones produced by the adenohypophysis.
6. Discuss the significant direct effects of growth hormone and prolactin on nonendocrine organs.
7. Present some forms of pituitary pathophysiology.

The **pituitary gland** (also called the **hypophysis**) is a small (about 0.5 g in weight) yet complex endocrine structure at the base of the forebrain (Fig. 5.1A and B). It is composed of an epithelial component, called the **adenohypophysis** or **anterior pituitary**, and a neural structure, called the **neurohypophysis**. The caudal end of the neurohypophysis is called the pars nervosa, or posterior pituitary. The anterior pituitary contains five cell types that secrete six hormones. The neurohypophysis acts as a site of release of multiple neurohormones. All endocrine functions of the pituitary gland are regulated by the **hypothalamus** and by **negative and positive feedback loops.**

EMBRYOLOGY AND ANATOMY

Microscopic examination of the pituitary reveals two distinct types of tissues: epithelial and neural (Fig. 5.1C and D). This dual nature of the gland is best understood by reviewing its development. During development, a caudal extension of the primitive forebrain (i.e., the diencephalon) grows toward the roof of the primitive oral cavity (Fig. 5.2). This neural downgrowth, called the **infundibulum**, secretes factors that induce the epithelium of the roof of the oral cavity to extend cranially toward the base of the developing brain. This extension of the oral ectoderm is

called **Rathke pouch.** As Rathke pouch moves upward, the following events occur:

1. Rathke pouch loses its contact with the oral cavity, and by doing so, becomes a ductless endocrine structure. Remnants of Rathke pouch may persist and can give rise to craniopharyngiomas.
2. Rathke pouch comes into direct contact with the infundibulum. The cells on the posterior side of the pouch lumen facing the infundibulum give rise to the **pars intermedia** in the fetus. These cells degenerate in the adult human pituitary. The cells on the anterior side of the pouch lumen facing away from the infundibulum expand considerably and give rise to the **pars distalis**. The pars distalis makes up almost all of the adenohypophysis in the adult and is also referred to as the **anterior pituitary**. A third division of Rathke pouch develops into the **pars tuberalis** and is composed of a thin layer of cells that wrap around the infundibular stalk at the superior end of the anterior pituitary. To summarize, the adenohypophysis (i.e., the **epithelial** portion of the pituitary, or anterior pituitary) develops from epithelial cells (the oral ectoderm) and is composed of the pars distalis, a thin layer called the *pars tuberalis*, and the pars intermedia, which is lost in adult humans.

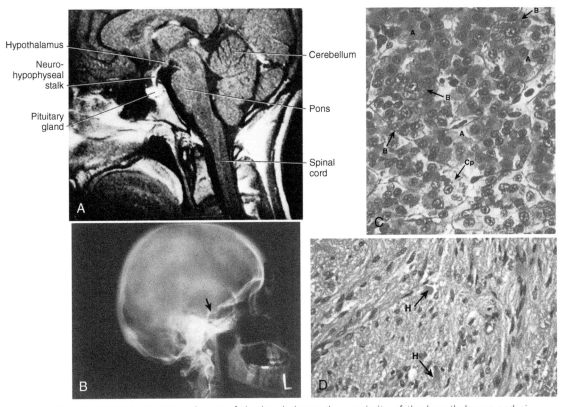

Fig. 5.1 (A) Magnetic resonance image of the head shows the proximity of the hypothalamus and pituitary gland and their connection by a neurohypophyseal (pituitary) stalk. (B) Pituitary gland is located in the sella turcica *(arrow)*. (C) Histology of pars distalis. (D) Histology of pars nervosa. *A,* Acidophil; *B,* basophil; *Cp,* chromophobe; *H,* Herring bodies. (A, Courtesy of Dr. Steven Weiner. From Berne RM, Levy MN, Koeppen BM, et al: *Physiology,* 5th ed., St. Louis, 2004, Mosby. B, Courtesy of Dr. C. Joe. C and D, From Young B, Lowe JS, Stevens A, et al: *Wheater's Functional Histology,* 5th ed., Edinburgh, 2006, Churchill Livingstone.)

3. The infundibular process expands at its lower end to give rise to a structure called the **pars nervosa**. The pars nervosa is also called the **posterior lobe of the pituitary** (or simply, the **posterior pituitary**). At the superior end of the infundibulum, a funnel-shaped swelling develops called the **median eminence**. The rest of the infundibular process, which extends from the medium eminence down to the pars nervosa, is called the *infundibulum.* To summarize, the neurohypophysis develops from a downgrowth of **neural tissue** at the base of the diencephalon (corresponding to the hypothalamus in the adult) and gives rise to the pars nervosa, the infundibulum, and the median eminence. The infundibulum and the pars tuberalis make up the **pituitary stalk**.

CLINICAL BOX 5.1

With development, the pituitary gland becomes encased in the sphenoid bone in a structure called the **sella turcica** (see Fig. 5.1B). The pituitary stalk emerges superiorly out of the sella turcica in the vicinity of the optic nerves and optic chiasm. Generally, cancers of the pituitary have only one way to expand, which is superiorly into the brain and against the **optic nerves**. Thus any increase in the size of the pituitary is often associated with **dizziness** or **vision problems**. The sella turcica is sealed off from the brain by a membrane called the **diaphragma sellae**. Defective development of the diaphragma sellae can allow cerebrospinal fluid to enter the sellar cavity and encroach on developing pituitary tissue. This can give rise to **empty sella syndrome,** which represents a reduction of pituitary tissue (but not always pituitary function) within the sella turcica.

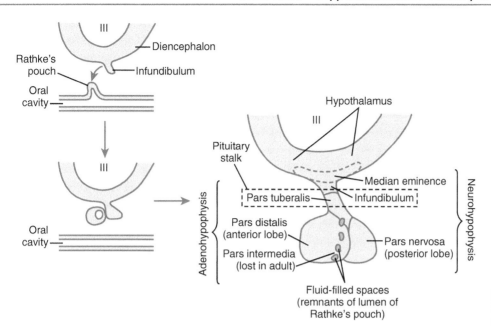

Fig. 5.2 Development of the pituitary gland from neural and epithelial sources.

Labels in figure:
III
Diencephalon
Rathke's pouch
Infundibulum
Oral cavity
Hypothalamus
Pituitary stalk
III
Median eminence
Pars tuberalis
Infundibulum
Pars distalis (anterior lobe)
Pars nervosa (posterior lobe)
Pars intermedia (lost in adult)
Fluid-filled spaces (remnants of lumen of Rathke's pouch)
Adenohypophysis
Neurohypophysis
Oral cavity
III

NEUROHYPOPHYSIS

The pars nervosa is a **neurovascular** structure that is the site of release of neurohormones adjacent to a rich bed of fenestrated capillaries. The peptide hormones that are released are **antidiuretic hormone (ADH)** (also called **vasopressin**) and **oxytocin**. The cell bodies of the neurons that project to the pars nervosa are located in the **supraoptic nuclei (SON)** and **paraventricular nuclei (PVN)** of the hypothalamus (in this context, a *nucleus* refers to a collection of neuronal cell bodies residing within the central nervous system [CNS]—a *ganglion* is a collection of neuronal cell bodies residing outside the CNS). The cell bodies of these neurons are described as **magnocellular** (i.e., large cell bodies) and are equipped with enough biosynthetic capacity to produce a short-lived peptide hormone that is released into and diluted by the peripheral circulation. The magnocellular neurons project axons down the infundibular stalk as the **hypothalamohypophyseal tracts**. These axons terminate in the pars nervosa (Fig. 5.3). In addition to axonal processes and termini from the SON and PVN, there are glial-like supportive cells called **pituicytes**. As is typical of endocrine organs, the posterior pituitary is extensively vascularized, and the capillaries are fenestrated, thereby facilitating diffusion of hormones into the vasculature.

Synthesis of Antidiuretic Hormone (Vasopressin) and Oxytocin

ADH and oxytocin are nonapeptides (9 amino acids) and are similar in structure, differing in only 2 amino acids (Fig. 5.4).

They have limited overlapping activity. ADH (vasopressin) and oxytocin are synthesized as preprohormones. Each prohormone harbors the structure of oxytocin or ADH, each of which is composed of 9 amino acids and a cosecreted peptide called either **neurophysin-II** (associated with ADH) or **neurophysin-I** (associated with oxytocin). These preprohormones are called **preprovasophysin** and **preprooxyphysin**. The N-signal peptide is cleaved while the peptide is transported into the endoplasmic reticulum. The prohormone is packaged in the endoplasmic reticulum and Golgi in a membrane-bound secretory granule in the cell bodies within the SON and PVN (Fig. 5.5). The secretory granules are conveyed intraaxonally through a "fast" (i.e., millimeters/hour) adenosine triphosphate (ATP)–dependent transport mechanism down the infundibular stalk to the axonal termini in the pars nervosa. During transit of the secretory granule, the prohormones are proteolytically cleaved, producing equimolar amounts of hormone and neurophysin. Secretory granules containing fully processed peptides are stored in the axonal termini. Axonal swellings due to the storage of secretory granules can be observed by light microscopy with certain stains and are termed **Herring bodies** (see Fig. 5.1D).

ADH and oxytocin are released at the pars nervosa in response to stimuli that are primarily detected at the cell bodies and their dendrites in the SON and PVN of the hypothalamus. The stimuli are primarily in the form of neurotransmitters released from hypothalamic interneurons. On sufficient stimulus, the neurons will depolarize

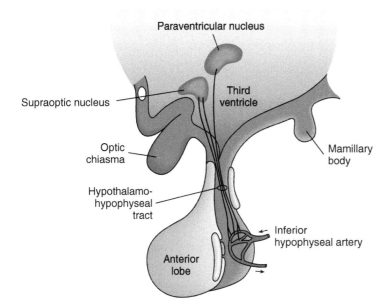

Fig. 5.3 Axonal projections from the paraventricular nuclei (PVN) and supraoptic nuclei (SON) to the pars nervosa.

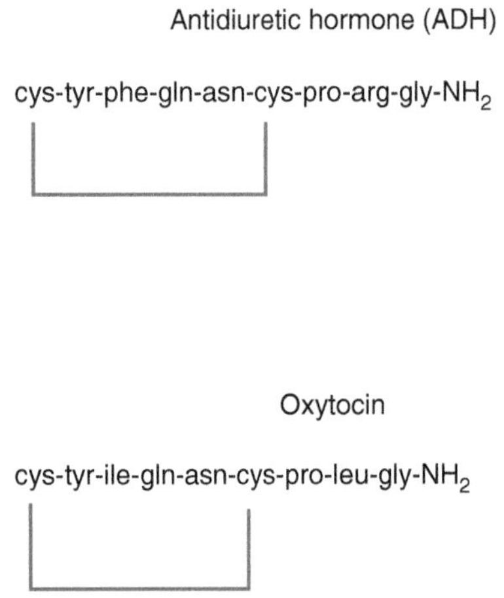

Antidiuretic hormone (ADH)

cys-tyr-phe-gln-asn-cys-pro-arg-gly-NH$_2$

Oxytocin

cys-tyr-ile-gln-asn-cys-pro-leu-gly-NH$_2$

Fig. 5.4 Structure of antidiuretic hormone and oxytocin.

and propagate an action potential down the axon. At the axonal termini, the action potential increases intracellular Ca^{2+} and results in a stimulus-secretion response, with the exocytosis of ADH or oxytocin, along with neurophysins, into the extracellular fluid (ECF) of the pars nervosa (see Fig. 5.5). Both hormones and neurophysins gain access to the peripheral circulation, and both can be measured in the blood.

CLINICAL BOX 5.2

There is no known biologic function for circulating neurophysins. However, several mutations in **familial diabetes insipidus** (in which ADH production is deficient) have been mapped to mutations within the neurophysin structure, suggesting that the sequence and structure of the neurophysin portion are important for the correct processing of the prohormone.

Because posterior pituitary hormones are synthesized in the hypothalamus rather than the pituitary, hypophysectomy (pituitary removal) does not necessarily permanently disrupt synthesis and secretion of these hormones. Immediately after hypophysectomy, secretion of the hormones decreases. However, over a period of weeks, the severed proximal end of the tract will show histologic modification, and pituicytes will form around the neuron terminals. Secretory vacuoles are visible, and secretion of hormone resumes from this proximal end. Secretion of hormone can actually potentially return to normal levels. In contrast, a lesion higher up on the pituitary stalk can lead to loss of the neuronal cell bodies in the PVN and SON.

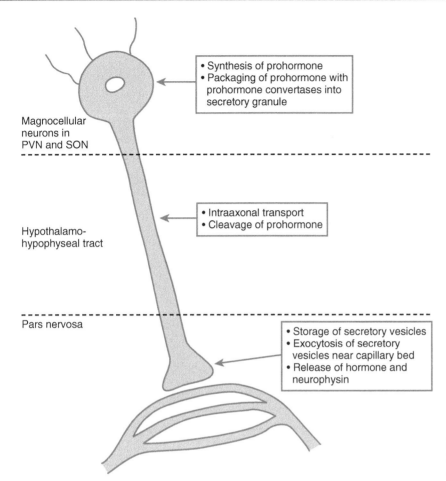

Magnocellular
neurons in
PVN and SON

- Synthesis of prohormone
- Packaging of prohormone with prohormone convertases into secretory granule

Hypothalamo-
hypophyseal tract

- Intraaxonal transport
- Cleavage of prohormone

Pars nervosa

- Storage of secretory vesicles
- Exocytosis of secretory vesicles near capillary bed
- Release of hormone and neurophysin

Fig. 5.5 Intraaxonal transport and processing of preprovasophysin and preprooxyphysin.

Antidiuretic Hormone

Actions of Antidiuretic Hormone

(Mosby Physiology Monograph Series: Chapter 9 in *Renal Physiology*, 6th Ed., BM Koeppen and BA Stanton)

The primary functions of ADH in humans are maintenance of normal osmolality of body fluids and maintenance of normal blood volume. The primary target cells of the ADH are the cells lining the distal renal tubule and the principal cells of the collecting ducts in the kidney. ADH binds to the **vasopressin-2 (V2) receptor** on the basal side of renal cells (Fig. 5.6). The V2 receptor is a G-protein–coupled receptor (GPCR) linked to the Gs-cAMP-PKA pathway. Signaling from the V2 receptor induces the insertion of vesicles containing the water channel protein, called **aquaporin-2**, into the apical membrane of the principal cells, thereby increasing water permeability of this membrane. ADH also increases the gene expression and new synthesis of aquaporin-2. While the basolateral side of the target cells constitutively expresses aquaporin-3 and -4, the ADH-induced increase in apical membrane aquaporin-2 enhances the transepithelial flow of water from the lumen toward the renal interstitium. Therefore, in the presence of ADH, urine flow decreases (**antidiuresis**), and urine osmolality approaches that of the medullary epithelium (about 1200 mOsm/kg). In the absence of ADH, urine flow increases (**diuresis**), and urine osmolality decreases.

ADH increases mesangial cell contraction, which lowers the filtration coefficient of the glomerular membrane and therefore decreases the glomerular filtration rate. This action will further decrease the volume of urine flow. ADH inhibits renin release, a response that could be beneficial in compensation for an increase in ECF osmolality.

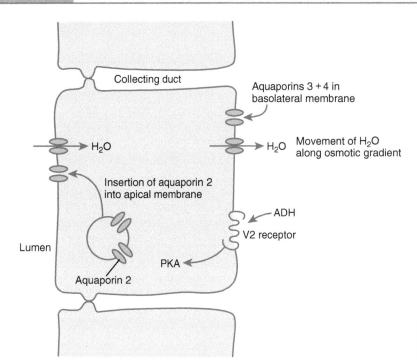

Fig. 5.6 Mechanism of antidiuretic hormone action on the kidney to promote water retention (i.e., antidiuresis).

As part of its role in the defense against the cardiovascular consequences of severe volume depletion, ADH levels increase to supraphysiologic levels (i.e., increase by greater than 100-fold) during **vasodilatory shock**. At these levels, ADH binds to the **V1 receptor** on vascular smooth muscle. The V1 receptor is coupled to a Gq–phospholipase C–intracellular Ca^{2+} signaling pathway, which increases vascular smooth muscle contraction. Thus the vasopressive actions of ADH become important during early states of vasodilatory shock.

Regulation of Antidiuretic Hormone Secretion

ADH is released in response to increased ECF osmolality or decreased blood volume and pressure. **Osmoreceptive neurons**, probably in the hypothalamus or circumventricular organs, innervate the magnocellular neurons of the PVN and SON. These osmoreceptive neurons respond to changes in ECF osmolality by shrinkage or swelling. Thus increased osmolarity indirectly stimulates the magnocellular cells and action potential frequency increases in the neuronal axons constituting the hypothalamohypophyseal tract, with a resultant increase in posterior pituitary ADH release. Because the actual stimulus is cellular dehydration, the response to the hyperosmolality depends on the nature of the solutes. Solutes such as sodium, sucrose, and mannitol that do not readily enter the osmoreceptor cells

are effective stimulators, whereas urea, to which the cells are more permeable, has about one third the potency of sodium. These effects may be demonstrated with the following relationship:

$$\uparrow ECF\ osmolality \rightarrow \uparrow ADH \rightarrow$$
$$\uparrow Renal\ water\ reabsorption \rightarrow \downarrow ECF\ osmolality$$

$$(5.1)$$

The regulatory system is sensitive to serum osmolality changes in the range of 280 to 295 mOsm/kg (Fig. 5.7). Within this range, a rise in as little as 1% in serum osmolality will stimulate a measurable increase in ADH secretion.

ADH release can also be stimulated by a drop in effective blood volume. The receptors for this stimulus are the **cardiovascular volume receptors**, including low-pressure receptors in the atria of the heart, great veins, and pulmonary vasculature and high-pressure receptors in the aortic arch and carotid sinus baroreceptors (Fig. 5.8). Although all of these volume receptors are capable of regulating ADH secretion, the predominant regulator appears to be the atrial volume receptors. The sensitivity of the system to volume change is low at small volume changes. However, volume change does become a significant stimulus when circulating blood volume decreases 8% to 10% or more

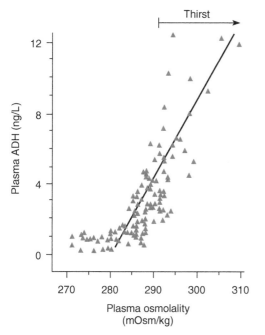

Fig. 5.7 Relation between plasma osmolality and plasma antidiuretic hormone. (Redrawn from Wilson JD, Foster DW, Kronenberg HM, et al, editors: *Williams' Textbook of Endocrinology,* 9th ed., Philadelphia, 1998, WB Saunders.)

(Fig. 5.9). This becomes the only mechanism of ADH stimulation during hemorrhage. A decrease in effective blood volume increases the sensitivity of ADH secretion to an increase in ECF osmolality.

Relationship Between Osmotic and Volume Stimuli

Vascular volume influences the sensitivity of the system to osmotic stimuli. At lower vascular volumes, the system becomes more sensitive to a rise in serum osmolality. In turn, as vascular volume increases, the sensitivity of ADH release to osmotic stimuli decreases.

Other Factors Altering Antidiuretic Hormone Secretion

Several drugs, including barbiturates, nicotine, and opiates, increase ADH secretion. Alcohol is an effective suppressor of ADH secretion. For this reason, consumption of alcoholic beverages can lead to dehydration rather than volume expansion. Nausea increases ADH secretion, affording a protective effect against imminent volume loss due to vomiting. The hormones atrial natriuretic peptide (ANP) and cortisol (see Chapter 7) inhibit ADH secretion.

Regulation of Thirst

The regulation of thirst and drinking behavior is an important component of body fluid balance regulation. Thirst is regulated by many of the same factors that regulate ADH

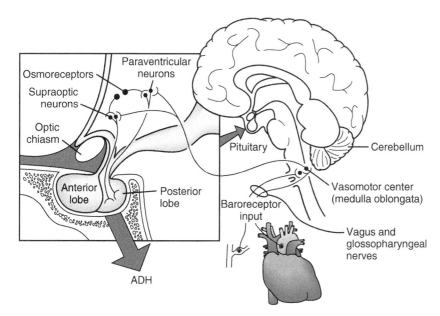

Fig. 5.8 Anatomy of the hypothalamus and pituitary gland (midsagittal section) depicting the pathways for antidiuretic hormone secretion. The *closed box* illustrates an expanded view of the hypothalamus and pituitary gland. (From Koeppen BM, Stanton BA: *Renal Physiology,* 3rd ed., St. Louis, 2001, Mosby.)

secretion. Increased serum osmolality, decreased vascular volume, and ADH secretion are effective stimuli for thirst. The osmoreceptors regulating thirst involve medial hypothalamic regions that approximate the osmoreceptors regulating ADH secretion. Angiotensin II is also thought to play a major role in the regulation of thirst. There are many components to the regulation of drinking, which include, in humans, chemical factors, social factors, and pharyngeal and gastrointestinal factors.

Degradation

ADH is predominantly destroyed by proteolysis in the kidney and liver. The circulating half-life of ADH is about 15 to 20 minutes.

CLINICAL BOX 5.3

A deficiency in ADH production results in **diabetes insipidus (DI)**. People with DI are unable to concentrate urine normally and, therefore, excrete a large volume of urine. These individuals can have urinary flow rates as high as 25 L/day. Thirst increases as a result of the dehydration caused by the high urinary flow. Diabetes insipidus differs from **osmotic diuresis** in that in the former, the urinary osmolality (or specific gravity) is much lower than plasma, whereas in the latter, the urinary osmolality approaches that of plasma.

Neurogenic (Pituitary-Hypothalamic) Diabetes Insipidus

Neurogenic DI is due to mutations in the **preprovasophysin gene** or to destruction of either the hypothalamus (e.g., by hypothalamic tumors) or the posterior pituitary (e.g., by metastatic disease). Thus excessive water is lost in the urine. People with neurogenic diabetes insipidus have a high urine volume and a low urinary osmolality (Table 5.1), accompanied by a high plasma osmolality with inappropriately low ADH levels. If fluids are withheld, these patients continue to produce an excessive urinary volume and a dilute urine. Note that the receptor for ADH (**vasopressin-2, or V2, receptor**) is intact and will respond to exogenous ADH administration. Thus ADH treatment will decrease urinary volume and increase urinary osmolality and will decrease plasma osmolality.

Nephrogenic Diabetes Insipidus

Individuals with **nephrogenic DI** have normal ADH production but lack a normal renal ADH response. The two primary defects in congenital nephrogenic DI are mutations in the **V2 receptor** and **aquaporin-2** (see Fig. 5.6). **Acquired nephrogenic DI** can occur from disruption of renal architecture with washout of the medullary gradient or by certain drugs (e.g., lithium) that impair the signaling pathway from the V2 receptor. Blood ADH levels are normal or elevated in patients with nephrogenic DI, and administration of exogenous ADH analogs does not decrease the urinary flow rate.

Psychogenic Diabetes Insipidus

Those with psychogenic DI are compulsive water drinkers. If water is withheld, the ADH secretion increases and urinary flow decreases, whereas osmolality increases. Individuals with this disorder respond to treatment with ADH.

Syndrome of Inappropriate Secretion of Antidiuretic Hormone

Many disorders can produce inappropriately high ADH concentrations relative to plasma osmolality. Some **neoplasms** produce ADH and release it into plasma. This is particularly common with pulmonary carcinomas, but it can occur in other types of tumors, including nonmalignant tumors. In addition, there are many other causes of the **syndrome of inappropriate secretion of antidiuretic hormone (SIADH)**. Pulmonary tuberculosis is often associated with SIADH, as are trauma, anesthesia, and pain. In SIADH, falling serum osmolality does not inhibit ADH secretion because control of ADH secretion is no longer linked to the normal regulatory mechanisms.

In an individual with SIADH who consumes a normal amount of water, water is retained because of the inappropriately high ADH levels. The resultant increase in blood volume and hence blood pressure increases renal glomerular filtration and therefore increases the loss of sodium in the urine. The **hypervolemia** stimulates release of **atrial natriuretic peptide (ANP)**, which promotes renal sodium loss. The person consequently becomes **hyponatremic** (low blood sodium) and has a low serum osmolality. The urine osmolality is inappropriately high (the free water clearance decreases). If water is restricted in an individual with this condition, serum sodium and osmolality will return to normal.

Oxytocin

The nonapeptide oxytocin is structurally similar to ADH, and there is some overlap in biologic activity. Although the major actions of oxytocin are on uterine motility and milk release, many other biologic actions have been proposed.

Oxytocin and Uterine Motility

Oxytocin stimulates contraction of the uterine myometrium. The magnitude of the oxytocin action depends on the phase of the menstrual cycle. Estrogens increase the uterine response to oxytocin, and progestins decrease the

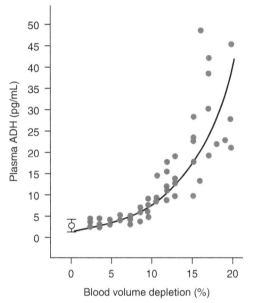

Fig. 5.9 Relation between blood volume and plasma antidiuretic hormone (ADH). (From Greenspan FS, Strewler GJ: *Basic and Clinical Endocrinology,* 5th ed., Norwalk, CT, 1997, Appleton & Lange.)

response. Although uterine responsiveness to oxytocin increases around the time of parturition, oxytocin is not thought to be a factor initiating labor. Oxytocin secretion does not increase until after labor has begun. Once labor begins, the stretching of the vagina and cervix stimulates oxytocin release, which facilitates labor. This is referred to as a **neuroendocrine reflex**, which in this case has a positive feedback nature. Whereas negative feedback loops confer stability, positive feedback loops confer instability—that is, "something has to give." In the case of labor, increasing labor contractions stimulate the cervix and vagina, stimulating more oxytocin, increasing labor contractions, and so on. The pregnancy becomes unstable and is terminated by the delivery of the baby.

Sexual intercourse can stimulate oxytocin release in both men and women. Although the exact role of oxytocin in men is not entirely understood, the increased release of oxytocin during intercourse in women may aid in sperm transport in the female reproductive tract by stimulating uterine motility.

Oxytocin and Milk Letdown

The role of oxytocin in the mammary glands during nursing is discussed in Chapter 11.

Degradation

Like ADH, oxytocin circulates unbound. It has a relatively short half-life of 3 to 5 minutes. Its degradation occurs primarily in the liver and kidney. However, it can also be degraded in other tissues, including the mammary glands and uterus.

Pathologic Conditions Involving Oxytocin

No known pathologic problems are associated with excess levels of oxytocin. Although a deficiency of oxytocin does not cause major problems, it can prolong labor and produce lactational difficulties as a result of poor milk ejection in some women. Oxytocin release is inhibited by several forms of stress.

TABLE 5.1 Analysis of Various Types of Diabetes Insipidus			
	Neurogenic	**Nephrogenic**	**Psychogenic**
Plasma osmolality	↑	↑	↓
Urine osmolality	↓	↓	↓
Plasma ADH	Low	Normal to high	Low
Urine osmolality after mild water deprivation	No change	No change	↑
Plasma ADH after water deprivation	No change	↑	↑
Urine osmolality after administration of ADH	↑	No change	↑

ADH, Antidiuretic hormone.

ADENOHYPOPHYSIS

Because the pars distalis makes up most of the adenohypophysis in the adult human, the terms adenohypophysis, pars distalis, and anterior pituitary are often used synonymously. The anterior pituitary is composed of five endocrine cell types that produce six hormones (Table 5.2). Because of the tinctorial characteristics of the cell types, the corticotropes, thyrotropes, and gonadotropes are referred to as pituitary basophils, whereas the somatotropes and lactotropes are referred to as pituitary acidophils (see Fig. 5.1C). All but one of these hormones are part of an endocrine axis.

Endocrine Axes

A major part of the endocrine system is organized into endocrine axes (Fig. 5.10), which contain three levels of hormonal output. The highest level of hormonal output is actually neurohormonal, and is made up of several hypothalamic nuclei, collectively referred to as the hypophysiotropic region of the hypothalamus, that regulate the adenohypophysis. These nuclei are distinguished from the magnocellular neurons of the PVN and SON that project to the pars nervosa in that they have small parvicellular neuronal cell bodies that project axons to the median eminence. Parvicellular neurons release neurohormones called releasing hormones at the median eminence (Fig. 5.11). The median eminence is like the pars nervosa in that it represents another neurovascular organ. Releasing hormones secreted from axonal endings at the median eminence enter a primary plexus of fenestrated capillaries. Hypothalamic-releasing hormones are then conveyed from the median eminence to a second capillary plexus located in the pars distalis by the hypothalamohypophyseal portal vessels (a "portal" vessel is defined as a vessel that begins and ends in capillaries without going through the heart). With one exception (see later) all releasing hormones are short-lived peptides (see Table 5.2) and reach significant levels only in the *private* portal system between the hypothalamus and the pituitary gland. At the secondary capillary plexus, the releasing hormones diffuse out of the vasculature and bind to their specific receptors on specific cell types within the anterior pituitary.

CLINICAL BOX 5.4

The neurovascular link (i.e., the pituitary stalk) between the hypothalamus and pituitary is somewhat fragile and can be disrupted by physical trauma, surgery, or hypothalamic disease. Damage to the stalk and subsequent functional isolation of the anterior pituitary result in the decline of all anterior pituitary tropic hormones except prolactin (see later in this chapter).

The cells of the anterior pituitary make up the second, intermediate level of an endocrine axis. The anterior pituitary secretes protein hormones that are referred to as tropic hormones—adrenocorticotropic hormone (ACTH), thyroid-stimulating hormone (TSH), follicle-stimulating hormone (FSH), luteinizing hormone (LH), growth hormone (GH), and prolactin (PRL) (see Table 5.2). With a few exceptions, tropic hormones bind their receptors on peripheral endocrine glands. Because of this arrangement, pituitary tropic hormones generally do not *directly* regulate physiologic responses.

The third level of an endocrine axis involves the peripheral endocrine organs, which include the thyroid gland, the adrenal cortex, the ovary, the testis, and the liver. These peripheral endocrine glands are stimulated by pituitary tropic hormones to secrete thyroid hormone, cortisol, estrogen, progesterone, testosterone, and insulin-like growth factor-I (IGF-I). Thus we refer to the following endocrine axes: hypothalamus-pituitary-adrenal axis, hypothalamus-pituitary-thyroid axis, hypothalamus-pituitary-ovary axis, hypothalamus-pituitary-testis axis, and hypothalamus-pituitary-liver axis. These axes, through the peripheral hormones they regulate, have a broad range of effects on growth, metabolism, homeostasis, and reproduction, as discussed in Chapters 6, 7, 9, and 10. The endocrine axes have the following important features:

1. The activity of a specific axis is normally maintained at a setpoint (which in truth is a normal range of activity). The setpoint is determined primarily by the integration of hypothalamic stimulation and peripheral hormone negative feedback. Importantly, the negative feedback is not exerted primarily by the physiologic responses regulated by a specific endocrine axis, but rather from the peripheral hormone acting on the pituitary and hypothalamus (see Fig. 5.10). Thus, if the level of a peripheral hormone drops, the secretion of hypothalamic-releasing hormones and pituitary tropic hormones will increase. As the level of peripheral hormone rises, the hypothalamus and pituitary will decrease secretion owing to negative feedback. Although some nonendocrine physiologic parameters (e.g., acute hypoglycemia) can regulate some endocrine axes, the axes function semiautonomously with respect to the physiologic changes they produce. This configuration means that a peripheral hormone (e.g., thyroid hormone) can evolve to regulate multiple organ systems, without those organ systems exerting competing negative feedback regulation on the hormone. Clinically, this partial autonomy means that multiple aspects of a patient's physiology are at the mercy of whatever derangements exist within a specific axis.

TABLE 5.2 Endocrine Cell Types of the Adenohypophysis

Cell Type	Corticotrope	Thyrotrope	Gonadotrope	Somatotrope	Lactotrope
Primary hypothalamic regulation	Corticotropin-releasing hormone (CRH) (41-aa peptide) stimulatory	Thyrotropin-releasing hormone (TRH) (tripeptide) stimulatory	Gonadotropin-releasing hormone (GnRH) (decapeptide) stimulatory	Growth hormone-releasing hormone (GHRH) (44-aa peptide) stimulatory and somatostatin (tetradecapeptide) inhibitory	Dopamine (catecholamine) inhibitory Prolactin (PRL) releasing factor (stimulatory)
Tropic hormone secreted	Adrenocorticotropic hormone (ACTH) (39-aa peptide)	Thyroid-stimulating hormone (TSH) (glycoprotein hormone)	Follicle-stimulating hormone and luteinizing hormone (FSH, LH) and (glycoprotein hormone)	Growth hormone (GH) (ca. 22-kDa protein)	Prolactin (ca. 23-kDa protein)
Receptor	MC2R (Gs-linked GPCR)	TSH receptor (Gs-linked GPCR)	FSH and LH receptors (Gs-linked GPCRs)	GH receptor (JAK/STAT-linked cytokine receptor)	PRL receptor (JAK/STAT-linked cytokine receptor)
Target endocrine gland	Zona fasciculata and zona reticularis of the adrenal cortex	Thyroid epithelium	Ovary (theca and granulosa[a]) Testis (Leydig and Sertoli)	Liver (but also direct actions—especially in terms of metabolic effects)	No endocrine target organ—not part of an endocrine axis
Peripheral hormone involved in negative feedback	Cortisol	Triiodothyronine (T$_3$)	Estrogen,[b] progesterone, testosterone, inhibin[c]	IGF-I	None

IGF-I, Insulin-like growth factor-I.

[a]Both follicular and luteinized thecal and granulosa cells.

[b]Estrogen can also have a positive feedback in women.

[c]Inhibin selectively inhibits FSH release from the gonadotrope.

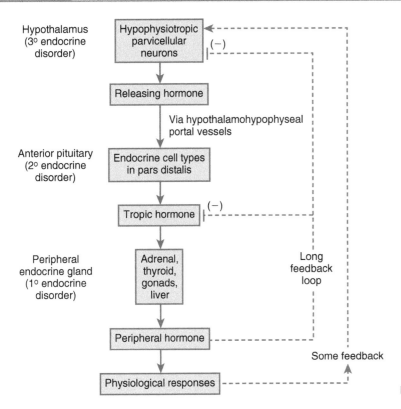

Fig. 5.10 Configuration of an endocrine axis.

2. Hypothalamic hypophysiotropic neurons often secrete in a **pulsatile** manner and are entrained to daily and seasonal rhythms through CNS inputs. Additionally, hypothalamic nuclei receive various neuronal inputs from higher and lower levels of the brain. These can be short term (e.g., various stresses/infections) or long term (e.g., onset of reproductive function at puberty). Thus the inclusion of the hypothalamus in an endocrine axis allows for the integration of a considerable amount of information in determining or changing the setpoint of that axis.

3. The loss of a peripheral hormone (e.g., thyroid hormone) may be due to a defect at the level of the peripheral endocrine gland (e.g., thyroid), the pituitary gland, or the hypothalamus, which are referred to as **primary, secondary, and tertiary endocrine disorders**, respectively (see Fig. 5.10). A thorough understanding of the feedback relationships within an axis allows the physician to determine where the defect lies. Primary endocrine deficiencies tend to be the most severe because they often involve complete absence of the peripheral hormone. Disorders can also be due to excessive secretion at the primary, secondary, or tertiary level of an axis. This is usually due to a hormone-producing tumor (e.g., Cushing disease is due to an ACTH-producing pituitary tumor).

CLINICAL BOX 5.5

Clinically, the inclusion of the hypothalamus within an endocrine axis means that a broad range of complex, neurogenic states can alter pituitary function. **Psychosocial dwarfism** is a striking example of this, in which children who are abused or under intense emotional stress have lower growth rates as a result of decreased growth hormone secretion by the pituitary gland.

Endocrine Function of the Anterior Pituitary

The anterior pituitary comprises the following endocrine cell types: **corticotropes, thyrotropes, gonadotropes, somatotropes, and lactotropes.** Each cell type is discussed subsequently in the context of hormonal production and action, hypothalamic regulation, and feedback regulation.

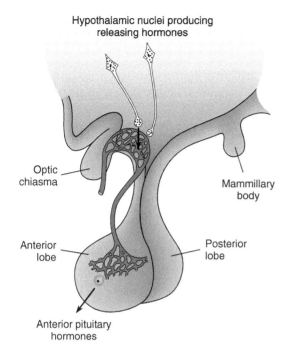

Hypothalamic nuclei producing
releasing hormones

Optic
chiasma

Mammillary
body

Anterior
lobe

Posterior
lobe

Anterior pituitary
hormones

Fig. 5.11 Hypophysiotropic hormones (also called hypothalamic releasing hormones) are secreted into hypophyseal portal circulation and then transported to anterior pituitary. (From Aron DC, Findling JW, Tyrrell JB, et al: Hypothalamus and pituitary. In Greenspan FS, Strewler GJ, editors: *Basic and Clinical Endocrinology*, 5th ed., Norwalk, CT, 1997, Appleton & Lange.)

Corticotropes

Corticotropes stimulate (i.e., are *tropic to*) the **adrenal cortex**, as part of the **hypothalamus-pituitary-adrenal (HPA) axis**. Corticotropes produce the hormone, **adrenocorticotropic hormone (ACTH; corticotropin)**, which stimulates two zones of the adrenal cortex (see Chapter 7).

ACTH is a 39-amino acid peptide that is synthesized as part of a larger prohormone, **proopiomelanocortin (POMC)**. Corticotropes are also referred to as **POMC cells** (note that POMC neurons were discussed in relation to appetite control in Chapter 3; these neurons release α-melanocyte-stimulating hormone [α-MSH] as their neurotransmitter). POMC harbors the peptide sequence for ACTH, α- and β-MSH, endorphins (endogenous opioids), and enkephalins (Fig. 5.12). However, the human corticotrope expresses only the **prohormone convertases** capable of producing ACTH as the sole active hormone secreted from these cells in humans. The other fragments that are cleaved from POMC and secreted by the corticotropes are the N-terminal fragment and β-lipotropic hormone (β-LPH). Neither of these fragments appear to play a physiologic role in humans.

ACTH circulates as an unbound hormone and has a short half-life of about 10 minutes. ACTH binds to the **melanocortin-2 receptor (MC2R)** on cells in the **adrenal cortex** (Fig. 5.13). MC2R is a GPCR coupled to the Gs-cAMP-PKA signaling pathway. ACTH acutely increases cortisol and adrenal androgen production but also increases expression of steroidogenic enzyme genes and, in the long-term, promotes growth and survival of two zones of the adrenal cortex (see Chapter 7).

CLINICAL BOX 5.6

At supraphysiologic levels (e.g., Addison disease with loss of negative feedback by cortisol), ACTH causes darkening of light-colored skin. Normally, keratinocytes express the *POMC* gene, but secrete α-MSH instead of ACTH. Keratinocytes secrete α-MSH in response to ultraviolet light, and α-MSH acts as a paracrine factor on neighboring melanocytes to darken the skin. α-MSH binds to the MC1R on melanocytes. However, at high levels, ACTH can also cross-react with the MC1R receptor on skin melanocytes (see Fig. 5.13). Thus darkening of skin is a clinical sign of excessive ACTH levels, especially in the presence of low cortisol.

ACTH is under stimulatory control by the hypothalamus. A subset of parvicellular hypothalamic neurons expresses the peptide, **procorticotropin-releasing hormone (pro-CRH)**. Pro-CRH is processed to an amidated 41-amino acid peptide, **CRH**. CRH binds to the CRH receptor, **CRH-R1**, on corticotropes. CRH-R1 is a GPCR linked to a Gs-cAMP-PKA signaling pathway. CRH acutely stimulates ACTH secretion and increases transcription of the *POMC* gene. The parvicellular neurons that express CRH also coexpress **ADH**. ADH binds to **V3 receptors** on corticotropes. The V3 receptor is GPCR linked to a Gq–phospholipase C signaling pathway. ADH potentiates the action of CRH on corticotropes.

ACTH secretion shows a pronounced diurnal pattern, with a peak in early morning and a nadir in late afternoon (Fig. 5.14). In addition, secretion of CRH, and hence secretion of ACTH, is pulsatile. There are multiple regulators of the HPA axis, and many of them are mediated through the CNS (Fig. 5.15). Many types of **stress**, both **neurogenic** (e.g., fear) and **systemic** (e.g., infection), stimulate ACTH secretion. The stress effects are mediated through CRH and vasopressin and the CNS. The response to many forms of severe stress can persist despite negative feedback from high cortisol levels. This means that the hypothalamus has the ability to alter the setpoint of the HPA axis in response to stress. Severe, chronic depression can cause

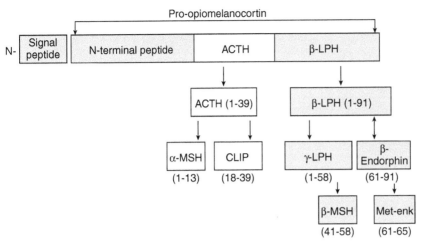

Fig. 5.12 The proopiomelanocortin gene transcript encodes the amino acid sequences of multiple bioactive compounds. Note that adrenocorticotropic hormone *(ACTH)* is the only bioactive peptide released by the human corticotrope. *α-MSH*, α-Melanocyte-stimulating hormone; *β-LPH*, β-lipotrophic hormone; *β-MSH*, β-melanocyte-stimulating hormone; *CLIP*, corticotropin-like intermediate peptide; *γ-LPH*, γ-lipotrophic hormone; *Met-enk*, metenkephalin.

such a resetting of the HPA axis due to hypersecretion of CRH and is, in fact, a factor in the development of **tertiary hypercortisolism** (i.e., excess cortisol production due to hypothalamic dysfunction). Because cortisol has profound effects on the immune system (see Chapter 7), the HPA axis and the immune system are closely coupled, and **cytokines**—particularly interleukin-1 (IL-1), IL-2, and IL-6—stimulate the HPA axis.

Cortisol exerts a negative feedback on the pituitary, where it suppresses *POMC* gene expression and ACTH secretion, and on the hypothalamus, where it decreases pro-*CRH* gene expression and CRH release. As mentioned earlier, ACTH has a long-term effect on the growth and survival of adrenocortical cells. This means that long-term administration of exogenous corticosteroids will cause the adrenal cortex to atrophy because of the negative feedback of the exogenous hormone on ACTH secretion. In such a patient, termination of exogenous corticosteroid therapy must be gradual in order to allow the adrenal cortex to regain its normal functional capacity.

Thyrotropes

Thyrotropes regulate thyroid function by secreting the hormone **TSH** (also called **thyrotropin**) as part of the **hypothalamus-pituitary-thyroid axis**. TSH is one of three **pituitary glycoprotein hormones** along with FSH and LH (see later in the text). TSH is a heterodimer composed of an α-subunit, called the **α-glycoprotein subunit (α-GSU)**, and a **β-subunit (β-TSH)** (Fig. 5.16). The α-GSU

is common to TSH, FSH, and LH, whereas the β-subunit is specific to the hormone (i.e., β-TSH, β-FSH, and β-LH are all unique).

Glycosylation (in particular, terminal sialylation) of the subunits increases their stability in the circulation. The half-lives of TSH, FSH, and LH (and an LH-like placental glycoprotein hormone, **human chorionic gonadotropin [hCG]**) are relatively long, ranging from tens of minutes to several hours. Glycosylation also serves to increase the affinity and specificity of the hormones for their receptors.

TSH binds to the **TSH receptor** on thyroid epithelial cells (Fig. 5.17). The TSH receptor is a GPCR linked to a Gs-cAMP-PKA signal transduction pathway. As discussed in Chapter 6, the production of thyroid hormones is a complex, multistep process. TSH stimulates essentially every aspect of thyroid function. TSH also has a strong tropic effect, stimulating hypertrophy, hyperplasia, and survival of thyroid epithelial cells. Indeed, in geographic regions of low iodide availability (iodide is required for thyroid hormone synthesis), TSH levels become elevated because of reduced negative feedback. Elevated TSH levels can produce noticeable growth of the thyroid, causing a bulge in the neck, called a **goiter**.

The pituitary thyrotrope is stimulated by the **thyrotropin-releasing hormone (TRH)**. TRH is produced by a subset of parvicellular hypothalamic neurons. TRH is a tripeptide, with cyclization of a glutamine at its N-terminus (pyroGlu), and an amidated C-terminus (similar to the structure of gastrin termini; see Chapter 2).

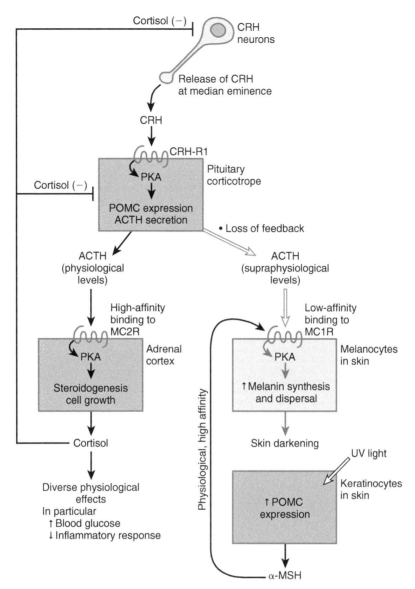

Fig. 5.13 Normal levels of adrenocorticotropic hormone *(ACTH)* act on the MC2R to increase cortisol. Supraphysiologic levels of ACTH (due to loss of cortisol) act on both the MC2R and the MC1R on melanocytes, causing skin darkening.

TRH is synthesized as a larger prohormone, which contains six copies of TRH within its sequence. TRH binds to the **TRH receptor** on the thyrotropes (see Fig. 5.17). The TRH receptor is a GPCR linked to a Gq–phospholipase C signaling pathway. TRH neurons are regulated by numerous CNS-mediated stimuli. TRH is released according to a diurnal rhythm (highest during overnight hours, lowest around dinnertime). TRH is regulated by various stresses, but unlike with CRH, stresses inhibit TRH secretion. These include physical and mental stress, starvation, and infection. The active form of thyroid hormone, triiodothyronine (T_3), negatively feeds back on both pituitary thyrotropes and TRH-producing neurons. T_3 represses both β-TSH expression and the sensitivity of thyrotropes to TRH. T_3 also inhibits TRH production and secretion.

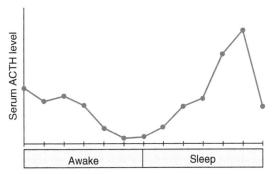

Fig. 5.14 Diurnal pattern for serum adrenocorticotropic hormone *(ACTH)*.

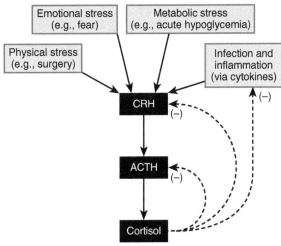

Fig. 5.15 Hypothalamic-pituitary-adrenal axis illustrating factors regulating secretion of corticotropin-releasing hormone *(CRH). ACTH*, Adrenocorticotropic hormone.

Gonadotropes

The **gonadotrope** is a dual hormone producer in that the same cell secretes **FSH** and **LH**. FSH and LH are also referred to as **gonadotropins** and have the same nomenclature in men and women, while being named for their actions in women. The gonadotrope regulates the function of gonads in both sexes. As such, the gonadotrope plays an integral role in the **hypothalamus-pituitary-testis axis** and the **hypothalamus-pituitary-ovary axis** (Fig. 5.18).

As discussed earlier, FSH and LH are pituitary glycoprotein hormones composed of a common α-GSU heterodimerized with a unique β-FSH or β-LH subunit. Importantly, FSH and LH are segregated to a large degree into different secretory granules and are not co-secreted in equimolar amounts (in contrast to ADH and neurophysin, for example). This allows for the modulation of the ratio of FSH/LH secretion by the gonadotropes. FSH and LH bind to their respective receptors, which are both GPCRs primarily coupled to Gs-cAMP-PKA signaling pathways. The actions of FSH and LH on gonadal function are complex, especially in women, and are discussed in detail in Chapters 9 and 10. In general, gonadotropins promote testosterone production in men and estrogen and progesterone secretion in women. FSH also increases the secretion of a TGF-β–related protein hormone, called **inhibin**, in both sexes.

FSH and LH secretion are regulated by one hypothalamic-releasing hormone, **gonadotropin-releasing hormone (GnRH)**. GnRH is a 10-amino acid peptide produced by a subset of parvicellular hypothalamic GnRH neurons. GnRH is produced as a larger prohormone, and as part of its processing to a decapeptide, is modified with a cyclized glutamine (pyroGlu) at its amino terminus and has an amidated carboxy terminus.

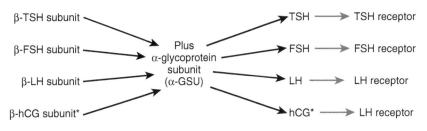

*hCG is human chorionic gonadotropin. hCG is made by the placenta, and binds to the LH receptor.

Fig. 5.16 Pituitary glycoprotein hormones. Human chorionic gonadotropin *(hCG)* is made by the placenta and binds to the luteinizing hormone *(LH)* receptor. *FSH*, Follicle-stimulating hormone; *TSH*, thyroid-stimulating hormone.

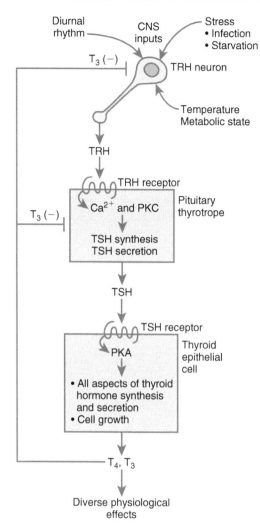

Fig. 5.17 Hypothalamus-pituitary-thyroid axis. *PKA*, Protein kinase A; *PKC*, protein kinase C; *TRH*, thyrotropin-releasing hormone; *TSH*, thyroid-stimulating hormone; T_4, tetraiodothyronine; T_3, triiodothyronine (active form of thyroid hormone).

CLINICAL BOX 5.7

During embryonic development, the GnRH neurons migrate to the mediobasal hypothalamus from the nasal placode. Patients with **Kallmann syndrome** have **tertiary hypogonadotropic hypogonadism**, often associated with loss of sense of smell (**anosmia**). This is due to a mutation in the *KAL* gene, which results in the failure of the GnRH neuronal precursors to properly migrate to the hypothalamus from the region of the nasal placode and to establish a neurovascular link to the pars distalis.

GnRH binds to the **GnRH receptor**, which is a GPCR coupled primarily to a Gq–phospholipase C signaling pathway. GnRH is released in a pulsatile manner, and both the pulsatile secretion and the frequency of the pulses have important effects on the gonadotrope. Continuous infusion of GnRH downregulates the GnRH receptor, resulting in a decrease in FSH and LH secretion. In contrast, pulsatile secretion does not desensitize the gonadotrope to GnRH, and FSH and LH secretion are normal. At a frequency of 1 pulse per hour, GnRH preferentially increases LH secretion (Fig. 5.19). At a slower frequency of 1 pulse per 3 hours, GnRH preferentially increases FSH secretion. The mechanism by which the frequency of GnRH secretion determines the ratio of FSH to LH levels in the blood is poorly understood but may involve multiple signaling pathways linked to the GnRH receptor, leading to differential synthesis or glycosylation, or both, of FSH versus LH.

GnRH secretion is inhibited by numerous drugs (e.g., opioids, selective serotonin reuptake inhibitors) and by intense exercise and mental stress (depression). GnRH secretion is also regulated by the program of puberty. During infancy and childhood, GnRH is under inhibitory signaling from the CNS. At puberty, this inhibition is lost, and GnRH levels increase. The hormone leptin, which acts as a gauge of adipose mass and thus energy supplies, plays a permissive role in puberty.

CLINICAL BOX 5.8

Anorexia nervosa is an eating disorder in which an extreme resistance to eating and a distorted body image in which they perceive themselves as overweight even in the face of emaciation develops in patients (usually girls in early adolescence). A diagnostic criterion for anorexia nervosa in postmenarchal girls is **amenorrhea**, as defined by the absence of three consecutive menstrual cycles. The amenorrhea is due to loss of **GnRH** secretion in response to an **extreme energy deficit**.

Gonadotropins increase sex steroid synthesis. In men, testosterone and estrogen negatively feed back at the level of the pituitary and the hypothalamus. Exogenous progesterone also inhibits gonadotropin function in men and could act as a possible male contraceptive agent. Additionally, inhibin negatively feeds back selectively on FSH secretion in men and women. In women, progesterone and testosterone negatively feed back on gonadotropic function at the level of hypothalamus and pituitary. At low doses, estrogen also exerts a negative feedback on FSH and LH secretion. However, high estrogen levels (e.g., 500 pg/mL) maintained for 3 days cause a surge of LH and, to a lesser extent, FSH secretion (see Chapter 10). This positive

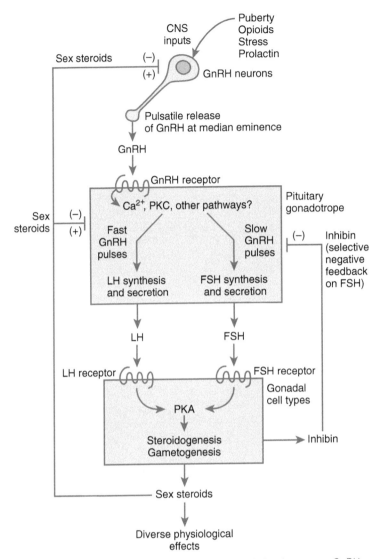

Fig. 5.18 Hypothalamus-pituitary-gonadal axis. *FSH*, Follicle-stimulating hormone; *GnRH*, gonadotropin-releasing hormone; *LH*, luteinizing hormone.

feedback is observed at the hypothalamus and pituitary. At the hypothalamus, GnRH pulse amplitude and frequency increase. At the pituitary, high estrogen levels greatly increase the sensitivity of the gonadotrope to GnRH by increasing GnRH receptor levels and by enhancing postreceptor signaling pathway components.

Somatotropes

The somatotropes produce GH (also called somatotropin). A major target of GH is the liver, where it stimulates the production of IGF-I. Thus the somatotrope is part of the hypothalamus-pituitary-liver axis (Fig. 5.20).

However, GH also has several direct actions at physiologic levels on nonendocrine organs (Box 5.1).

GH is a 191-amino acid protein that is similar to PRL and human placental lactogen (hPL), and there is some overlap in activity among these hormones. Multiple forms of GH are seen in serum, thereby constituting a "family of hormones," with the 191-amino acid (22-kDa) form representing about 75% of the circulating GH. The GH receptor is a member of the cytokine-GH-PRL-erythropoietin receptor family and, as such, is linked to the JAK/STAT signaling pathway. Human GH can also act as an agonist for the PRL receptor.

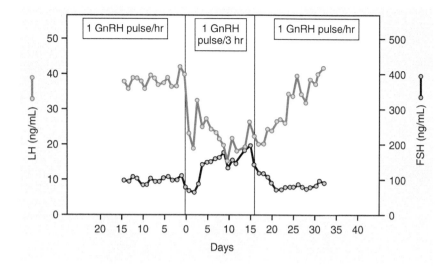

Fig. 5.19 Frequency encoded regulation of follicle-stimulating hormone *(FSH)* and luteinizing hormone *(LH)*. A higher frequency of GnRH pulses preferentially stimulates LH secretion, whereas a slower frequency preferentially stimulates FSH secretion. (From Larsen PR, Kronenberg HM, Melmed S, et al, editors: *Williams Textbook of Endocrinology,* 10th ed., Philadelphia, 2003, Saunders; and Koeppen BM, Stanton BA, editors: *Berne & Levy Physiology,* 6th ed., Philadelphia, 2010, Mosby, p 719.)

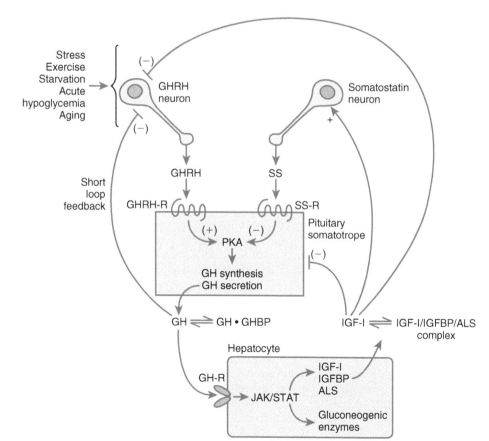

Fig. 5.20 Hypothalamus-pituitary-liver axis. *ALS,* Acid labile subunit; *GHBP,* growth hormone–binding protein; *GHRH,* growth hormone–releasing hormone; *IGF-I,* insulin-like growth factor-I; *IGFBP,* insulin-like growth factor–binding protein; *SS,* somatostatin.

BOX 5.1   Metabolic Actions of Growth Hormone

Carbohydrates
- Increase blood glucose
- Decrease peripheral insulin sensitivity
- Increase hepatic output of glucose
- Administration results in increased serum insulin levels

Proteins
- Increase tissue amino acid uptake
- Increase incorporation into proteins
- Decrease urea production
- Produce positive nitrogen balance

Lipids
- Promotes lipolysis
- Can be ketogenic after long-term administration, particularly if insulin is deficient

Insulin-like Growth Factor
- Stimulates IGF production
- Stimulates growth
- Is mitogenic

About 50% of the 22-kDa form of GH in serum is bound to the N-terminal portion (the extracellular domain) of the GH receptor, called **GH-binding protein (GHBP)**. GHBP reduces renal clearance and thus increases the biologic half-life of GH, which is nevertheless only about 20 minutes. The liver and kidney are major sites of hormone degradation.

GH secretion is under dual control by the hypothalamus (see Fig. 5.20). The hypothalamus predominantly stimulates GH secretion through the peptide, **growth hormone–releasing hormone (GHRH)**. GHRH is a member of the vasoactive intestinal peptide (VIP)-secretin-glucagon family and is processed into a 44-amino acid peptide with an amidated C-terminus from a larger prohormone. GHRH binds to the **GHRH receptor**, which is coupled to a Gs-cAMP-PKA signaling pathway. GHRH enhances GH secretion and *GH* gene expression. The hypothalamus inhibits pituitary GH synthesis and release through the peptide **somatostatin**. Somatostatin is a cyclic tetradecapeptide that is found in many locations in the body (see Chapter 2). Somatostatin in the anterior pituitary inhibits GH and TSH release. Somatostatin binds to the **somatostatin receptor**, which lowers cyclic adenosine monophosphate (cAMP) through a Gi-linked signaling pathway.

The primary negative feedback on the somatotrope is exerted by IGF-I. GH stimulates IGF-I production by the liver, and IGF-I then inhibits GH synthesis and secretion at the pituitary and hypothalamus by a classic long feedback loop. In addition, GH exerts negative feedback on GHRH release through a short feedback loop. GH also increases somatostatin release.

GH secretion, like that of ACTH, shows prominent diurnal rhythms, with peak secretion occurring in the early morning just before awakening (see Fig. 5.20). Its secretion is stimulated during deep, slow-wave sleep (stages III and IV). GH secretion is lowest during the day. This rhythm is entrained to sleep-wake patterns rather than light-dark patterns, so a phase shift occurs in people who work night shifts. As is typical of anterior pituitary hormones, GH secretion is pulsatile. The levels of GH in serum vary widely (0 to 30 ng/mL, with most values usually falling between 0 and 3). Because of this marked variation, serum GH values are of minimal clinical value unless the sampling time is known. Alternatively, IGF-I may be measured because its secretion is regulated by GH, and IGF-I has a relatively long circulating half-life that buffers pulsatile and diurnal changes in secretion.

GH secretion is also regulated by several different physiologic states (see Fig. 5.20). GH is classified as one of the stress hormones and is increased by neurogenic and physical stress. As discussed later, GH promotes lipolysis, increases protein synthesis, and antagonizes the ability of insulin to reduce blood glucose. It is not surprising, therefore, that hypoglycemia is a stimulus for GH secretion, and GH is classified as a **hyperglycemic hormone**. Although its secretion is not regulated by minor variations in serum glucose levels, its release is stimulated by falling glucose levels or by hypoglycemia. Falling blood glucose levels are such an effective stimulus that insulin-induced hypoglycemia has been used as a provocative test for the ability to secrete GH. However, this test is not commonly done because of safety concerns. A rise in certain serum amino acids also serves as an effective stimulus for GH secretion. Arginine is one of these amino acids, and the GH response to arginine infusion may be used to evaluate GH secretion. In contrast, an increase in blood glucose or free fatty acids inhibits GH secretion. Obesity also inhibits GH secretion, in part because of insulin resistance (relative hyperglycemia) and increased circulating free fatty acids. Conversely, exercise is an effective stimulator of GH secretion. GH is also increased during starvation. Other hormonal regulators of GH include estrogen, androgens, and thyroid hormone, which enhance GH secretion; they have direct effects on IGF-I secretion and bone maturation as well.

GH secretion is also regulated by **ghrelin**, which is primarily produced by the stomach (see Chapter 3). Ghrelin is expressed in response to an empty stomach during fasting. GH is also secreted during fasting in response to decreased

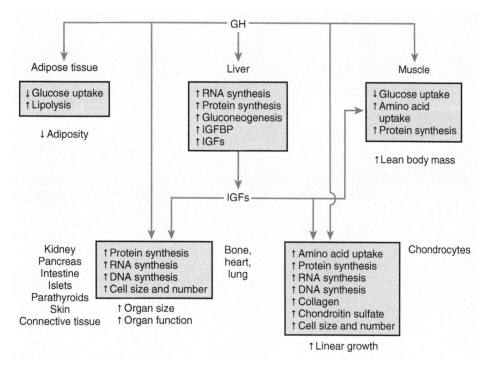

Fig. 5.21 Biologic actions of GH. (From Koeppen BM, Stanton BA editors: *Berne & Levy Physiology*, 6th ed., Philadelphia, 2010, Mosby.)

nutrient levels, especially hypoglycemia. Thus ghrelin not only promotes eating but also reinforces the secretion of GH. GH, in turn promotes lipolysis in adipose tissue and opposes the actions of insulin on glucose uptake by muscle and adipose tissue (see later in the text).

Direct Versus Indirect Actions of Growth Hormone

Direct Actions of Growth Hormone on Metabolism

GH acts directly on the liver, muscle, and adipose tissue to regulate energy metabolism (Fig. 5.21). It shifts metabolism to lipid use for energy, thereby conserving carbohydrates and proteins.

GH is a protein anabolic hormone that increases cellular amino acid uptake and incorporation into protein and represses proteolysis. Consequently, it produces nitrogen retention (a positive nitrogen balance) and a decreased urea production. The muscle wasting that occurs concomitant with aging has been proposed to be caused, at least in part, by the decrease in GH secretion that occurs with aging.

GH is a lipolytic hormone. It activates hormone-sensitive lipase and therefore mobilizes neutral fats from adipose tissue. As a result, serum fatty acid levels rise after GH administration. More fats are used for energy production. Fatty acid uptake and oxidation increase in skeletal muscle and liver. GH can be ketogenic as a result of the increase in fatty acid oxidation (the ketogenic effect of GH is not seen when insulin levels are normal). If insulin is given along with GH, the lipolytic effects of GH are abolished.

GH alters carbohydrate metabolism. Many of its actions may be secondary to the increase in fat mobilization and oxidation; an increase in serum free fatty acids inhibits glucose uptake and utilization in skeletal muscle and adipose tissue. After GH administration, blood glucose rises. The hyperglycemic effects of GH are mild and slower than those of glucagon and epinephrine. The increase in blood glucose results, in part, from decreased glucose uptake and use in skeletal muscle and adipose tissue. Liver glucose output increases, and this is probably not a result of glycogenolysis. In fact, glycogen levels can rise after GH administration. However, the increase in fatty acid oxidation and, hence, the rise in liver acetyl coenzyme A (acetyl CoA) stimulate gluconeogenesis, followed by increased glucose production from substrates such as lactate and glycerol.

GH antagonizes the action of insulin at the postreceptor level in skeletal muscle and adipose tissue (but not liver). Hypophysectomy (removal of the pituitary gland) can improve diabetic management because GH, like cortisol, decreases insulin sensitivity. Because GH produces insulin insensitivity, it is considered a **diabetogenic hormone**. When secreted in excess, GH can cause insulin resistance and ultimately type 2 diabetes. Normal levels of GH are required for normal pancreatic function and insulin secretion. In the absence of GH, insulin secretion declines.

Effects of Growth Hormone on Growth

GH promotes the growth of bones and visceral organs. GH administration increases skeletal and visceral growth; children without GH show growth stunting or dwarfism. GH results in increased cartilage growth, long-bone length, and periosteal growth. These effects are due in part to direct effects of GH on the growth plate to increase recruitment of proliferating chondrocytes. In addition, both systemic (from liver) and locally produced IGF-I are important regulators of bone growth (see Fig. 5.21).

Insulin-like Growth Factors

IGFs are multifunctional hormones that regulate cellular proliferation, differentiation, and cellular metabolism. These protein hormones resemble insulin in structure and function. The two hormones in this family, IGF-I and IGF-II, are produced in many tissues and have autocrine, paracrine, and endocrine actions. Both hormones are structurally similar to proinsulin, with IGF-I having 42% structural homology with proinsulin. IGFs and insulin cross-react with each other's receptors, and IGFs in high concentration mimic the metabolic actions of insulin. Both IGF-I and IGF-II act through **type 1 IGF receptors**. However, IGF-II also binds to the **type 2 IGF–mannose-6-phosphate receptor**. This receptor does not resemble the insulin receptor and does not have intrinsic tyrosine kinase. Binding to these receptors probably facilitates internalization and degradation of the growth factor. IGFs stimulate glucose and amino acid uptake and protein and DNA synthesis. They were initially called somatomedins because they mediate GH (somatotropin) action on cartilage and bone growth. IGF-II is the major form produced in the fetus and its expression is regulated by genomic imprinting with the paternal allele being expressed. IGF-I is the major form produced in most adult tissues and will be discussed further. Initially, IGF-I was thought to be exclusively produced by the liver in response to GH, but it is now known that IGF-I is produced in many tissues and that many of its actions are autocrine or paracrine. The liver is the predominant source of circulating IGF-I (see Fig. 5.20).

Essentially all circulating IGF-I is transported in serum bound to **insulin-like growth factor–binding proteins (IGFBPs)**. IGFBPs bind to IGF-I and then associate with another protein, called **acid labile subunit (ALS)**. GH stimulates the hepatic production of IGF-I, IGFBPs, and ALS (see Fig. 5.20). The IGFBP–ALS–IGF-I complex mediates transport and bioavailability of IGF-I. Although IGFBPs generally inhibit IGF-I action, they greatly increased its biologic half-life (up to 12 hours). IGFBP proteases degrade IGFBP and probably play a role locally in generating free (i.e., active) IGF-I. This is of interest in the context of IGF-responsive cancers (e.g., prostate cancer), which may overexpress one or more IGFBP proteases.

IGF-I has profound effects on bone and cartilage (see Fig. 5.21). It stimulates the growth of bones, cartilage, and soft tissue and regulates essentially all aspects of the metabolism of the cartilage-forming cells, called *chondrocytes*. IGF-I is mitogenic. During puberty, the setpoint of the hypothalamic-pituitary-liver access is increased by the onset of sex steroid production, resulting in increased levels of GH and IGF-I. This accounts for the acceleration of long bone growth at this time. Although appositional growth of long bones continues after closure of the epiphyses, growth in length ceases. IGF-I stimulates osteoblast replication and collagen and bone matrix synthesis. Serum IGF-I levels correlate well with growth in children.

Interaction of Role of Growth Hormone, Insulin-like Growth Factor, and Insulin in Different Metabolic States

When ample supplies of nutrients are available, the high serum amino acid levels stimulate GH and insulin secretion, and the high serum glucose levels stimulate insulin secretion. The high serum GH, insulin, and nutrient supplies stimulate IGF production, and these conditions are appropriate for growth.

However, if the diet is high in calories but low in amino acids, the conditions change. Whereas the high carbohydrate availability results in high insulin availability, the low serum amino acid levels inhibit GH and IGF production. These conditions allow dietary carbohydrates and fats to be used, but conditions are unfavorable for tissue growth.

During fasting, when nutrient availability decreases, serum GH levels rise, and serum insulin levels fall (because of hypoglycemia). Importantly, GH does not stimulate hepatic IGF-I production in the absence of insulin. This means that during starvation, with very low levels of insulin, IGF-I secretion is effectively inhibited because nutritional conditions are not favorable for growth. Under these circumstances, the decrease in IGF-I reduces negative feedback on GH. The consequent rise in GH secretion is beneficial because it promotes fat mobilization while minimizing tissue protein loss. In the absence of insulin, peripheral tissue glucose use decreases, thereby conserving glucose for essential tissues such as brain.

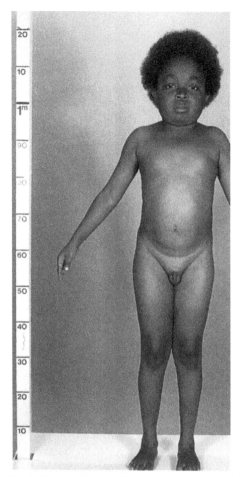

Fig. 5.22 A 17-year-old boy with growth hormone deficiency associated with hypopituitarism. The patient has short stature for his age (note scale bar) and underdeveloped genitalia. (From Besser GM, Thorner MO: *Clinical Endocrinology*, London, 1994, Mosby-Wolfe.)

Pathologic Conditions Involving Growth Hormone

GH is necessary for growth before adulthood. Deficiencies can produce dwarfism, and excesses can produce gigantism. Normal growth requires not only normal levels of GH but also normal levels of thyroid hormones, sex steroids, and insulin.

Growth Hormone Deficiency

If GH deficiency occurs before puberty, growth is severely impaired (Fig. 5.22). Individuals with this condition are relatively well proportioned and have normal intelligence. If the anterior pituitary deficiency is limited to GH, life span should be unaffected. They are sometimes obese because GH-induced lipolysis is lost. If they have

panhypopituitarism (all anterior pituitary hormones are deficient) so that gonadotropins are deficient, they may not mature sexually and remain infertile. People with GH deficiency show few metabolic abnormalities other than a tendency toward hypoglycemia, insulinopenia, and increased insulin sensitivity. There are multiple potential sites of impairment. GH secretion may be reduced, GH-stimulated IGF production may decrease, or IGF action may be deficient. Laron syndrome is characterized by GH resistance due to a genetic defect in the expression of the GH receptor, so that response to GH is impaired. Hence, although the serum GH levels are normal to high, they do not produce IGF-I in response to GH. Interestingly, type 2 diabetes does not develop in patients with Laron syndrome despite increased adiposity.

Growth Hormone Deficiency in Adults

GH deficiency in adults is only currently becoming recognized as a pathologic syndrome. If the GH deficiency occurs after the epiphyses close, growth is not impaired. A GH deficiency is one of many possible causes of hypoglycemia. Recent studies have shown that extended deficiencies of GH lead to body composition changes. The percentage of the body weight represented by fat increases, whereas the percentage of lean body mass protein decreases. In addition, muscle weakness and early exhaustion are symptoms of GH deficiency.

GH levels decrease in senescence, and muscle loss that occurs with aging may result in part from an age-related decline in GH production. However, normal aging is not considered GH deficiency and should not be treated with exogenous GH, because the risks greatly outweigh the benefits.

Growth Hormone Excess Before Puberty

Excessive GH production before puberty results in gigantism. Individuals with this condition can reach heights greater than 8 ft. The GH excess results in an increase in body weight as well as height. Many complications are associated with gigantism. These individuals frequently have glucose intolerance and hyperinsulinemia. Overt clinical diabetes mellitus can develop, but ketoacidosis is rare. They have cardiovascular problems, including cardiac hypertrophy (all viscera increase in size); they are more susceptible to infections than normal; and they rarely live past their 20s. Hypersecretion of GH generally results from pituitary tumors; tumor growth eventually compresses other components of the anterior pituitary, decreasing secretion of other anterior pituitary hormones.

Fig. 5.23 shows Robert Wadlow, who was known as the Alton Giant. At 1 year, he weighed 62 lb. His adult size was 8 ft, 11 in and 475 lb. Note the long extremities.

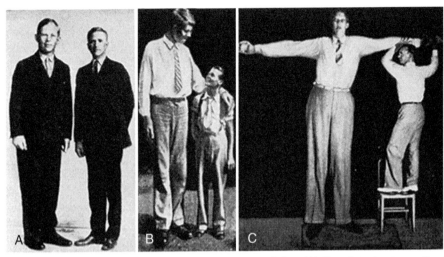

Fig. 5.23 A notable example of growth hormone excess was Robert Wadlow, later known as the "Alton Giant." Although he weighed only 9 lb at birth, he grew rapidly, and by 6 months of age, he weighed 30 lb. At 1 year of age, he weighed 62 lb. Growth continued throughout his life. A. Robert with his father at age 10. B. Robert with a pal at age 16. C. Shortly before his death at age 22 years from cellulitis of the feet, he was 8 ft, 11 in tall and weighed 475 lb. (A and B, from Fadner F: *Biography of Robert Wadlow,* Boston, MA, 1944, Bruce Humphreys. C, Courtesy Dr. C. M. Charles and Dr. C. M. MacBryde.)

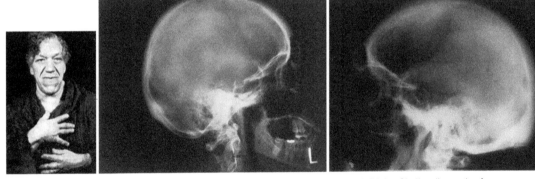

Fig. 5.24 Left, Severe acromegaly. Middle, Radiograph of a normal skull. Right, Skull radiograph of a woman with acromegaly. The sella turcica is enlarged as a result of growth of the pituitary adenoma. The skull is thicker than normal, and protrusion of the frontal ridge with enlargement of frontal sinuses is evident. (Left, From Clinico-pathologic conference: acromegaly, diabetes, hypermetabolism, proteinuria, and heart failure. *Am J Med* 20:133, 1956; Middle and right, Courtesy of Dr. C. Joe.)

The androgen deficiency secondary to the gonadotropin deficiency caused delayed puberty, resulting in late closure of the epiphyses and contributing to long bone growth.

Acromegaly

Excessive GH secretion after the epiphyses close results in appositional bone growth, but not a further lengthening of long bones. Cartilage and membranous bones continue to grow, and gross deformities can result. In addition, soft tissue growth increases, and the abdomen protrudes as a result of visceral enlargement. Brain weight increases, with a resultant decrease in ventricular size. There is an increase in the growth of the nose, ears, and mandible, with the mandibular enlargement producing prognathism and widely spaced teeth (Fig. 5.24). The calvarium thickens, and the frontal sinuses enlarge, resulting in protrusion of the frontal ridge of the orbit of the eye. The characteristic enlargement of the hands and feet is the basis for the name **acromegaly** (*acro*, end or extremity; *megaly*, enlargement). The excessive bone and cartilage growth can produce carpal tunnel syndrome and joint problems. The voice deepens because of laryngeal growth. Acromegaly usually results from a **functional tumor of the somatotropes**. Because it is generally slow in onset, patients typically do not seek medical help for 13 to 14 years. Unfortunately, by that time, they often have permanent physical deformities, including coarsening of facial features (see Fig. 5.24). People with gigantism eventually exhibit acromegaly if the condition is not corrected before puberty. A person with untreated acromegaly has a shortened life expectancy.

Lactotropes

The **lactotrope** produces the hormone, prolactin (PRL), which is a 199-amino acid single-chain protein. The lactotrope differs from the other endocrine cell types of the adenohypophysis in two major ways.

- The lactotrope is not part of an endocrine axis. This means that PRL acts directly on nonendocrine cells to induce physiologic changes.
- The production and secretion of PRL is predominantly under inhibitory control by the hypothalamus through the neurotransmitter, **dopamine**. Thus disruption of the pituitary stalk and the hypothalamohypophyseal portal vessels (e.g., due to surgery or physical trauma) results in an increase in PRL levels, but a decrease in ACTH, TSH, FSH, LH, and GH.

PRL circulates unbound to serum proteins and thus has a relatively short half-life of about 20 minutes. As is typical of protein hormones, there is heterogeneity of circulating forms of PRL, and the 199-amino acid form represents only 60% to 80% of the PRL measured by radioimmunoassays. Normal basal serum concentrations are similar in men and women.

PRL release is normally under tonic inhibition by the hypothalamus. This is exerted by dopaminergic tracts that secrete dopamine at the median eminence. Dopamine binds to the D2 receptor, which is linked to a Gi signaling pathway. There is also evidence for the existence of a prolactin-releasing factor (PRF). The exact nature of this compound is not known, although many factors, including TRH and hormones in the glucagon family (secretin, glucagon, VIP, and gastroinhibitory peptide [GIP]), can stimulate PRL release.

The regulation of PRL secretion during pregnancy and lactation is discussed in Chapter 11.

Drugs that interfere with dopamine synthesis or action increase PRL secretion. Many commonly prescribed antihypertensive drugs and tricyclic antidepressant drugs are dopamine inhibitors. **Bromocriptine** is a dopamine agonist that can be used to inhibit PRL secretion. Somatostatin, TSH, and GH also inhibit PRL secretion.

The **PRL receptor** belongs to the cytokine-GH-PRL-erythropoietin receptor superfamily. Therefore PRL acts through a JAK/STAT signaling pathway (see Chapter 1). Many different actions have been proposed for PRL; which actions are seen often depends on the dose of hormone used and the species studied. In humans, the predominant physiologic role of PRL is the regulation of essentially every aspect of postnatal breast development and function, as discussed in Chapter 11.

> ## CLINICAL BOX 5.9
>
> PRL-secreting tumors (**prolactinomas**) account for about 70% of all anterior pituitary tumors. Furthermore, many drugs interfere with dopamine production or action and hence increase PRL release. For these reasons, **hyperprolactinemia** is a common disorder in humans. Hyperprolactinemia in women is associated with **oligomenorrhea** or **amenorrhea and infertility**. GnRH release, the gonadotrope response to GnRH, and the ovarian response to LH all decrease. In the early stages of the pathologic condition, PRL suppresses follicular maturation, leading to an inadequate corpus luteum and a short luteal phase. While the hyperprolactinemia persists, the preovulatory estrogen peak is lost, thereby lengthening the cycle and leading to oligomenorrhea and anovulatory cycles. Hyperprolactinemia can produce **infertility in men**. Although breast enlargement in men can occur, true **gynecomastia** (inappropriate growth of breasts) and **galactorrhea** (inappropriate flow of milk) are rare.

The primary symptoms causing men and postmenopausal women with PRL-secreting tumors to seek medical attention may be those resulting from compression by the pituitary mass. These patients may experience **severe headaches** or **visual disturbances** that can include bitemporal hemianopia (defect in vision in the temporal half of the field of vision in both eyes). Both men and women may suffer from decreased libido and signs of hypogonadism.

Dopamine agonists not only inhibit PRL production but also repress lactotrope growth and proliferation. Thus dopamine agonists can be used as an antitumor drug in the case of dopamine-responsive prolactinomas.

Hypopituitarism

Panhypopituitarism

There are many causes of hypopituitarism, which can involve either hypothalamic or pituitary problems. The deficiencies can be variable for the different anterior pituitary hormones. The symptoms of hypopituitarism are slow in onset and are reflected in deficiencies in the target organs of the anterior pituitary. Hypogonadism, hypothyroidism, hypoadrenalism, and growth impairment (in children) may be present. People with panhypopituitarism tend to have sallow complexions because of the ACTH deficiency, and they become particularly sensitive to the actions of insulin because of the decreased secretion of the insulin antagonists GH and cortisol. They are prone to experience hypoglycemia, particularly when stressed. Hypogonadism is manifested by amenorrhea in women, impotence in men, and loss of libido in both men and women. Some of the clinical manifestations of hypothyroidism are cold, dry skin, constipation, hoarseness, and bradycardia. The myxedema (nonpitting edema) associated with severe hypothyroidism is rare. Adrenal insufficiency caused by the ACTH deficiency can result in weakness, mild postural hypotension, hypoglycemia, and a loss of pubic and axillary hair. The only symptom associated with the PRL deficiency is the incapacity for postpartum lactation. Finely wrinkled skin is characteristic of a deficiency of both gonadotropin and GH. The GH deficiency can also lead to fasting hypoglycemia in adults and children. In children, growth is impaired, and the relative increase in adipose tissue and decrease in muscle mass may produce a chubby appearance. The symptoms of the endocrine deficiencies are not as severe as they are in primary thyroid, adrenal, and gonadal deficiencies.

Growth

Normal growth is a complex process that requires normal endocrine function. There are definitive patterns for normal growth. The most rapid growth occurs during fetal development, when both IGF-I and IGF-II play critical roles in placental and fetal growth. Postnatally, the most rapid growth occurs in the neonate, when growth falls under the control of GH and IGF-I. The next period of rapid growth occurs at puberty. It is during late puberty that the rising sex steroids, in concert with GH and IGF-I, produce the growth spurt. Ultimately, estrogen stimulates closure (fusion) of the growth plate in both males and females, and hence causes the termination of long-bone growth.

BOX 5.2 Causes of Retarded Growth In Children

- GH deficiency
  - IGF-I deficiency
  - Impaired IGF-I action
- Thyroid deficiency
- Insulin deficiency
- Cortisol excess
- Malnutrition, undernutrition
- Psychosocial growth retardation
- Constitutional delay
- Chronic disease
- Genetic disorders characterized by short stature

GH, Growth hormone; *IGF-I*, insulin-like growth factor-I.

The roles of GH, IGF-I and sex steroids in growth regulation have been emphasized. However, appropriate levels of thyroid hormones, insulin, and cortisol are also required for normal growth. The growth deficiencies associated with hypothyroidism are discussed in Chapter 6. Causes of growth deficits in children are listed in Box 5.2. In the absence of normal insulin levels, intermediary metabolism is impaired, and IGF production decreases. Hypercortisolism is associated with growth impairment. Growth is stunted if nutrition is not adequate. In either starvation or malnutrition, IGF-I production is low, and growth is slowed. Chronic illnesses also impair growth. Upon resolution of either prolonged illness or malnutrition, children will often display a well-known but poorly understood period of accelerated growth known as "catch-up growth."

Another cause of growth impairment is psychosocial short stature (formerly psychosocial dwarfism). Infants who are not stimulated and nurtured or children who are raised in an abusive environment can demonstrate poor growth. These children have an immature appearance and often have unusual eating and drinking habits. Pituitary function in these children is suppressed. However, when such children are removed from the adverse environment, normal pituitary function and growth resume.

In many cases, short stature in childhood is merely a result of a constitutional delay of growth and puberty. This is not a pathologic condition but a genetic variation that may have been exhibited by one or both parents. These children typically show delayed skeletal age and pubertal development, but demonstrate rapid growth during puberty and typically catch up to attain a normal adult stature.

SUMMARY

1. The pituitary gland (also called the *hypophysis*) is derived from a neural structure (the infundibulum) and an epithelial structure (Rathke pouch). The infundibulum develops into the neurohypophysis, which includes the median eminence, infundibular stalk, and pars nervosa (also called the *posterior pituitary*). Rathke pouch develops into the adenohypophysis (also called *anterior pituitary*), which includes the pars distalis, pars tuberalis, and pars intermedia (the pars intermedia is lost in the adult human). The pituitary gland sits in a pocket of the sphenoid bone, called the *sella turcica*, at the base of the forebrain.

2. Magnocellular hypothalamic neurons in the paraventricular and supraoptic nuclei project axons down the infundibular stalk and terminate in the pars nervosa. The pars nervosa is a neurovascular organ, wherein neurohormones are released and diffuse into the vasculature.

3. Two neurohormones, antidiuretic hormone (ADH; also called *vasopressin*) and oxytocin, are synthesized in the hypothalamus in the magnocellular neuronal cell bodies. ADH and oxytocin are transported intraaxonally down the hypothalamohypophyseal tracts to the pars nervosa. Stimuli perceived by the cell bodies and dendrites in the hypothalamus control the release of ADH and oxytocin at the pars nervosa.

4. The primary action of ADH is to promote water reuptake at the distal nephron and collecting duct. ADH also has vasopressive actions, which are important during vasodilatory shock.

5. Diabetes insipidus (DI) is a disease in which either there is deficient ADH (central DI) or deficient response to ADH at the kidney (nephrogenic DI). DI is associated with increased urine flow, dehydration, and increased thirst. The syndrome of inappropriate ADH secretion (SIADH) is characterized by high ADH levels, which increase volume and blood pressure, and a low serum osmolarity.

6. Oxytocin acts on the breast to cause milk letdown during nursing and on the uterus to cause muscular contractions during labor.

7. The adenohypophysis secretes several tropic hormones, which are part of the endocrine axes. An endocrine axis includes the hypothalamus, the pituitary, and a peripheral endocrine gland. The setpoint of an axis is largely controlled by the negative feedback of the peripheral hormone on the pituitary and hypothalamus.

8. The adenohypophysis contains five endocrine cell types: corticotropes, thyrotropes, gonadotropes, somatotropes, and lactotropes. Corticotropes secrete ACTH, thyrotropes secrete TSH, gonadotropes secrete FSH and LH, somatotropes secrete GH, and lactotropes secrete PRL.

9. The predominant control exerted by the hypothalamus on the anterior pituitary is mediated by releasing hormones. These small peptides are carried through the hypophyseal portal system to the anterior pituitary, where they control synthesis and release of the pituitary hormones ACTH, TSH, FSH, LH, and GH. PRL is under predominantly inhibitory control by the hypothalamus through the catecholamine dopamine.

10. GH stimulates growth directly and through regulation of the growth-promoting hormone IGF-I. GH also has metabolic actions. It raises blood glucose by decreasing peripheral tissue utilization. It is protein anabolic and lipolytic.

11. The predominant action of PRL in humans is the initiation and maintenance of lactation.

12. Normal growth is a complex process that requires normal endocrine function. Consequently, growth deficiencies are associated with many endocrine disorders in children.

SELF-STUDY PROBLEMS

1. Explain the origins of the neurohypophysis and adenohypophysis.
2. How is a portion of the neurohypophysis critical to the normal function of the anterior pituitary?
3. Is ADH secretion more sensitive to changes in volume or changes in osmolality? Explain.
4. Describe the production of ADH in terms of hormone synthesis, processing, and secretion. Where do each of these steps occur?
5. How does SIADH result in hyponatremia?
6. Name two proteins that are mutated in congenital nephrogenic diabetes insipidus.
7. Cushing disease is hypercortisolism due to hypothalamic-independent excessive ACTH production by corticotropes. Is this a primary, secondary, or tertiary endocrine disorder and why?
8. McCune-Albright syndrome is a genetically mosaic condition in which some cells express a Gs protein with an activating mutation. Explain why this can lead to excessive growth of somatotropes and high GH levels.

9. Explain why GH is referred to as a diabetogenic hormone.
10. How does stress (in any form) affect the secretion of the following elements: CRH, TRH, GnRH, and GHRH?
11. Compare the actions of GH secreted after consumption of a balanced meal with the actions of GH stimulated by hypoglycemia during fasting.
12. How is skin darkening related to primary hypocortisolism?
13. What is the effect of hypoglycemia on GH and IGF-I secretion?
14. Explain the relationship of GH and IGF-I with respect to:
    a. IGF-I secretion
    b. Feedback regulation of the GH/IGF-I axis
    c. Bone and organ growth

KEYWORDS AND CONCEPTS

Acid labile subunit (ALS)
Acidophils
Acromegaly
Adenohypophysis
Adrenocorticotropic hormone (ACTH)
α-Glycoprotein subunit (α-GSU)
Anterior pituitary
Antidiuretic hormone
Corticotrope
Corticotropin-releasing hormone (CRH)
Cortisol
Diabetes insipidus
Dopamine
Empty sella syndrome
Endocrine axis
Follicle-stimulating hormone (FSH)
GH-binding protein (GHBP)
Ghrelin
Gigantism
Gonadotrope
Gonadotropin-releasing hormone (GnRH)
Growth hormone (GH)
Growth hormone–releasing hormone (GHRH)
Hypophysis
Hypothalamohypophyseal portal vessels
Hypothalamohypophyseal tract
IGF-binding protein (IGFBP)
Infundibulum
Insulin-like growth factor-I (IGF-I)
KAL gene
Kallmann syndrome
Lactational amenorrhea
Lactotrope
Laron syndrome
Luteinizing hormone (LH)
Magnocellular neurons
Median eminence

Melanocortin-2 receptor (MC2R)
Milk ejection (letdown)
Neuroendocrine reflex
Neurohypophysis
Neurophysin
Oxytocin
Panhypopituitarism
Paraventricular nucleus (PVN)
Pars (distalis; intermedia; nervosa; tuberalis)
Parvicellular neurons
Pituicyte
Pituitary gland
Positive feedback
Posterior lobe of the pituitary
Primary endocrine disorder
Progesterone
Prolactin (PRL)
Prolactin-releasing factor (PRF)
Proopiomelanocortin (POMC)
Rathke pouch
Secondary endocrine disorder
Sella turcica
Somatostatin
Somatotrope
Supraoptic nucleus (SON)
Syndrome of inappropriate secretion of antidiuretic hormone (SIADH)
Tertiary endocrine disorder
Testosterone
Thyroid hormone
Thyroid-stimulating hormone (TSH)
Thyrotrope
Thyrotropin
Thyrotropin-releasing hormone (TRH)
Tropic hormones
Vasopressin-2 (V2) receptor

The Thyroid Gland

OBJECTIVES

1. Explain the mechanisms of thyroid hormone synthesis.
2. Describe the regulation of thyroid function and the actions of thyroid hormones.
3. Compare and contrast the functions of thyroxine and triiodothyronine.
4. Discuss the peripheral conversion of thyroid hormones by deiodinases.
5. Draw the regulatory feedback loop for the regulation of thyroid function.
6. Understand the etiology, major symptoms, and pathophysiology of the symptoms for Graves disease, Hashimoto thyroiditis, sporadic congenital hypothyroidism, and cretinism.

The thyroid gland produces the prohormone, tetraiodothyronine (T_4), and the active hormone, triiodothyronine (T_3). The synthesis of T_4 and T_3 requires iodine, which can be a limiting factor in some parts of the world. Much of T_3 is also made by peripheral conversion of T_4 to T_3. T_3 acts primarily through a nuclear receptor that regulates gene expression. T_3 is critical for normal brain and skeletal development, and has broad effects on metabolism and cardiovascular function in the adult.

ANATOMY AND HISTOLOGY OF THE THYROID GLAND

The thyroid gland is composed of right and left lobes that sit anterolaterally to the trachea (Fig. 6.1). Normally, the lobes of the thyroid gland are connected by a midventral isthmus. The functional unit of the thyroid gland is the thyroid follicle, a spherical structure about 200 to 300 μm in diameter ringed by a single layer of thyroid epithelial cells (Fig. 6.2). The epithelium sits on a basal lamina, surrounded by a rich capillary supply. The apical side of the follicular epithelium faces the lumen of the follicle. The lumen is filled with colloid composed of thyroglobulin, which is secreted and iodinated by the thyroid epithelial cells. The size of the epithelial cells and the amount of colloid are dynamic features that change with the activity of the gland. The thyroid gland contains another type of cell in addition to follicular cells. Scattered within the gland are parafollicular cells, or C cells. These cells are the source of the polypeptide hormone calcitonin, whose function is unclear in humans.

CLINICAL BOX 6.1

Although parafollicular C cells and calcitonin may be of minimal importance in normal humans, C cells can give rise to **medullary thyroid carcinoma**. Medullary cancer is an aggressive form of thyroid cancer, and metastasis to lungs, liver, bone, or other organs drastically reduces survival. Although most medullary cancer is sporadic, about one fifth of cases are familial. The familial forms are due to activating mutations of the **RET protooncogene**, a tyrosine kinase receptor that interacts with coreceptors and is activated by glial-derived neurotrophic factor and related proteins. Familial medullary thyroid cancer can occur independently of other endocrine glands or as part of a **multiple endocrine neoplasia (MEN)** syndrome, which in this case also involves adrenal medulla chromaffin cells (pheochromocytoma), parathyroid glands, and/or ganglioneuromas. These cancers remain differentiated enough to secrete **calcitonin**, and assay of calcitonin in the blood is useful in assessing treatment and possible recurrence during follow-up. Medullary thyroid cancer is treated by total thyroidectomy and removal of regional lymph nodes. Effective chemotherapy regimens that target the tyrosine kinase receptor, c-ret, have also been developed.

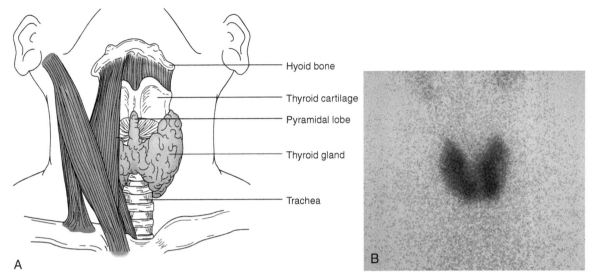

Hyoid bone

Thyroid cartilage

Pyramidal lobe

Thyroid gland

Trachea

A

B

Fig. 6.1 (A) Anatomy of the thyroid gland. (B) Image of pertechnetate uptake by a normal thyroid gland. (Modified from Drake RL, Vogl W, Mitchell AWM: *Gray's Anatomy for Students,* Philadelphia, 2005, Churchill Livingstone.)

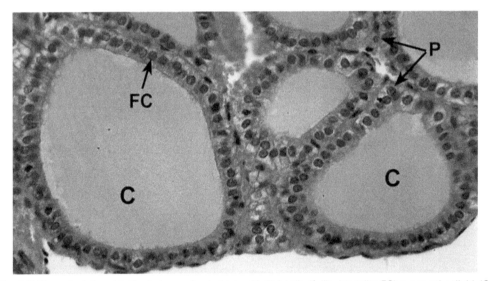

Fig. 6.2 Normal rat thyroid. Single layer of cuboidal epithelial cells (follicular cells; FC) surround colloid *(C)*. Parafollicular cells *(P)* produce calcitonin (see Chapter 4).

PRODUCTION OF THYROID HORMONES

The secretory products of the thyroid gland are **iodothyronines** (Fig. 6.3), a class of hormones resulting from the coupling of two iodinated tyrosine molecules. About 90% of the thyroid output is **3,5,3′,5′-tetraiodothyronine** (thyroxine, or T_4). T_4 is a prohormone. About 10% is **3,5,3′-triiodothyronine** (T_3), which is the active form of thyroid hormone. Less than 1% of thyroid output is

3,3′,5′-triiodothyronine (reverse T_3, or rT_3), which is inactive. Normally, these three products are secreted in the same proportions at which they are stored in the gland.

Because the primary product of the thyroid gland is T_4, yet the active form of thyroid hormone is T_3, the thyroid axis relies heavily on **peripheral conversion** through the action of **thyronine-specific deiodinases** (see Fig. 6.3).

Type 1 deiodinase, which is expressed in the plasma membrane of liver and kidney cells, is a low-affinity enzyme

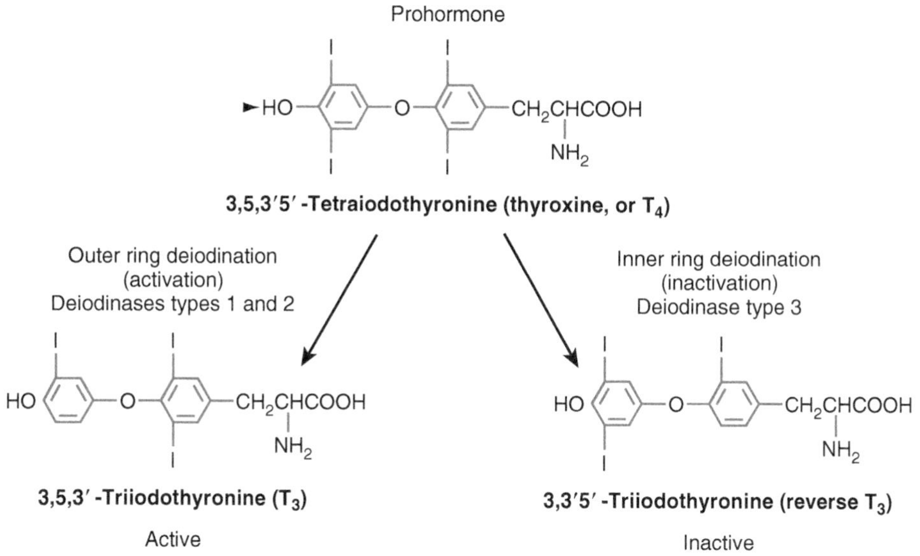

Fig. 6.3 Structure of iodo-thyronines, T_4, T_3, and reverse T_3.

capable of both outer- and inner-ring deiodination of T_4. Current evidence suggests that type 1 deiodinase may function primarily as a scavenger enzyme that removes iodine from sulfated thyroid hormones before they are excreted in bile or urine. However, in hyperthyroidism, type 1 deiodinase is a major contributor to elevated circulating T_3 levels in this disease.

Type 2 deiodinase, on the other hand, is a high-affinity ($Km = 1$ nM) outer-ring deiodinase that converts T_4 to T_3. It is localized intracellularly in the endoplasmic reticulum and expressed in several cell types, including glial cells of the central nervous system (CNS), the pituitary gland, brown fat, placenta, and skeletal muscle (albeit at low levels). Cell types that express the type 2 deiodinase are able to customize the levels of available T_3 in their local environment. For example, the brain can maintain constant intracellular levels of T_3 by upregulating type 2 deiodinase in hypothyroidism, when free T_4 falls to low levels. Importantly, type 2 deiodinase is also present in the thyrotropes of the pituitary, where it acts as a "thyroid axis sensor" by integrating total circulating free T_3 and T_4. T_3 in the thyrotrope, which either enters the cell as T_3 or is converted from T_4 by the type 2 deiodinase, represents the feedback signal that regulates thyroid-stimulating hormone (TSH) secretion (see later). Brown fat is able to increase heat production in response to adrenergic stimulation of local T_3 production by the type 2 deiodinase (discussed later). In addition to local production of T_3, type 2 deiodinase generates most of the circulating pool of T_3 in humans under euthyroid conditions.

Finally, there also exists an "inactivating" deiodinase, called type 3 deiodinase. Type 3 deiodinase is a high-affinity, inner-ring deiodinase that converts T_4 to the inactive rT_3. Type 3 deiodinase is increased during hyperthyroidism, which helps to blunt the overproduction of T_4. All forms of iodothyronines are further deiodinated, eventually to noniodinated thyronine (Table 6.1).

Iodide Balance

Because of the unique role of iodide (iodide, or I^-, is the water-soluble ionized form of diatomic iodine, or I_2) in thyroid physiology, a description of thyroid hormone synthesis requires some understanding of iodide turnover (Fig. 6.4). The average dietary intake of iodide is 400 µg in the United States, compared with a minimum daily requirement of 150 µg for adults, 90 to 120 µg for children, and 200 µg for pregnant women. In the steady state, virtually the same amount, 400 µg, is excreted in the urine. Iodide is actively concentrated in the thyroid gland, salivary glands, gastric glands, lacrimal glands, mammary glands, and choroid plexus. About 70 to 80 µg of iodide is taken up daily by the thyroid gland. The total iodide content of the thyroid gland averages around 7500 µg, virtually all of which is in the form of iodothyronines. In the steady state, 70 to 80 µg of iodide, or about 1% of the total, is released from the gland daily. Of this amount, 75% is secreted as thyroid hormone, and the remainder is secreted as free iodide. The large ratio (100:1) of iodide stored in the form of hormone to the amount turned over daily protects against iodide deficiency for about 2 months. Iodide is also conserved by a marked reduction in the renal excretion of iodide as the concentration in serum falls.

TABLE 6.1   Average Thyroid Hormone Turnover

	T_4	T_3	rT_3
Daily production (μg)	90	35	35
From thyroid (%)	100	25	5
From T_4 (%)	—	75	95
Extracellular pool (μg)	850	40	40
Plasma concentration			
Total (μg/dL)	8.0	0.12	0.04
Free (ng/dL)	2.0	0.28	0.20
Half-life (days)	7	1	0.8
Metabolic clearance (L/day)	1	26	77
Fractional turnover per day (%)	10	75	90

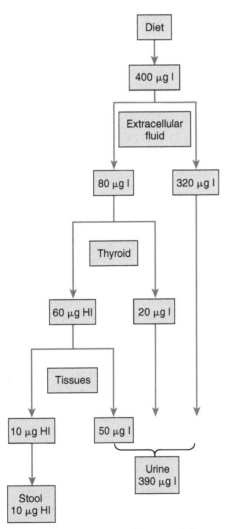

Fig. 6.4 Iodine distribution and turnover in humans.

Overview of Thyroid Hormone Synthesis

To understand thyroid hormone synthesis and secretion, one must appreciate the directionality of each process as it relates to the polarized thyroid epithelial cell (Fig. 6.5). Synthesis of thyroid hormone requires two precursors, thyroglobulin and iodide. Iodide is transported across cells from the basal (vascular) side to the apical (follicular luminal) side of the thyroid epithelium. Amino acids are assembled by translation into thyroglobulin, which is then secreted from the apical membrane into the follicular lumen. Thus synthesis involves a basal-to-apical movement of precursors into the follicular lumen (see Fig. 6.5; *black arrows*). Actual synthesis of iodothyronines occurs enzymatically in the follicular lumen close to the apical membrane of the epithelial cells (see later). Secretion involves fluid phase endocytosis of iodinated thyroglobulin and apical-to-basal movement of the endocytic vesicles and their fusion with lysosomes. Thyroglobulin is then enzymatically degraded, which results in the release of thyroid hormones from the thyroglobulin peptide backbone. Finally, thyroid hormones move across the basolateral membrane, probably through a specific transporter, and ultimately into the blood. Thus secretion involves an apical-to-basal movement (see Fig. 6.5; *orange arrows*). There are also scavenger pathways within the epithelial cell that reuse iodine and amino acids after enzymatic digestion of thyroglobulin (see Fig. 6.5; *open arrows*).

Synthesis of Iodothyronines Within a Thyroglobulin Backbone

Iodide is transported into the gland against chemical and electrical gradients by a Na⁺-I symporter (NIS) located in the basolateral membrane of thyroid epithelial cells. Normally, a thyroid-to-plasma free iodide ratio of 30 is maintained. This so-called iodide trap is highly expressed in the thyroid gland, but NIS is also expressed at lower levels in the placenta, salivary glands, and actively lactating breast. One iodide ion is transported uphill against

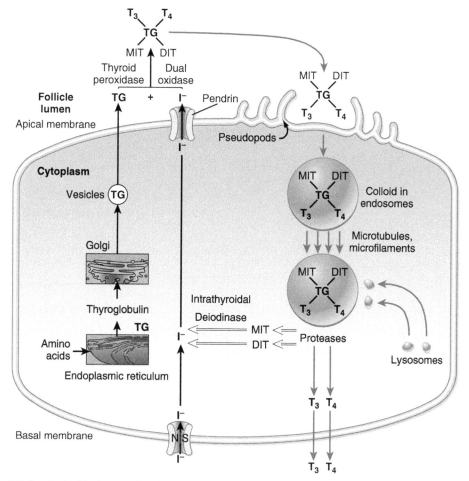

Fig. 6.5 Synthesis *(black arrows)* and secretion *(orange arrows)* of thyroid hormones by the thyroid epithelial cell. *Open arrows* denote pathways involved in the conservation of iodine and amino acids.

an iodide gradient, whereas two sodium ions move down the electrochemical gradient from the extracellular fluid into the thyroid cell. The energy source for this secondary active transporter is provided by a Na^+, K^+-ATPase in the plasma membrane. Expression of the *NIS* gene is inhibited by iodide and stimulated by TSH (see later in the text). Numerous inflammatory cytokines also suppress *NIS* gene expression. A reduction in dietary iodide intake depletes the circulating iodide pool and greatly enhances the activity of the iodide trap. When dietary iodide intake is low, the rates of thyroid uptake of iodide can reach 80% to 90%.

The steps in thyroid hormone synthesis are shown in Fig. 6.6. After entering the gland, iodide rapidly moves to the apical plasma membrane of the epithelial cells. From there, iodide is transported into the lumen of the follicles by a sodium-independent iodide-chloride transporter, named **pendrin**.

> ### CLINICAL BOX 6.2
>
> **Pendred syndrome** refers to a condition caused by an autosomal recessive mutation in the pendrin gene (referred to as *PDS* or *SLC26A4*). Because iodide is not efficiently transported into the follicular lumen, **hypothyroidism** develops in patients. Some patients exhibit enlarged thyroid glands called **goiters**. This form of hypothyroidism can be treated with replacement thyroxine. Unfortunately, pendrin is also expressed in the inner ear and is required for normal structural development of the inner ear. Thus patients with Pendred syndrome experience hearing loss in infancy or early childhood.

Once in the follicular lumen, iodide (I^-) is immediately oxidized and incorporated into tyrosine residues within the primary structure of thyroglobulin. Thyroglobulin is continually synthesized, exocytosed into the follicular lumen

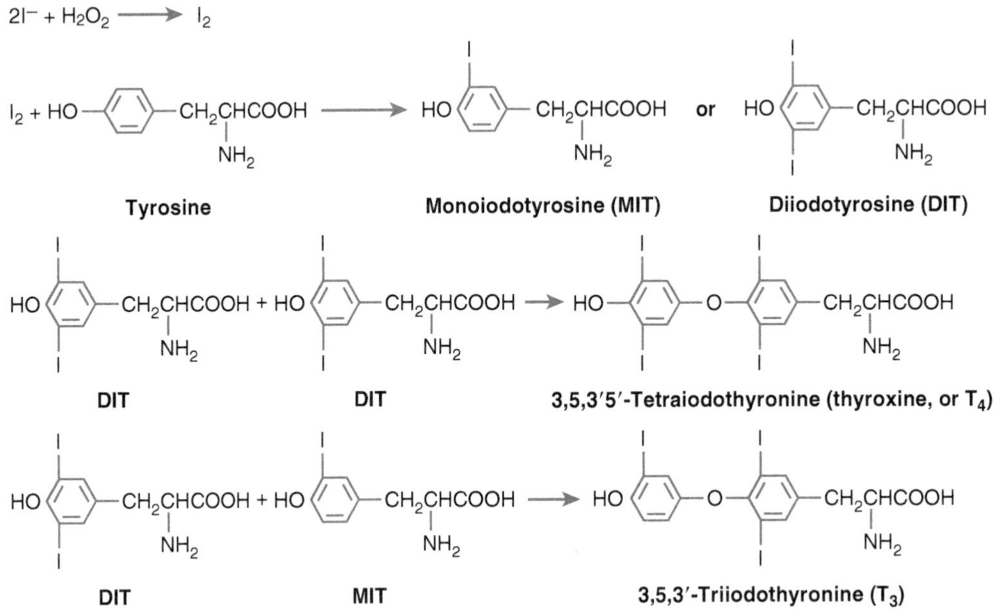

Fig. 6.6 Reactions involved in the generation of iodide, MIT, DIT, T_3, and T_4.

and iodinated to form either monoiodotyrosine (MIT) or diiodotyrosine (DIT) (see Fig. 6.6). After iodination, two DIT molecules are coupled to form T_4, or one MIT and one DIT molecule are coupled to form T_3. The coupling occurs between iodinated tyrosines that remain part of the primary structure of thyroglobulin. This entire sequence of reactions is catalyzed by thyroid peroxidase (TPO), an enzyme complex that spans the apical membrane. The immediate oxidant (electron acceptor) for the reaction is hydrogen peroxide (H_2O_2). H_2O_2 is generated in the thyroid gland by an enzyme called dual oxidase (Duox) that is also localized to the apical membrane.

When iodide availability is restricted, the formation of T_3 is favored. This response provides more active hormone per molecule of organified iodide. The proportion of T_3 is also increased when the gland is hyperstimulated by TSH or other activators.

Secretion of Thyroid Hormones

After thyroglobulin has been iodinated, it is stored in the lumen of the follicle as colloid (see Fig. 6.2). Release of the T_4 and T_3 into the bloodstream requires endocytosis and lysosomal degradation of thyroglobulin (see Fig. 6.5; *orange arrows*). Enzymatically released T_4 and T_3 then leave the basal side of the cell and enter the blood.

The MIT and DIT molecules, which also are released during proteolysis of thyroglobulin, are rapidly deiodinated within the follicular cell by an enzyme called intrathyroidal deiodinase (see Fig. 6.5; *open arrows*). This deiodinase is specific for MIT and DIT and cannot use T_4 and T_3 as substrates. The iodide is then recycled into T_4 and T_3 synthesis. Amino acids from the digestion of thyroglobulin reenter the intrathyroidal amino acid pool and can be reused for protein synthesis. Only minor amounts of intact thyroglobulin leave the follicular cell under normal circumstances.

CLINICAL BOX 6.3

Because of its ability to **trap** and incorporate iodine into thyroglobulin (called **organification**), the activity of the thyroid can be assessed by **radioactive iodine uptake (RAIU)**. For this, a tracer dose of ^{123}I is administered, and the RAIU is measured by placing a gamma detector on the neck after 4 to 6 hours and after 24 hours. In the United States, where the diet is relatively rich in iodine, the RAIU is about 15% after 6 hours and 25% after 24 hours (Fig. 6.7). Abnormally high RAIU (> 60%) after 24 hours indicates hyperthyroidism. Abnormally low RAIU (< 5%) after 24 hours indicates hypothyroidism. In individuals with extreme chronic stimulation of the thyroid (Graves disease–associated thyrotoxicosis), iodide is trapped, organified, and released as hormone very rapidly. In these cases of elevated turnover, the 6-hour RAIU will be very high, but the 24-hour RAIU will be lower (Fig. 6.8). A number of anions, such as thiocyanate

CLINICAL BOX 6.3—cont'd

(SCN^-), perchlorate ($HClO_4^-$), and pertechnetate (TcO^{4-}), are inhibitors of iodide transport through the NIS. If iodide cannot be rapidly incorporated into tyrosine (**organification defect**) after its uptake by the cell, administration of one of these anions will, by blocking further iodide uptake, cause a rapid release of the iodide from the gland (see Fig. 6.8). This release occurs as a result of the high thyroid-to-plasma concentration gradient of iodide.

The thyroid can be imaged using the iodine isotopes ^{123}I or ^{131}I, or the iodine mimic, pertechnetate (^{99m}Tc), followed by imaging with a rectilinear scanner or gamma camera. Imaging can display the size and shape of the thyroid (see Fig. 6.1B), as well as heterogeneities of active versus inactive tissue within the thyroid gland. Such heterogeneities

are often due to the development of **thyroid nodules**, which are regions of enlarged follicles with evidence of regressive changes indicating cycles of stimulation and involution. So-called **hot nodules** (i.e., nodules that display a high RAIU on imaging) are usually not cancerous but may lead to thyrotoxicosis (hyperthyroidism; see later in the text.) **Cold nodules** are 10 times more likely to be cancerous than hot nodules. Such nodules can be sampled to assess for pathology by **fine-needle aspiration biopsy**.

The thyroid can also be imaged by **ultrasonography**, which is superior in resolution to RAIU imaging. Ultrasonography is used to guide the physician during fine-needle aspiration biopsy of a nodule. Highest resolution of the thyroid gland is achieved with **magnetic resonance imaging**.

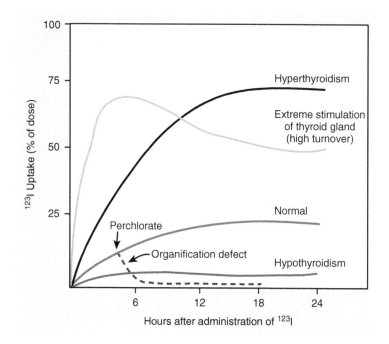

Fig. 6.7 Thyroid gland iodothyronine uptake curves for normal, hypothyroid, hyperthyroid, and organification defective states.

TRANSPORT AND METABOLISM OF THYROID HORMONES

Secreted T_4 and T_3 circulate in the bloodstream almost entirely bound to proteins. Normally, only about 0.04% of total plasma T_4 and 0.4% of total plasma T_3 exist in the free state (see Table 6.1). Free T_3 is biologically active and mediates thyroid hormone effects on peripheral tissues as well as in negative feedback on the pituitary and hypothalamic (see later). The major binding protein is **thyroxine-binding**

globulin (**TBG**). TBG is synthesized in the liver and binds one molecule of T_4 or T_3.

About 70% of circulating T_4 and T_3 is bound to TBG; 10% to 15% is bound to another specific thyroid-binding protein, called **transthyretin (TTR)**. **Albumin** binds 15% to 20%, and 3% is bound to lipoproteins. Ordinarily, only alterations in TBG concentration significantly affect total plasma T_4 and T_3 levels. Two important biologic functions have been ascribed to TBG. First, it maintains a large circulating **reservoir** of T_4 that buffers any acute changes in thyroid gland function.

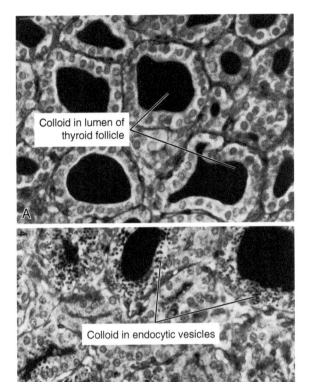

Fig. 6.8 Normal and hyperactive thyroid glands. Note the colloid present in the lumen of thyroid follicles in a normal thyroid gland (*top panel*). In hyperthyroidism, colloid is turning over rapidly, with many follicles depleted of colloid , which can be seen in endocytic vesicles within the follicular cells (*bottom panel*).

Second, the binding of plasma T_4 and T_3 to proteins prevents the loss of these relatively small hormone molecules in the urine and thereby helps conserve iodide. TTR, in particular, provides thyroid hormones to the CNS.

CLINICAL BOX 6.4

There are several transporters that mediate thyroid hormone transport across cell membranes **Thyroid hormone transporters** include sodium taurocholate cotransporting polypeptide (NCTP), organic anion transporting polypeptide (OATP), L-type amino acid transporter (LAT), and the monocarboxylate transporters (MCT). These transporters show specificity with respect to T_4 versus T_3 binding and cell-specific expression. MCT8 is required for neuronal uptake of thyroid hormones. Mutations in MCT8 are linked to severe psychomotor deficits (Allan-Herndon-Dudley syndrome) that cannot be treated with exogenous T_3 or T_4.

Regulation of Thyroid Function

The most important regulator of thyroid gland function and growth is the **hypothalamic-pituitary-thyroid axis** (see Chapter 5). TSH stimulates every aspect of thyroid function. TSH has early, intermediate, and long-term actions on the thyroid epithelium. Immediate actions of TSH involve induction of pseudopod extension, endocytosis of colloid, and formation of colloid droplets in the cytoplasm, which represent thyroglobulin within endocytic vesicles. Shortly thereafter, iodide uptake and TPO activity increase. Concurrently, TSH stimulates glucose entry into the hexose monophosphate shunt pathway, which generates the NADPH that is needed for the peroxidase reaction. TSH also stimulates the proteolysis of thyroglobulin and the release of T_4 and T_3 from the gland. Intermediate effects of TSH on the thyroid gland occur after a delay of hours to days and involve protein synthesis and the expression of numerous genes, including those encoding NIS, thyroglobulin, and TPO. Sustained TSH stimulation leads to the long-term effects of hypertrophy and hyperplasia of the follicular cells. Capillaries proliferate, and thyroid blood flow increases. These actions, which underlie the growth-promoting effects of TSH on the gland, are supported by the local production of growth factors. A noticeably enlarged thyroid gland is called a **goiter**.

CLINICAL BOX 6.5

Goiter can develop in response to multiple imbalances and disease within the hypothalamus-pituitary-thyroid axis, occurring in the context of a hypothyroid, euthyroid (normal), or hyperthyroid status. These imbalances include the following elements:

Primary Hypothyroidism
- Lack of adequate iodine in the diet (nontoxic goiter, endemic goiter)
- Benign nodules or mutation of growth-related gene (nontoxic goiter)
- Sporadic hypothyroidism of unknown etiology (nontoxic goiter)
- Chronic thyroiditis (Hashimoto disease; autoimmune-induced deficiency in thyroid function)

Hyperthyroidism
- Excessive stimulation of the TSH receptor by an autoantibody (Graves disease)
- Excessive secretion of TSH from a TSH-producing tumor (i.e., secondary hyperthyroidism)
- Thyroid hormone–producing (toxic) adenoma (nodular) or toxic multinodular goiter
- An inactivating mutation in thyroid receptor β-2 (TRβ2; see later)

The regulation of thyroid hormone secretion by TSH is under exquisite negative feedback control. Circulating thyroid hormones act on the pituitary gland to decrease TSH secretion, primarily by repressing TSHβ subunit gene expression. The pituitary gland expresses the high-affinity type 2 deiodinase. Thus small changes in free T_4 in the blood result in significant changes in intracellular T_3 in the pituitary thyrotrope. Because the diurnal variation of TSH secretion is small, thyroid hormone secretion and plasma concentrations are relatively constant. Only small nocturnal increases in secretion of TSH and release of T_4 occur. Thyroid hormones also feed back on the hypothalamic TRH-secreting neurons. In these neurons, T_3 inhibits the expression of the prepro-*TRH* gene.

Another important regulator of thyroid gland function is iodide itself, which has a biphasic action. At relatively low levels of iodide intake, the rate of thyroid hormone synthesis is directly related to iodide availability. However, if the intake of iodide exceeds 2 mg/day, the intraglandular concentration of iodide reaches a level that suppresses Duox activity and the *NIS* and *TPO* genes, and thereby the mechanism of hormone biosynthesis. This autoregulatory phenomenon is known as the **Wolff-Chaikoff effect**. As the intrathyroidal iodide level subsequently falls, *NIS* and *TPO* genes are de-repressed, and the production of thyroid hormone returns to normal. In unusual instances, the inhibition of hormone synthesis by iodide can be great enough to induce thyroid hormone deficiency. The temporary reduction in hormone synthesis by excess iodide can also be used therapeutically in hyperthyroidism, especially before thyroid surgery to prevent **thyroid storm** (thyrotoxicosis) during the procedure.

Thyroid hormones increase oxygen use, energy expenditure, and heat production. Therefore it is logical to expect that the availability of active thyroid hormone correlates with changes in the body's caloric and thermal status. In fact, ingestion of excess calories, particularly in the form of carbohydrate, increases the production and plasma concentration of T_3 as well as the individual's metabolic rate. On the other hand, serious illness, injury or starvation leads to inactivation of thyroid hormone by type 3 deiodinase, outer-ring deiodinase activity declines. Moreover, central input depresses the function of the thyroid hormone axis, causing TSH levels to drop below those expected given the reduced level circulating thyroid hormones. This has been termed *nonthyroidal illness syndrome* or *sick euthyroid syndrome*, because this does not reflect thyroid pathology, but represents an adaptation to illness or injury allowing energy to be conserved for fighting infection, to support reparative processes, or to prolong the availability of nutrients.

CLINICAL BOX 6.6

Graves disease represents the most common form of **hyperthyroidism**; it occurs most frequently between the ages of 20 and 50 years and is 10 times more common in women than in men. Graves disease is an autoimmune disorder in which autoantibodies are produced against the TSH receptor. The nature of specific autoantibodies depends on the epitope that they are directed against. The most critical type is called the **thyroid-stimulating immunoglobulin (TSI)**. The hyperthyroidism is often accompanied by a diffuse goiter due to hyperplasia and hypertrophy of the gland. The follicular epithelial cells become tall columnar cells, and the colloid shows a scalloped periphery indicative of rapid turnover.

The primary clinical state found in Graves disease is **thyrotoxicosis**—the state of excessive thyroid hormone in the blood and tissues. The patient with thyrotoxicosis presents one of the most striking pictures in clinical medicine. The large increase in metabolic rate is accompanied by the highly characteristic symptom of weight loss despite an increased intake of food. The increased heat production causes discomfort in warm environments, excessive sweating, and a greater intake of water. The increase in adrenergic activity is manifested by a rapid heart rate, palpitations, hyperkinesis, tremor, anxiety, and irritability. Weakness is caused by a loss of muscle mass as well as by an impairment of muscle function. Other symptoms include a labile emotional state, breathlessness during exercise, and difficulty in swallowing or breathing due to compression of the esophagus or trachea by the enlarged thyroid gland (goiter). The most common cardiovascular sign is sinus tachycardia. There is an increased cardiac output associated with widened pulse pressure due to a positive inotropic effect coupled with a decrease in vascular resistance. Major clinical signs in Graves disease are **exophthalmos** (abnormal protrusion of the eyeball; Fig. 6.9) and **periorbital edema** due to recognition by the anti-TSH receptor antibodies of a similar epitope within the orbital fibroblasts.

Graves disease is diagnosed by an elevated serum free and total T_4 or T_3 level (i.e., thyrotoxicosis) and the clinical signs of diffuse goiter and ophthalmopathy. In most cases, the thyroid uptake of iodine or pertechnetate is excessive and diffuse. Serum TSH levels are low, because the hypothalamus and the pituitary gland are inhibited by the high levels of T_4 and T_3. Assaying TSH levels, and for the presence of circulating TSI, will distinguish Graves disease (a primary endocrine disorder) from a rare adenoma of the pituitary thyrotrophs (a secondary endocrine

Continued

CLINICAL BOX 6.6—cont'd

disease). The latter etiology generates elevated TSH levels unaccompanied by TSI.

Treatment of Graves disease is usually removal of the thyroid tissue, followed by lifelong replacement therapy with T₄. Thyroid tissue can be ablated by either the radiation effects of ^{131}I or by surgery. Surgical removal of the gland rarely but potentially precipitates a massive release of hormone, causing a thyroid storm, which causes potentially life-threatening tachycardia, arrhythmia, and heart failure. An alternative to removal of thyroid tissue is administration of **antithyroid drugs** that inhibit TPO activity.

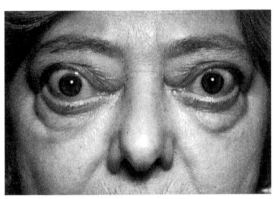

Fig. 6.9 Severe exophthalmos of Graves disease. Note lid retraction, periorbital edema, and proptosis. (From Hall R, Evered DC: *Color Atlas of Endocrinology,* 2nd ed., London, 1990, Mosby-Wolfe.)

Mechanism of Thyroid Hormone Action

Free T₄ and T₃ enter cells by a carrier-mediated, energy-dependent process. The transport of T₄ is rate limiting for the intracellular production of T₃. Within the cell, most, if not all, of the T₄ is converted to T₃ (or rT₃). Many of the T₃ actions are mediated through its binding one of members of the **thyroid hormone receptor (TR) family**. The TR family belongs to the nuclear hormone receptor superfamily of transcription factors. TRs bind to a specific DNA sequence, termed a thyroid-response element (TRE), usually as a heterodimer with retinoid X receptor (RXR). As discussed in Chapter 1, gene activation by T₃ involves (1) the unliganded TR/RXR bound to a TRE and recruiting corepressor proteins that deacetylate DNA in the vicinity of the regulated gene; (2) binding of T₃ and the dissociation of corepressor proteins; and (3) recruitment of coactivator proteins that, in part, acetylate DNA and activate the gene in question (see Fig. 1.24 in Chapter 1). However, T₃ also represses gene expression, indicating that other mechanisms exist, probably in a cell type–specific and gene-specific manner.

In humans, there are two TR genes, *THRA* and *THRB,* located on chromosomes 17 and 3, respectively, that encode the classic nuclear thyroid hormone receptors. THRA encodes TRα, which is alternatively spliced to form two main isoforms. TRα1 is a bona fide TR, whereas the other isoform does not bind T₃. THRB encodes TRβ1 and TRβ2, both of which are high-affinity receptors for T₃. The tissue distribution of TRα1 and TRβ1 is widespread. TRα1 is especially expressed in cardiac and skeletal muscle, and TRα1 is the dominant TR that transduces thyroid hormone actions on the heart. By contrast, TRβ1 is expressed more in the brain, liver, and kidneys. TRβ2 expression is restricted to the pituitary and critical areas of the hypothalamus, as well as the cochlea and retina. T₃-bound TRβ2 is responsible for inhibiting the expression of the prepro-*TRH* gene in the paraventricular neurons of the hypothalamus and of the β-subunit *TSH* gene in pituitary thyrotropes. Thus negative feedback effects of thyroid hormone on both TRH and TSH secretion are largely mediated by TRβ2. T₃ also downregulates *TRβ2* gene expression in the pituitary gland.

CLINICAL BOX 6.7

An understanding of TR subtypes and tissue expression is of more than academic interest because inactivating mutant genes have been found increasingly to be causes of clinical syndromes manifested by **resistance to thyroid hormone (RTH) syndrome**. The most common mutations occur in the pituitary-hypothalamus-specific TRβ2 subtype. In these patients, there is incomplete negative thyroid hormone feedback at the hypothalamic-pituitary level. Thus T₄ levels are elevated, but TSH is not suppressed. When the resistance is purely at the hypothalamic-pituitary level, the patient may exhibit signs of hyperthyroidism due to excess effects of high thyroid hormone levels on peripheral tissue, particularly on the heart through TRα1. These individuals have clinical signs such as goiter, short stature, decreased weight, tachycardia, hearing loss, monochromatic vision, and decreased IQ.

As an additional example, the beneficial effect of thyroid hormones on the serum lipoprotein profile have been attributed to TRβ2 actions in the liver. There has therefore been ongoing interest in TRβ2 as a potential therapeutic target for development of TRβ2-specific ligands as a means to prevent atherosclerosis and cardiovascular disease.

Physiologic Effects of Thyroid Hormone

Thyroid hormone acts on essentially all cells and tissues, and imbalances in thyroid function represent one of the most common endocrine diseases. Thyroid hormone has many direct actions, but it also acts in subtle ways to optimize the actions of several other hormones and neurotransmitters. One way to categorize the most prevalent actions of thyroid hormone is to recall the 4 Bs: brain, bone, BMR and β-adrenergic—referring to CNS development, skeletal development, basal metabolic rate, and sympathomimetic actions on the cardiovascular system.

Cardiovascular Effects

Perhaps the most clinically important actions of thyroid hormone are those on cardiovascular physiology. T_3 increases cardiac output, ensuring sufficient oxygen delivery to the tissues (Fig. 6.10). The resting heart rate and the stroke volume are increased. The speed and force of myocardial contractions are enhanced (positive chronotropic and inotropic effects, respectively), and the diastolic relaxation time is shortened (positive lusitropic effect). Systolic blood pressure is modestly augmented, and diastolic blood pressure is decreased. The resultant widened pulse pressure reflects the combined effects of the increased stroke volume and the reduction in total peripheral vascular resistance that result from blood vessel dilation in skin, muscle, and heart. These effects in turn are partly secondary to the increase in tissue production of heat and metabolites that thyroid hormone induces (see later). In addition, however, thyroid hormone decreases systemic vascular resistance by dilating resistance arterioles in the peripheral circulation. Total blood volume is increased by activating the renin-angiotensin-aldosterone axis and thereby increasing renal tubular sodium reabsorption (see Chapter 7).

The cardiac inotropic effects of T_3 are both direct (Fig. 6.11) and indirect, through enhanced responsiveness to catecholamines (see Chapter 7). Myocardial calcium uptake is increased, which enhances contractile force. Thyroid hormone inhibits expression of the **Na-Ca antiporter,** thereby increasing intramyocellular Ca^{2+} concentrations. T_3 increases the velocity and strength of myocardial contraction. T_3 promotes the expression of the faster and stronger α-isoform and represses the slower, weaker β-isoform of cardiac myosin heavy chain. T_3 also increases the **ryanodine Ca^{2+} channels** in the sarcoplasmic reticulum, promoting Ca^{2+} release from the sarcoplasmic reticulum during systole. The **calcium adenosine triphosphatase (ATPase) of the sarcoplasmic reticulum (SERCA)** is increased by T_3, which facilitates sequestration of calcium during diastole and shortens the relaxation time.

CLINICAL BOX 6.8

Thyroid hormone levels in the normal range are necessary for optimal cardiac performance. **Hypothyroidism** in humans reduces stroke volume, left ventricular ejection fraction, cardiac output, and the efficiency of cardiac function. The latter defect is shown by the fact that the stroke work index [(stroke volume/left ventricular mass) × peak systolic blood pressure] is decreased even more than is myocardial oxidative metabolism. The rise in systemic vascular resistance may contribute to this cardiac debility. On the other hand, **hyperthyroidism** increases cardiac output and reduces peripheral resistance, generating a widened pulse pressure. T_3 increases UCP2 and UCP3 in cardiac muscle, which uncouples ATP production from oxygen use during the β-oxidation of free fatty acids. This can cause high-output cardiac failure. When hyperthyroidism develops in aging individuals, the cardiac effects of thyroid hormone may include rapid atrial arrhythmias, flutter, and fibrillation.

Effects on Basal Metabolic Rate

Thyroid hormones increase the basal metabolic rate (BMR), defined as the basal rate of oxygen consumption and heat production. A deficiency in thyroid hormone availability causes cold intolerance, whereas hyperthyroidism is associated with heat intolerance associated with compensatory increases in heat loss through thyroid hormone–mediated increases in blood flow, sweating, and ventilation. Thyroid hormone–regulated thermogenesis occurs primarily in skeletal muscle, which represents 30% to 40% of body mass, and in brown fat. The best understood mechanism occurs in brown fat, where expression of the type 2 deiodinase is upregulated by adrenergic stimulation, leading to increased generation of T_3. Thyroid hormone, in turn, stimulates expression of uncoupling protein-1 (UCP1), which uncouples the mitochondrial proton gradient from ATP production, with the energy stored in the gradient dissipated as heat. Recent studies have demonstrated that adult humans have more brown fat than previously recognized, but the relative contribution of brown fat to thermogenesis in adult humans remains unclear. In skeletal muscle, multiple mechanisms of thyroid hormone–induced thermogenesis have been proposed, including maintenance of the sodium gradient by the Na/K ATPase, increased calcium pumping by SERCA, and uncoupling of ATP production in mitochondria. Thyroid hormone increases expression of SERCA in skeletal muscle and increases expression of the UCP1 homologue UCP3 in skeletal muscle. However, the precise

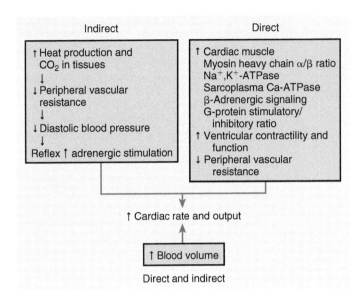

Indirect

Direct

↑ Heat production and
  CO$_2$ in tissues
↓
↓ Peripheral vascular
  resistance
↓
↓ Diastolic blood pressure
↓
Reflex ↑ adrenergic stimulation

↑ Cardiac muscle
  Myosin heavy chain α/β ratio
  Na$^+$,K$^+$-ATPase
  Sarcoplasma Ca-ATPase
  β-Adrenergic signaling
  G-protein stimulatory/
    inhibitory ratio
↑ Ventricular contractility and
  function
↓ Peripheral vascular
  resistance

↑ Cardiac rate and output

↑ Blood volume

Direct and indirect

Fig. 6.10 Mechanisms by which thyroid hormone increases cardiac output. The indirect mechanisms are probably quantitatively more important.

role of UCP3 in skeletal muscle thermogenesis remains to be determined.

Increased oxygen use ultimately depends on an increased supply of substrates for oxidation. T$_3$ augments glucose absorption from the gastrointestinal tract and increases glucose turnover (glucose uptake, oxidation, and synthesis). In adipose tissue, thyroid hormone enhances lipolysis by increasing the number of β-adrenergic receptors (see later in the text). Thyroid hormone also enhances clearance of chylomicrons. Thus lipid turnover (free fatty acid release from adipose tissue and oxidation) is augmented in hyperthyroidism.

Protein turnover (release of muscle amino acids, protein degradation, and to a lesser extent, protein synthesis and urea formation) is also increased by thyroid hormones. T$_3$ potentiates the respective stimulatory effects of epinephrine, norepinephrine, glucagon, cortisol, and growth hormone on gluconeogenesis, lipolysis, ketogenesis, and proteolysis of the labile protein pool. The overall metabolic effect of thyroid hormone has been aptly described as accelerating the response to starvation.

T$_3$ regulates lipoprotein metabolism and cholesterol synthesis and clearance. Hypothyroidism is associated with an increase in TG-rich lipoproteins and low-density lipoprotein and a decrease in high-density lipoproteins.

The metabolic clearance of adrenal and gonadal steroid hormones, some B vitamins, and some administered drugs is also increased by thyroid hormone.

Respiratory Effects

T$_3$ stimulates oxygen use and also enhances oxygen supply. Appropriately, T$_3$ increases the **resting respiratory rate, minute ventilation,** and the **ventilatory responses** to hypercapnia and hypoxia. These actions maintain a normal arterial Po$_2$ when O$_2$ use is increased, and a normal Pco$_2$ when CO$_2$ production is increased. T$_3$ promotes erythropoietin production, hemoglobin synthesis, and absorption of folate and vitamin B$_{12}$ from the gastrointestinal tract. Hypothyroidism in women is also associated with loss of iron due to excessive uterine bleeding (menorrhagia; see later). Thus hypothyroidism may be accompanied by various types of **anemia.**

Skeletal Muscle Function

Normal function of skeletal muscles also requires optimal amounts of thyroid hormone. This requirement may also be related to the regulation of energy production and storage. In hyperthyroidism, glycolysis and glycogenolysis are increased, and glycogen and creatine phosphate are reduced. The inability of muscle to take up and phosphorylate creatine leads to increased urinary excretion of creatine. Muscle pain and weakness can occur in both hypothyroidism and hyperthyroidism.

Effects on the Autonomic Nervous System and Catecholamine Action

There is synergism between catecholamines and thyroid hormones. Thyroid hormones are synergistic with

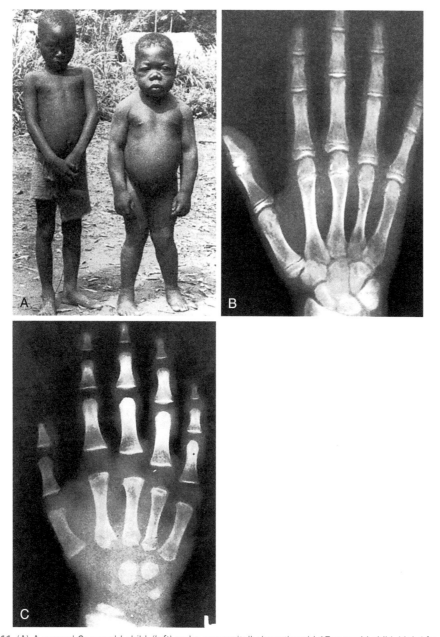

Fig. 6.11 (A) A normal 6-year-old child *(left)* and a congenitally hypothyroid 17-year-old child *(right)* from the same village in an area of endemic hypothyroidism. Note especially the short stature, obesity, malformed legs, and dull expression of the hypothyroid child. Other features are a prominent abdomen, a flat and broad nose, a hypoplastic mandible, dry and scaly skin, delayed puberty, muscle weakness and cognitive disability. Hand radiographs of a 13-year-old normal child (B) and a 13-year-old hypothyroid child (C). Note that the hypothyroid child has a marked delay in development of the small bones of the hands, in ossification centers at either end of the fingers, and in the ossification center of the distal end of the radius. (A, From Delange FM: Endemic cretinism. In Braverman LE, Utiger RD, editors: *Werner and Ingbar's the Thyroid*, 7th ed., Philadelphia, 1996, Lippincott-Raven. B, From Tanner JM, Whitehouse RH, Marshall WA, et al: *Assessment of Skeletal Maturity and Prediction of Adult Height (TW2 method)*, New York, 1975, Academic Press. C, From Andersen HJ: Nongoitrous hypothyroidism. In Gardner LI, editor: *Endocrine and Genetic Diseases of Childhood and Adolescence*, Philadelphia, 1975, Saunders.)

catecholamines in increasing metabolic rate, heat production, heart rate, motor activity, and CNS excitation. T_3 enhances sympathetic nervous system activity by increasing the number of β-adrenergic receptors in heart muscle and by increasing the generation of intracellular second messengers, such as cyclic adenosine monophosphate (cAMP).

Effects on Growth and Maturation

Another major effect of thyroid hormone is to promote growth and maturation. A small but crucial amount of thyroid hormone crosses the placenta, and the fetal thyroid axis becomes functional at midgestation. Thyroid hormone is extremely important for normal neurologic development and for proper bone formation in the fetus. Insufficient fetal thyroid hormone causes congenital hypothyroidism (formerly known as *cretinism*) in the infant, characterized by irreversible mental retardation and short stature.

Effects on Bone, Hard Tissues, and Dermis

Thyroid hormone stimulates endochondral ossification, linear growth of bone, and maturation of the epiphyseal bone centers. T_3 enhances the maturation and activity of chondrocytes in the cartilage growth plate, in part by increasing local growth factor production and action. Although thyroid hormone is not required for linear growth until after birth, it is essential for normal maturation of growth centers in the bones of the developing fetus. T_3 also stimulates adult bone remodeling.

The progression of tooth development and eruption depends on thyroid hormone, as does the normal cycle of growth and maturation of the epidermis, its hair follicles, and nails. The normal degradative processes in these structural and integumentary tissues are also stimulated by thyroid hormone. Thus either too much or too little thyroid hormone can lead to hair loss and abnormal nail formation.

Thyroid hormone alters the structure of subcutaneous tissue by inhibiting the synthesis, and increasing the degradation, of mucopolysaccharides (glycosaminoglycans) and fibronectin in the extracellular connective tissue. In hypothyroidism, the skin is thickened, cool, and dry, and the face becomes puffy because of the accumulation of subcutaneous glycosaminoglycans and other matrix molecules (myxedema).

Effects on the Nervous System

Thyroid hormone regulates the timing and pace of CNS development. Thyroid hormone deficiency in utero and in early infancy decreases growth of the cerebral and cerebellar cortex, proliferation of axons, branching of dendrites, synaptogenesis, myelinization, and cell migration. Irreversible brain damage results when thyroid hormone deficiency is not recognized and treated promptly after birth. The structural defects described earlier are paralleled by biochemical abnormalities. Decreased thyroid hormone levels reduce: cell size; RNA and protein content; tubulin- and microtubule-associated protein; protein and lipid content of myelin; local production of critical growth factors; and the rates of protein synthesis.

Thyroid hormone also enhances wakefulness, alertness, responsiveness to various stimuli, auditory sense, awareness of hunger, memory, and learning capacity. Normal emotional tone also depends on proper thyroid hormone availability. Furthermore, the speed and amplitude of peripheral nerve reflexes are increased by thyroid hormone, as is the motility of the gastrointestinal tract.

CLINICAL BOX 6.9

Hypothyroidism in the fetus or early childhood leads to congenital hypothyroidism. Affected individuals present with severe intellectual disability, short stature with incomplete skeletal development (see Fig. 6.11), coarse facial features, and a protruding tongue. The most common cause of hypothyroidism in children is iodide deficiency. Iodide is not plentiful in the environment, and deficiency of iodide is a major cause of hypothyroidism in certain mountainous regions of South America, Africa, and Asia as well as in some developed countries. This tragic form of **hypothyroidism** can be easily prevented by public health programs that add iodide to table salt or that provide yearly injections of a slowly absorbed iodide preparation. **Congenital defects** are a less common cause of neonatal and childhood hypothyroidism. In most cases, the thyroid gland simply does not develop (**thyroid gland dysgenesis**). Less frequent causes of childhood hypothyroidism are mutations in genes involved in thyroid hormone production (e.g., genes for NIS, TPO, thyroglobulin, and pendrin) and blocking antibodies to the TSH receptor (see later). The severity of neurologic and skeletal defects is closely linked to the time of diagnosis and replacement treatment with thyroid hormone (T_4), with early treatment resulting in normal cognitive ability and subtle neurologic deficits. Hypothyroid babies usually appear normal at birth because of maternal thyroid hormones.

CLINICAL BOX 6.9—cont'd

However, in geographic areas of endemic iodide deficiency, the mother may be hypothyroid and unable to make up for the fetal defects. **Neonatal screening** (T_4 or TSH levels) has played a major role in the detection and prevention of severe congenital hypothyroidism. If hypothyroidism at birth remains untreated for only 2 to 4 weeks, the central nervous system will not develop normally in the first year of life. Developmental milestones, such as sitting, standing, and walking, will be late, and severe irreversible cognitive disabilities can result.

Effects on Reproductive Organs and Endocrine Glands

In both women and men, thyroid hormone plays an important, permissive role in the regulation of reproductive function. The normal ovarian cycle of follicular development, maturation, and ovulation; the homologous testicular process of spermatogenesis; and the maintenance of the healthy pregnant state are all disrupted by significant deviations of thyroid hormone levels from the normal range. In part, these deleterious effects may be caused by alterations in the metabolism or availability of steroid hormones. For example, thyroid hormone stimulates hepatic synthesis and release of sex steroid–binding globulin.

Thyroid hormone also has significant effects on other parts of the endocrine system. Pituitary production of growth hormone is increased by thyroid hormone, whereas that of prolactin is decreased. Adrenocortical secretion of cortisol (see Chapter 7), as well as the metabolic clearance of this hormone, is stimulated, but plasma free cortisol levels remain normal. The ratio of estrogens to androgens (see Chapter 9) is increased in men (in whom breast enlargement may occur with hyperthyroidism). Decreases in both parathyroid hormone and in 1,25-dihydroxyvitamin D production are compensatory consequences of the effects of thyroid hormone on bone resorption (see Chapter 4).

Kidney size, renal plasma flow, glomerular filtration rate, and transport rates for a number of substances are also increased by thyroid hormone.

CLINICAL BOX 6.10

Hypothyroidism in adults who do not have iodide deficiency most often results from idiopathic atrophy of the gland, which is thought to be preceded by a chronic autoimmune inflammatory reaction. In this form of **lymphocytic (Hashimoto) thyroiditis**, the antibodies that are produced may block hormone synthesis or thyroid gland growth, or they may have cytotoxic effects. Other causes of hypothyroidism include iatrogenic causes (e.g., radiochemical damage or surgical removal for treatment of hyperthyroidism), nodular goiters, and pituitary or hypothalamic disease.

The clinical picture of hypothyroidism in adults is in many respects the exact opposite of that seen in hyperthyroidism. The lower-than-normal metabolic rate leads to weight gain without an appreciable increase in caloric intake. The decreased thermogenesis lowers body temperature and causes intolerance to cold, decreased sweating, and dry skin. Adrenergic activity is decreased, and therefore bradycardia may occur. Movement, speech, and thought are all slowed, and lethargy, sleepiness, and a lowering of the upper eyelids (ptosis) occur. An accumulation of mucopolysaccharides—extracellular matrix—in the tissues also causes an accumulation of fluid. This nonpitting **myxedema** produces puffy features (Fig. 6.12): an enlarged tongue; hoarseness; joint stiffness; effusions in the pleural, pericardial, and peritoneal spaces; and pressure on peripheral and cranial nerves, entrapped by excess ground substance. Constipation, loss of hair, menstrual dysfunction, and anemia are other symptoms. In adults lacking thyroid hormone, positron emission tomography demonstrates a generalized reduction in cerebral blood flow and glucose metabolism. This abnormality may explain the psychomotor impairment and depressed affect exhibited by hypothyroid individuals.

Replacement therapy with T_4 is the standard of care in adults who require thyroid replacement therapy. Generally, T_3 is not needed because it will be generated by deiodinases from the administered T_4. Furthermore, due to the short half-life of T_3, more frequent dosing is required, making it is challenging to maintain constant physiologic levels of active hormone. Nevertheless, studies are ongoing to determine whether there may be a subset of patients who would benefit from replacement with a combination of T_3 and T_4.

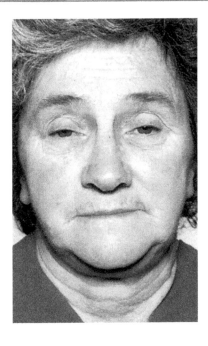

Fig. 6.12 Adult hypothyroidism. Note puffy face, puffy eyes, frowzy hair, and dull, apathetic appearance. (From Hall R, Evered DC: *Color Atlas of Endocrinology*, 2nd ed., London, 1990, Mosby-Wolfe.)

SUMMARY

1. The thyroid gland is situated in the ventral neck, composed of right and left lobes anterolateral to the trachea and connected by an isthmus.

2. The thyroid gland is the source of tetraiodothyronine (thyroxine, T_4) and triiodothyronine (T_3).

3. The basic endocrine unit in the gland is a follicle that consists of a single spherical layer of epithelial cells surrounding a central lumen that contains colloid or stored hormone.

4. Iodide is taken up into thyroid cells by a sodium iodide symporter in the basolateral plasma membrane.

5. T_4 and T_3 are synthesized from tyrosine and iodide by the enzyme complex, thyroid peroxidase. Tyrosine is incorporated in peptide linkages within the protein thyroglobulin. After iodination, two iodotyrosine molecules are coupled to yield the iodothyronines.

6. Secretion of stored T_4 and T_3 requires retrieval of thyroglobulin from the follicle lumen by endocytosis. To support hormone synthesis, iodide is conserved by recycling the iodotyrosine molecules that escape coupling within thyroglobulin.

7. More than 99.5% of the T_4 and T_3 circulates bound to the following proteins: thyroid-binding globulin (TBG), transthyretin, and albumin. Only the free fractions of T_4 and T_3 are biologically active.

8. T_4 functions as a prohormone whose disposition is regulated by three types of deiodinases. Monodeiodination of the outer ring yields 75% of the daily production of T_3, which is the principal active hormone. Alternatively, monodeiodination of the inner ring yields reverse T_3, which is biologically inactive. Proportioning of T_4 between T_3 and reverse T_3 regulates the availability of active thyroid hormone.

9. Thyroid-stimulating hormone (TSH; thyrotropin) acts on the thyroid gland through its plasma membrane receptor and cAMP to stimulate all steps in the production of T_4 and T_3. These steps include iodide uptake, iodination and coupling, and retrieval from thyroglobulin. TSH also stimulates glucose oxidation, protein synthesis, and growth of thyroid epithelial cells.

10. TSH is increased by hypothalamic TRH. T_3 negatively feeds back on TSH and, to a lesser extent, TRH.

11. T_3 binds to thyroid hormone receptor (TR) subtypes that exist linked to thyroid regulatory elements (TREs) in target DNA molecules. As a result, induction or repression of gene expression increases or decreases a large number of enzymes, as well as structural and functional proteins.

12. Thyroid hormone increases and is a major regulator of the basal metabolic rate. Additional important

actions of thyroid hormone are to increase heart rate, cardiac output, and ventilation, and to decrease peripheral resistance. The corresponding increase in heat production leads to increased sweating. Substrate mobilization and disposal of metabolic products are enhanced. As part of normal cardiopulmonary function, T_3 is required for erythrocyte production and function.

13. T_3 is absolutely required for normal development and function of the CNS. In the absence of the hormone, as in congenital hypothyroidism, brain development and cognitive ability may be severely impaired. In the adult, T_3 optimizes normal brain function. Hypothyroidism and hyperthyroidism can cause erratic behavior and depression.

14. T_3 also regulates skeletal development and is crucial to normal growth. In hypothyroidism, growth is retarded and the bones fail to mature. In adults, T_3 increases the rates of bone resorption and degradation of skin and hair. T_3 is required for normal muscle function and normal integrity of the skin, nails, and hair.

15. T_3 regulates several organs within the endocrine system. T_3 is required for normal reproductive function, including fertility, normal menstrual cycling and blood loss, ovulation, spermatogenesis, and erectile function.

SELF-STUDY PROBLEMS

1. Explain how the thyroid status of a patient presenting with a goiter can be hyperthyroid, hypothyroid, or euthyroid.
2. Explain how a thyroid hormone receptor mutation can result in a deficiency in cardiac function without any change in TSH.
3. Draw predicted radioactive iodine uptake (RAIU) curves that would be associated with inactivating mutations of the following genes compared with normal:
   a. TSH-R
   b. Thyroid peroxidase
   c. NIS
4. Why do serum T_4 levels approximately double in pregnancy? Are pregnant women hyperthyroid?
5. Describe the peripheral transport and metabolism of T_4 and its importance in maintaining a euthyroid state.
6. Explain how a patient's thyroid status may be altered when battling a severe illness.
7. How does T_3 affect cardiac function?
8. Why is it critically important to screen thyroid function in newborn infants?

KEYWORDS AND CONCEPTS

Basal metabolic rate (BMR)
Colloid
Congenital hypothyroidism
Diiodotyrosine (DIT)
Euthyroid
Exophthalmos
Extrathyroidal pools
Follicular cells
Glycosaminoglycan (GAG)
Goiter
Graves disease
Hashimoto thyroiditis
Hyperthyroid
Hypothyroid
Iodide
Iodide trap
Iodothyronine
Iodotyrosine
Monoiodotyrosine (MIT)
Myxedema
Organification
Radioactive iodide uptake (RAIU)
Reverse T_3 (rT_3)
Subacute thyroiditis
Thyroglobulin (TG)
Thyroid peroxidase (TPO)
Thyroid-responsive element
Thyrotropin, thyroid-stimulating hormone (TSH)
Thyrotropin-releasing hormone (TRH)
Thyroxine (T_4)
Thyroxine-binding globulin (TBG)
Transthyretin (TTR)
Triiodothyronine (T_3)
Wolff-Chaikoff effect

The Adrenal Gland

OBJECTIVES

1. Discuss the anatomy of the adrenal gland, including the vascular supply and cortical zonation.
2. Diagram the synthesis and regulated release of catecholamines in the chromaffin cell.
3. Explain the action of catecholamines on different adrenergic receptors and the integrated effects of catecholamines during exercise.
4. Outline the differences between the steroidogenic pathways in each zone of the adrenal cortex.

5. Describe the physiologic actions of cortisol, aldosterone, dehydroepiandrosterone sulfate (DHEAS), and other adrenal androgens.
6. Describe the regulation of the zona fasciculata and zona reticularis by the pituitary.
7. Describe the regulation of the zona glomerulosa by the renin–angiotensin II system.
8. Describe the pathophysiology of adrenal hormone excess and underproduction.

In the adult, the adrenal glands emerge as fairly complex endocrine structures (Box 7.1) that produce two structurally distinct classes of hormones: steroids and catecholamines. The catecholamine hormone, epinephrine, acts as a rapid responder to stresses such as hypoglycemia and exercise to regulate multiple parameters of physiology, including energy metabolism and cardiac output. Stress is also a major secretogogue of the longer-acting steroid hormone, cortisol, which regulates glucose use, immune and inflammatory homeostasis, cardiovascular tone, and numerous other processes. The adrenal glands also regulate salt and volume homeostasis through the steroid hormone, aldosterone. The adrenal gland secretes a large amount of the androgen precursor, dehydroepiandrosterone sulfate

(DHEAS), which plays a major role in fetoplacental estrogen synthesis and as a substrate for peripheral androgen synthesis in women.

ANATOMY

The adrenal glands are bilateral structures located immediately superior to the kidneys (ad, toward; renal, kidney) (Fig. 7.1A). In humans, they are also referred to as the suprarenal glands because they sit on the superior pole of each kidney. The adrenal glands are similar to the pituitary, in that they are derived from both neuronal tissue and epithelial (or epithelial-like) tissue. The outer portion of the adrenal gland, called the adrenal cortex, develops from mesodermal cells in the vicinity of the superior pole of the developing kidney. These cells form cords of epithelioid endocrine cells. The cells of the cortex develop into steroidogenic cells and produce mineralocorticoids, glucocorticoids, and adrenal androgens (Fig. 7.2; see Fig. 7.1C).

Soon after the cortex forms, neural crest–derived cells that are associated with the sympathetic ganglia—called chromaffin cells because they stain with chromium stains—migrate into the cortical cells and become encapsulated by them. Thus the chromaffin cells establish the inner portion of the adrenal gland, which is called the adrenal medulla (see Fig. 7.1C). The chromaffin cells of the adrenal medulla have the potential of developing into

BOX 7.1   Overview

The adrenal gland is a hybrid gland consisting of a cortex and a medulla. The hormones of the adrenal gland are important regulators of metabolism and serve an important role in adaptation to stress. The hormone aldosterone is critical to normal salt balance and, hence, water balance. Because of the antiinflammatory and immunosuppressive actions of adrenal corticosteroids, synthetic analogs are widely used in the treatment of disorders ranging from skin rashes to arthritis.

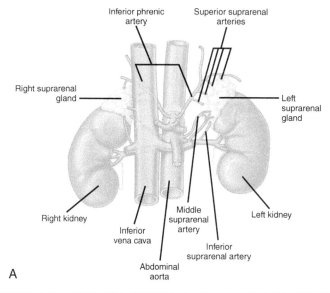

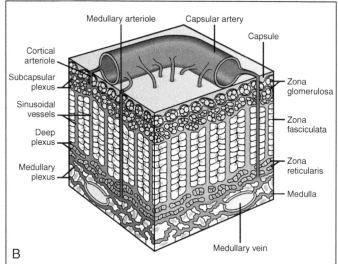

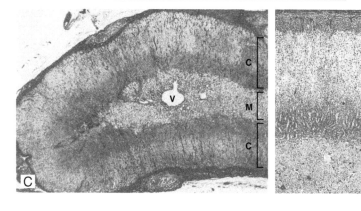

Fig. 7.1 (A) Anatomy of human adrenal glands. Adrenals sit on superior poles of kidneys and thus are also referred to as suprarenal glands. Adrenal glands receive a rich arterial supply from the inferior, middle, and superior suprarenal arteries. In contrast, adrenals are drained by a single suprarenal vein. (B) Blood flow through the adrenal gland. Capsular arteries give rise to sinusoidal vessels that carry blood centripetally through the cortex to the medulla. (C) *Left*, Low magnification of adrenal histology. *Right*, histologic zonation of adrenal gland. *C*, Cortex, *G*, zona glomerulosa, *F*, zona fasciculata, *M*, medulla, *R*, zona reticularis, *V*, central vein. (A, From Drake RL, Vogl W, Mitchell AWM: *Gray's Anatomy for Students*, Philadelphia, 2005, Churchill Livingstone. B, From Stevens A, Lowe J: *Human Histology*, 3rd ed., Philadelphia, 2005, Mosby. C, From Young B, Lowe JS, Stevens A, et al: *Wheater's Functional Histology*, Philadelphia, 2006, Churchill Livingstone.)

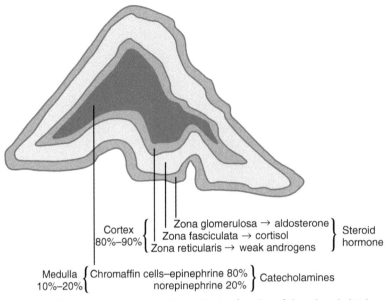

Cortex 80%–90% {
Zona glomerulosa → aldosterone
Zona fasciculata → cortisol
Zona reticularis → weak androgens
} Steroid hormone

Medulla 10%–20% { Chromaffin cells–epinephrine 80%
norepinephrine 20% } Catecholamines

Fig. 7.2 Zonation and corresponding endocrine function of the adrenal gland.

postganglionic sympathetic neurons. They are innervated by cholinergic preganglionic sympathetic neurons and can synthesize the catecholamine neurotransmitter, norepinephrine, from tyrosine. However, the cells of the adrenal medulla are exposed to high local concentrations of cortisol from the cortex. Cortisol inhibits neuronal differentiation of the medullary cells so that they fail to form dendrites and axons. Additionally, cortisol induces the expression of an additional enzyme, phenylethanolamine-N-methyl transferase (PNMT), in the catecholamine biosynthetic pathway. This enzyme adds a methyl group to norepinephrine, producing the catecholamine hormone, epinephrine, which is the primary hormonal product of the adrenal medulla (see Fig. 7.2).

The high local concentration of cortisol in the medulla is maintained by the vascular configuration within the adrenal gland. The outer connective tissue capsule of the adrenal gland is penetrated by a rich arterial supply coming from three main arterial branches (i.e., the inferior, middle, and superior suprarenal arteries; see Fig. 7.1A). These give rise to the following two types of blood vessels that carry blood from the cortex to the medulla (see Fig. 7.1B):

1. Relatively few medullary arterioles that provide high oxygen and nutrient blood directly to the medullary chromaffin cells
2. Relatively numerous cortical sinusoids, into which cortical cells secrete steroid hormones (including cortisol)

Both vessel types fuse to give rise to the medullary plexus of vessels that ultimately drain into a single suprarenal vein.

Thus secretions of the adrenal cortex percolate through the chromaffin cells, bathing them in high concentrations of cortisol before leaving the gland.

ADRENAL MEDULLA

Together, the two adrenal medullae weigh about 1 g. As described, the adrenal medulla is similar to a sympathetic ganglion without postganglionic processes. Instead of being secreted near a target organ and acting as neurotransmitters, adrenomedullary catecholamines are secreted into the blood and act as hormones. About 80% of the cells of the adrenal medulla secrete epinephrine, and the remaining 20% secrete norepinephrine. Although circulating epinephrine is derived entirely from the adrenal medulla, only about 30% of the circulating norepinephrine comes from the medulla. The remaining 70% is released from postganglionic sympathetic nerve terminals and diffuses into the vascular system. Because the adrenal medulla is not the sole source of catecholamine production, this tissue is not essential for life.

Synthesis of Epinephrine

The enzymatic steps in the synthesis of epinephrine are shown in Fig. 7.3. Synthesis begins with the sodium-linked transport of the amino acid, tyrosine, into the chromaffin cell cytoplasm and the subsequent hydroxylation of tyrosine by the rate-limiting enzyme, tyrosine hydroxylase, to produce dihydroxyphenylalanine (DOPA). DOPA is

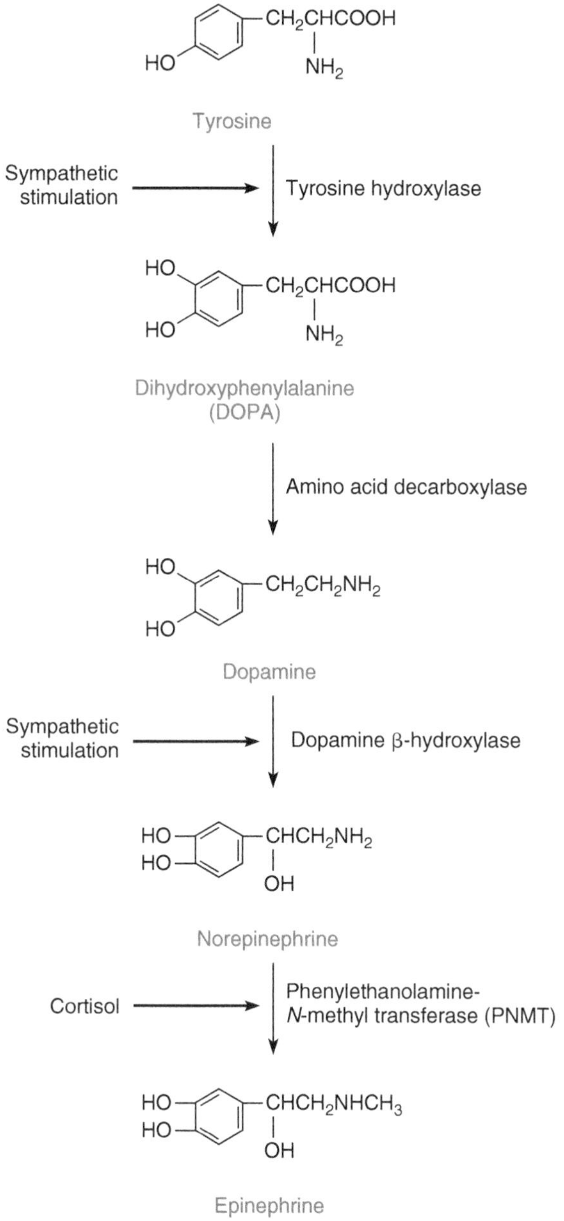

Fig. 7.3 Enzymatic steps and sites of regulation in the synthesis of catecholamines.

converted to dopamine by the cytoplasmic enzyme, aromatic amino acid decarboxylase, and is then transported into the secretory vesicle (also called the **chromaffin granule**). Within the granule, dopamine is converted to **norepinephrine** by the enzyme, dopamine β-hydroxylase. This is an efficient reaction, so essentially all of chromaffin granule dopamine is converted to norepinephrine. In most

adrenomedullary cells, essentially all of the norepinephrine diffuses out of the chromaffin granule by facilitated transport and is methylated by the cytoplasmic enzyme, **PNMT**, to form **epinephrine.** Epinephrine is then transported back into the granule by vesicular monoamine transporters (VMATs).

Multiple molecules of epinephrine, and to a lesser extent norepinephrine, are stored in the chromaffin granule complexed with adenosine triphosphate (ATP), Ca^{2+}, and proteins called **chromogranins**. These multimolecular complexes are thought to decrease the osmotic burden of storing individual molecules of epinephrine within chromaffin granules. Chromogranins play a role in the biogenesis of secretory vesicles and the organization of components within the vesicles. Circulating chromogranins can be used as a marker of sympathetic paraganglion-derived tumors (paragangliomas). Chromaffin cells also synthesize several secretory peptides, including adrenomedullin and enkephalins, which can have local, subtle effects on sympathetic input and adrenomedullary response.

Secretion of epinephrine and norepinephrine from the adrenal medulla is regulated primarily by descending sympathetic signals in response to various forms of stress, including emotional stress (fear, anger), exercise, hypoglycemia, and surgery. The primary autonomic centers that initiate sympathetic responses reside in the hypothalamus and brainstem, and they receive inputs from the cerebral cortex, the limbic system, and other regions of the hypothalamus and brainstem.

The chemical signal for catecholamine secretion from the adrenal medulla is **acetylcholine (ACh)**, which is secreted from preganglionic sympathetic neurons and binds to **nicotinic receptors** on chromaffin cells. Nicotinic receptors lead to depolarization of the chromaffin cell membrane followed by opening of voltage sensitive Ca^{2+} channels. ACh signaling increases the activity of the rate-limiting enzyme, tyrosine hydroxylase, in chromaffin cells (see Fig. 7.3). ACh also increases the activity of dopamine β-hydroxylase and stimulates exocytosis of the chromaffin granules. Synthesis of epinephrine and norepinephrine is closely coupled to secretion so that the levels of intracellular catecholamines do not change significantly, even in the face of changing sympathetic activity. As discussed earlier, cortisol regulates epinephrine production by maintaining adequate expression of the *PNMT* gene in chromaffin cells (see Fig. 7.3).

Mechanism of Action of Catecholamines

Catecholamines act through membrane GPCRs (see Chapter 1). The individual types of adrenergic receptors were first classified based on their pharmacology, and this

TABLE 7.1	Catecholamine Receptors	
Receptor Type	**Primary Mechanism of Action**	**Examples of Tissue Distribution**
α_1	$\uparrow IP_3$, DAG	Vascular smooth muscle
α_2	$\downarrow cAMP$	Pancreatic β cells
β_1	$\uparrow cAMP$	Heart
β_2	$\uparrow cAMP$	Liver
β_3	$\uparrow cAMP$	Adipose

cAMP, Cyclic adenosine monophosphate; *DAG*, diacylglycerol; *IP₃*, inositol triphosphate.

classification scheme has been supported by genetics and molecular cloning. Adrenergic receptors are generally classified as α- and β-adrenergic receptors, and these are further divided into α_1 and α_2 receptors and β_1, β_2, and β_3 receptors (Table 7.1). These receptors can be characterized according to the following elements:

1. The relative potency of endogenous and pharmacologic agonists and antagonists. For example, the synthetic isoproterenol is more potent than either epinephrine or norepinephrine on cardiac β_1 adrenergic receptors. A large number of synthetic selective and nonselective adrenergic agonists and antagonists now exist.
2. Downstream signaling pathways. Table 7.1 shows the primary pathways that are coupled to the different adrenergic receptors. This is an oversimplification because differences in signaling pathways for a given receptor have been linked to duration of agonist exposure and cell type.
3. Location and relative density of receptors. Importantly, different receptor types predominate in different tissues. For example, although both α_2 and β_2 receptors are expressed by islet β cells, the predominant response to a sympathetic discharge is mediated by α_2 receptors.

Physiologic Actions of Adrenomedullary Catecholamines

Because the adrenal medulla is directly innervated by the autonomic nervous system, adrenomedullary responses are very rapid. Because of the involvement of several centers in the central nervous system (CNS), most notably the cerebral cortex, adrenomedullary responses can precede onset of the actual stress (i.e., they can be anticipated). In many cases, the adrenomedullary output, which is primarily epinephrine, is coordinated with sympathetic nervous activity as determined by the release of norepinephrine from postganglionic sympathetic neurons. However, some stimuli (e.g., hypoglycemia) evoke a stronger adrenomedullary response than a sympathetic nervous response, and vice versa.

Many organs and tissues are affected by a sympathoadrenal response. An informative example of the major physiologic roles of catecholamines is the sympathoadrenal response to exercise. Exercise is similar to the fight-or-flight response, but without the subjective element of fear. Exercise increases circulating levels of both norepinephrine and epinephrine. The overall goal of the sympathoadrenal system during exercise is to meet the increased energy demands of skeletal and cardiac muscle while maintaining sufficient oxygen and glucose supply to the brain. The response to exercise includes three of the following major physiologic actions of norepinephrine and epinephrine (Fig. 7.4):

1. Increased blood flow to the muscles is achieved by the integrated actions of norepinephrine and epinephrine on the heart, veins, and lymphatics, and the nonmuscular (e.g., splanchnic) and muscular arteriolar beds. Norepinephrine and epinephrine act on β_1 receptors at the heart to increase the rate (chronotropy) and strength (inotropy) of contractions and facilitate ventricular relaxation during diastole (lusitropy). Catecholamines also induce vasoconstriction through α-adrenergic receptors of high-capacity vessels (veins and lymphatics), thereby increasing venous return to the heart. All these effects increase **cardiac output**. Catecholamines shunt blood away from the gastrointestinal (GI) tract through vasoconstriction of splanchnic arterioles (α receptors) and increase blood flow to skeletal muscle by inducing vasodilation of muscle arteriolar beds through β_2 receptors.
2. Epinephrine promotes **glycogenolysis** in muscle through β_2 receptors. Exercising muscle can also use free fatty acids (FFAs), and epinephrine and norepinephrine act through β_2 and β_3 receptors, respectively, to promote **lipolysis** in adipose tissue. The actions just described increase circulating levels of lactate and glycerol, which can be used by the liver as gluconeogenic substrates to increase glucose. Epinephrine does, in fact, increase blood glucose by increasing hepatic glycogenolysis and gluconeogenesis through β_2 receptors. The promotion of

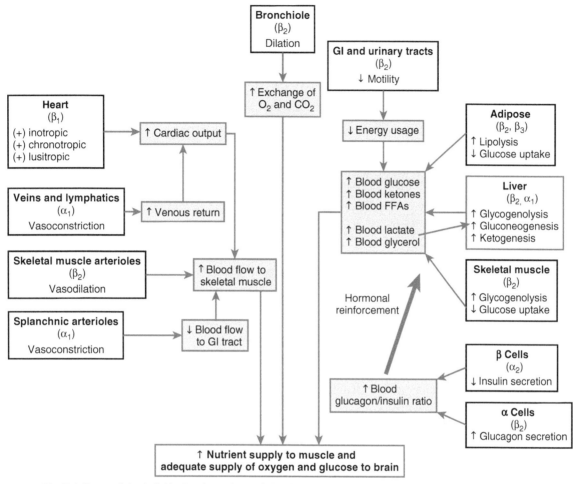

Fig. 7.4 Some of the individual actions of catecholamines that contribute to the integrated sympathoadrenal response to exercise.

lipolysis in adipose tissue is also coordinated with an epinephrine-induced increase in hepatic **ketogenesis**. Finally, the effects of catecholamines on metabolism are reinforced by the fact that they stimulate glucagon secretion (β_2 receptors) and inhibit insulin secretion (α_2 receptors). Efficient production of ATP during normal exercise (i.e., a 1-hr workout) also requires efficient exchange of gases with an adequate supply of oxygen to exercising muscle. Epinephrine promotes this by relaxation of bronchiolar smooth muscle through β_2 receptors.

3. Catecholamines decrease energy demand by visceral smooth muscle. In general, a sympathoadrenal response decreases overall motility of the smooth muscle in the GI tract and urinary tract, thereby conserving energy where it is not needed.

Metabolism of Catecholamines

In general, the duration of circulating epinephrine actions is longer than those of norepinephrine released from an autonomic neuron. There are two primary enzymes involved in the degradation of catecholamines: monoamine oxidase (MAO) and catechol-O-methyltransferase (COMT). Although MAO is the predominant enzyme in neuronal mitochondria, both enzymes are found in many nonneuronal tissues, including liver and kidney. The neurotransmitter norepinephrine is degraded by MAO and COMT after uptake of the compound into the presynaptic terminal. This mechanism is also involved in the catabolism of circulating adrenal catecholamines. However, the predominant fate of adrenal catecholamines is methylation by COMT in nonneuronal tissues such as the liver and kidney. The metabolism of catecholamines is shown in

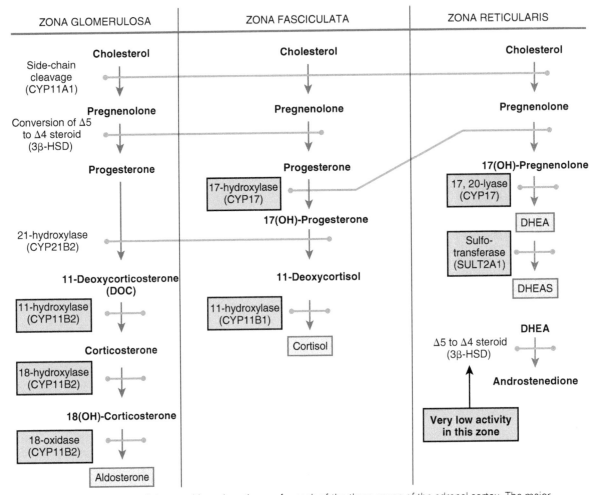

Fig. 7.5 Summary of the steroidogenic pathways for each of the three zones of the adrenal cortex. The major products of each zone are shown in *orange boxes*. Zone-specific enzymes are in *gray boxes*.

Fig. 7.5. Urinary vanillylmandelic acid (VMA) and metanephrine are sometimes used clinically to assess the level of catecholamine production in a patient. Much of the urinary VMA and metanephrine is derived from neuronal, rather than adrenal, catecholamines.

hyperadrenal medullary function and are often used as an example to demonstrate the functions of the adrenal medulla (Box 7.2). For unknown reasons, the symptoms of excessive catecholamine secretion are often sporadic rather than continuous. The symptoms include hypertension, headaches (from hypertension), sweating, anxiety, palpitations, and chest pain. In addition, patients with this disorder may experience orthostatic hypotension (despite the tendency for hypertension). This occurs because hypersecretion of catecholamines can decrease the postsynaptic response to norepinephrine as a result of downregulation of the receptors. Consequently, the baroreceptor response to the blood shifts that occur on standing is blunted.

CLINICAL BOX 7.1

A **pheochromocytoma** is a neuroendocrine tumor that produces excessive quantities of epinephrine and norepinephrine. **Paragangliomas** are derived from nonadrenal sympathetic ganglia and secrete only norepinephrine. Although pheochromocytomas are not common tumors, they are the most common source of

BOX 7.2 Biologic Actions of Cortisol

- Metabolic
- Hyperglycemic
- Glycogenic
- Gluconeogenic
- Lipolytic
- Protein catabolic
- Insulin antagonist in muscle and adipose tissue
- Inhibits bone formation, stimulates bone resorption
- Necessary for vascular response to catecholamines
- Antiinflammatory
- Suppresses immune system
- Inhibits antidiuretic hormone secretion and action
- Stimulates gastric acid secretion
- Necessary for integrity and function of gastrointestinal tract
- Stimulates red blood cell production
- Alters mood and behavior
- Permissive for calorigenic, lipolytic effects of catecholamine

ADRENAL CORTEX

The cortex of the adult human adrenal shows distinct zonation with respect to histologic appearance, steroidogenesis, and regulation. The adrenal cortex is made up of three zones: the outer zona glomerulosa, the middle zona fasciculata, and the inner zona reticularis (see Fig. 7.2). Each zone expresses a distinct complement of steroidogenic enzymes, resulting in the production of a different steroid hormone as the major endocrine product for each zone as summarized in Fig. 7.5. Recall from Chapter 1 that steroid hormones are derived from cholesterol, which is enzymatically modified in a cell type–specific manner. This means that the steroidogenic endocrine cells are characterized by the steroidogenic enzymes they express, as well as their final hormonal product. Associated with the production of a different steroid hormone, each zone has unique aspects concerning its regulation and the configuration of feedback loops. Recall also from Fig. 1.5 (Chapter 1) that the last steroid molecule within a steroidogenic pathway is what leaves the cell and enters the blood. This means that in the face of a loss of a steroidogenic enzyme within a pathway, the primary steroidlike product released from the gland is the substrate for that missing enzyme, because all subsequent reactions of the pathway cease to occur. An understanding of the steroidogenic pathways for each steroid hormone and steroidogenic cell type is required to understand the consequences of specific mutations in genes encoding steroidogenic enzymes and in states of dysregulation of specific steroidogenic pathways.

Zona Fasciculata

The Zona Fasciculata Makes Cortisol

The largest and most actively steroidogenic zone is the middle zona fasciculata (see Figs. 7.1B and 7.2). The zona fasciculata produces the glucocorticoid hormone, cortisol. This zone is composed of straight cords of large cells. These cells have a foamy cytoplasm because they are filled with lipid droplets that represent stored cholesterol esters. Although the cells make some cholesterol de novo from acetate, they are very efficient at capturing cholesterol from the blood circulating in the form of low-density lipoprotein (LDL) particles (delivery by high-density lipoprotein [HDL] is minimal in humans). Free cholesterol is then esterified by the enzyme acyl CoA cholesterol transferase (ACAT) and stored in lipid droplets (Fig. 7.6). The stored cholesterol is continually turned back into free cholesterol by hormone-sensitive lipase (HSL), a process that is increased by adrenocorticotropic hormone (ACTH; see later in the text).

Free cholesterol is modified by five reactions within a steroidogenic pathway to form cortisol. However, cholesterol is stored in the cytoplasm, and the first enzyme of the pathway, CYP11A1, is located on the inner mitochondrial membrane (see Fig. 7.6). Thus the rate-limiting reaction in steroidogenesis is the transfer of cholesterol from the outer mitochondrial membrane (OMM) to the inner mitochondrial membrane and its conversion to pregnenolone (P5). Although several proteins appear to be involved, one protein, called steroidogenic acute regulatory protein (StAR protein), is indispensable in the process of transporting cholesterol to the inner mitochondrial membrane (see Fig. 7.6). StAR is associated with the OMM and phosphorylation by ACTH-Gs-cAMP-PKA signaling increasing StAR activity.

CLINICAL BOX 7.2

Endocytosed LDL particles are enzymatically digested by lysosomal enzymes. Free cholesterol, but not cholesterol esters, is transported out of the lysosome and enters the cellular cholesterol pool. Cholesterol esters are cleaved by lysosomal acid lipase (LAL) encoded by the *LIPA* gene. Mutations in the *LIPA* gene cause cholesterol ester storage disease and the more severe variant, Wolman disease. Wolman disease affects numerous organs and is ultimately fatal. With respect to the adrenal cortex, Wolman disease causes adrenal insufficiency due to the inability of cells to use LDL cholesterol for steroidogenesis. This underscores the importance of LDL cholesterol for steroidogenesis.

The Niemann-Pick disease C transporters (NPC1 and NCP2) are required for transport of free cholesterol out of the lysosome after receptor-mediated endocytosis of the LDL receptor. NPC disease is caused by a mutation in either the *NPC1* gene or, at a much lower frequency, the **NPC2** gene. NPC disease leads to progressive neurodegeneration and death within the first decade of life.

StAR protein is encoded by the **StarD1** gene. Inactivating mutations in *StarD1* cause cells of the **adrenal cortex** and **gonads** to become excessively laden with lipid ("lipoid") because cholesterol cannot be accessed by CYP11A1 within the mitochondria and used for hormone synthesis. Loss of cortisol increases ACTH, causing adrenal hypertrophy. Thus mutations in *StarD1* lead to **lipoid congenital adrenal hyperplasia.** Elevated ACTH also increases cholesterol synthesis and transport of cholesterol into the cell cytoplasm through

LDL receptor–mediated endocytosis, worsening the engorgement of the cell with lipid. Affected individuals make a small amount of **cortisol, aldosterone,** or **gonadal steroid hormones** as a result of StAR-independent transport. Aldosterone insufficiency represents the most serious deficit because it leads to salt wasting, reduced blood volume, and hypotension (especially orthostatic). Hypoaldosteronism also causes hyperkalemia and metabolic acidosis (see later in the text). Hypocortisolism is especially a serious threat in the face of infection, trauma, surgery, or extended fasting (see later in the text).

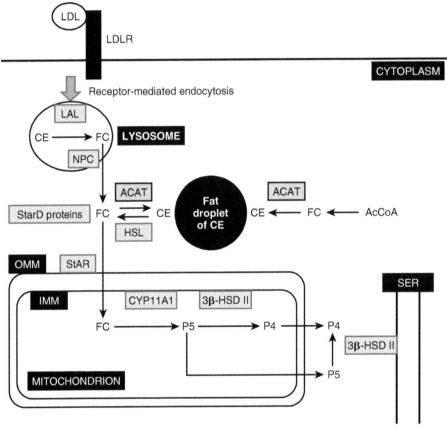

Fig. 7.6 Events involved in the first two reactions, which convert cholesterol to pregnenolone *(P5)* and then P5 to progesterone *(P4)*, in the steroidogenic pathway in zona fasciculata cells. Cholesterol is made de novo from acetyl CoA *(AcCoA)* to a limited extent *(not shown)*, and a significant amount of cholesterol is imported from low-density lipoprotein particles *(LDL)* through receptor-mediated endocytosis of the LDL receptor *(LDLR)*. Within endolysosomes, cholesterol esters *(CE)* released from LDL particles are converted to free cholesterol *(FC)*. Free cholesterol is transported out of the lysosome by Niemann-Pick C1 (NPC1) and NPC2 proteins. Free cholesterol *(FC)* is converted to the storage form of CEs by the enzyme, acyl CoA cholesterol acyltransferase *(ACAT)*. CEs coalesce to form lipid droplets in the cytoplasm. FC is mobilized for steroidogenesis by hormone-sensitive lipase *(HSL)* and transported to the outer mitochondrial membrane *(OMM)* by one or more cytoplasmic carrier proteins of the *StarD* gene family. FC must then be transported from the OMM to the inside of the inner mitochondrial membrane *(IMM)* where CYP11A1 (also called P-450 side-chain cleavage enzyme) is localized. The critical protein that carries out this transport is steroidogenic acute regulatory *(StAR)* protein. The second reaction that converts P5 to progesterone (P4) can occur in the mitochondria or at the cytoplasmic surface of the smooth endoplasmic reticulum (SER) by 3β-hydroxysteroid dehydrogenase type II *(3β-HSDII)*.

The pathway by which cortisol is synthesized involves three enzymes that are not specific to the adrenal and two enzymes that are specifically adrenocortical in their expression. Four of these enzymes belong to the cytochrome P-450 monooxidase gene family and thus are referred to as *CYPs*. The fifth enzyme is 3β-hydroxysteroid dehydrogenase type 2 (3β-HSD2).

The steroidogenic pathway from cholesterol to cortisol is as follows (refer to Fig. 1.4 in Chapter 1 for structure of cholesterol and numbering of cholesterol carbons):

- **Reaction 1.** The side chain of cholesterol (carbons 22 to 27) is removed by **CYP11A1** (also called **P-450 side-chain cleavage**) to generate a C21 steroid intermediate, pregnenolone (Fig. 7.7). Generating a C21 intermediate is a key step because cortisol (as well as aldosterone and progesterone) is a 21-carbon steroid.
- **Reactions 2a/b and 3a/b.** The next two enzymes compete with each other for pregnenolone, so they will be presented as reactions 2a and 2b. The products of reactions 2a and 2b are then modified by the reciprocal enzymes in reactions 3a and 3b, to generate the final product, **17-hydroxyprogesterone** (see Fig. 7.7).
- **Reaction 2a.** Pregnenolone is a substrate for the enzyme, **3β-HSD2**, which converts the hydroxyl group on the 3 carbon to a ketone and moves the double bond

from the 5 to 6 (Δ5) position to the 4 to 5 (Δ4) position. All active steroid hormones must be converted to Δ4 structures. This reaction converts **pregnenolone** (also called **P5**, because it is a Δ5 steroid) to **progesterone** (also called **P4**, because it is a Δ4 steroid).

- **Reaction 3a.** Progesterone is then hydroxylated to **17-hydroxyprogesterone** by **CYP17**. 17-Hydroxylation is an indispensable step for the formation of cortisol (and sex steroids). We will see that the presence or absence of CYP17 plays an important role in defining the nature of steroidogenic tissue.
- **Reaction 2b.** Pregnenolone can also be hydroxylated by CYP17 to **17-hydroypregnenolone** (this is called the **Δ5 pathway**). Because of the high level of 3β-HSD2 activity, reaction 2b is less important than reaction 2a (previous text.)
- **Reaction 3b.** 17-Hydroxypregnenolone can then be converted to **17-hydroxyprogesterone** by **3β-HSD**. Note that **CYP17** has two separate activities: a **17-hydroxylase function, and a 17,20-lyase function.** This latter function removes the 20 and 21 carbons, reducing the steroid to a 19-carbon precursor of active androgens. The zona fasciculata does not express cofactors that promote the 17,20-lyase

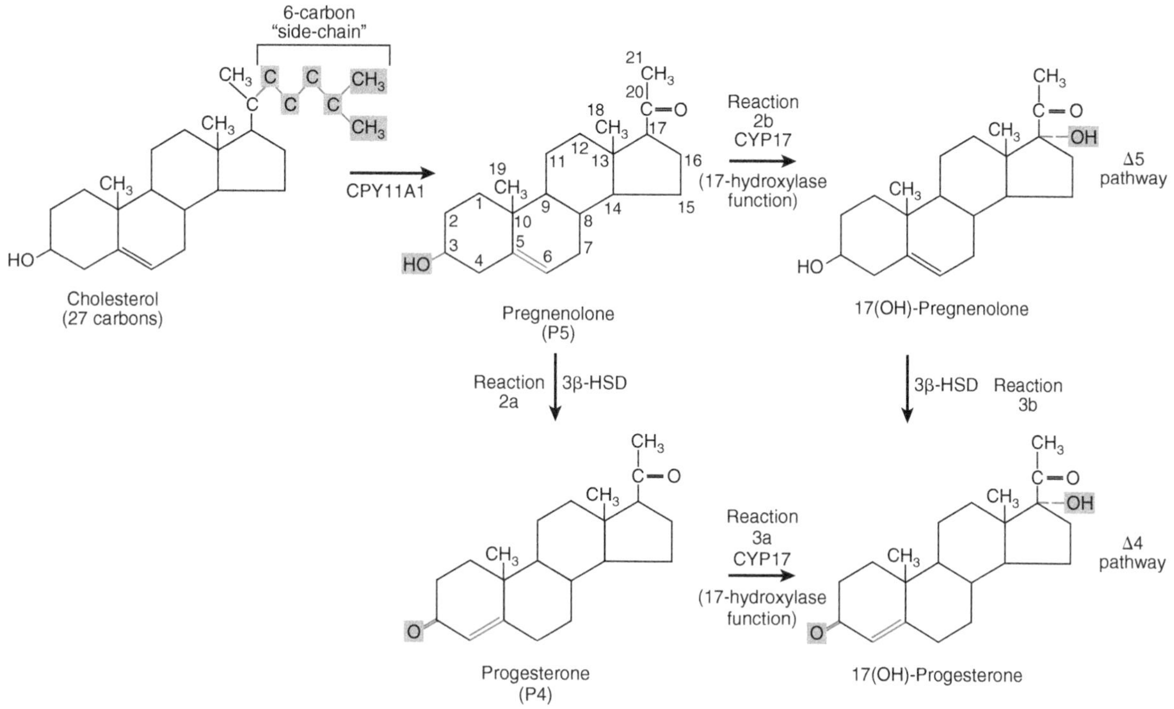

Fig. 7.7 Reaction 1, catalyzed by CYP11A1, in making cortisol. Reactions 2a/b and reactions 3a/b, involving CYP17 (17-hydroxylase function) and 3β-hydroxysteroid dehydrogenase (3β-HSD), in making cortisol.

activity of CYP17 and therefore does not produce significant amounts of androgen precursors. Instead, 17-hydroxyprogesterone is efficiently funneled into the cortisol-specific pathway, which involves two subsequent hydroxylations by adrenocortical-specific enzymes.

- **Reactions 4 and 5.** 17-Hydroxyprogesterone is hydroxylated on the 21 carbon by **CYP21**, producing **11-deoxycortisol.** 11-Deoxycortisol is then efficiently hydroxylated on the 11 carbon by **CYP11B1,** producing **cortisol** (Fig. 7.8). Note that **progesterone** (the product of reaction 2a) can also enter this

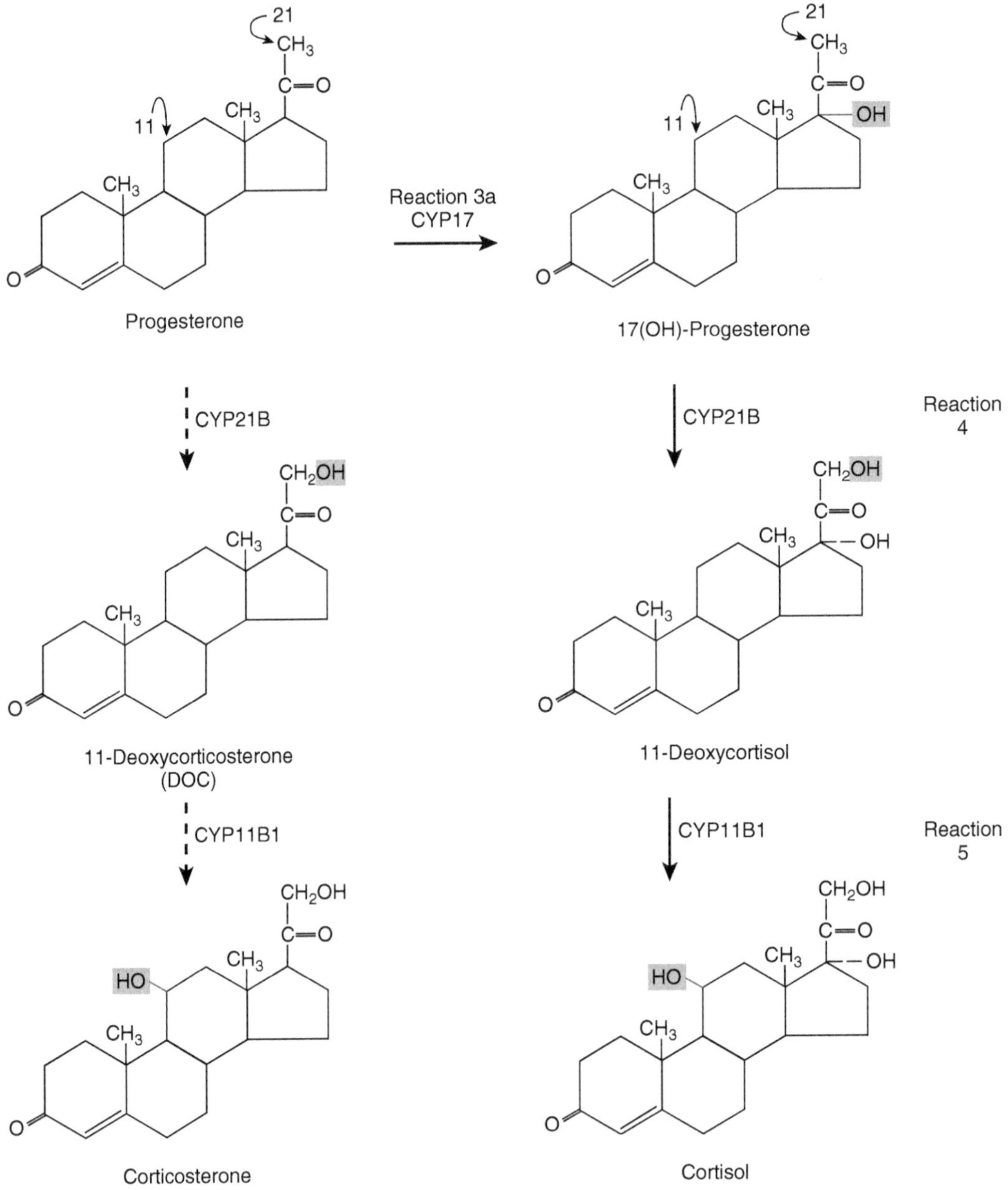

Fig. 7.8 Reactions 4 and 5, involving CYP21 and CYP11B1, that carry out the last two steps of the synthesis of cortisol. Also shown is the minor pathway leading to the synthesis of corticosterone in the zona fasciculata.

pathway of 21- and 11-hydroxylations, producing deoxycorticosterone (DOC) and corticosterone, respectively (see Fig. 7.5). However, CYP17 activity is robust in the human zona fasciculata, so DOC and corticosterone are normally minor products.

Transport and Metabolism of Cortisol

Cortisol is transported in blood predominantly bound to proteins. These are primarily corticosteroid-binding globulin (CBG) (also called transcortin), which binds about 90%, and albumin, which binds 5% to 7%, of the circulating hormone. As stated for thyroid hormones in Chapter 6, it is the unbound (free) form of the hormone that can enter a cell, bind to its receptor and exert biologic effects within target cells. It is also the free form of cortisol that feeds back on the pituitary and hypothalamus. Thus changes in CBG levels are usually counteracted by changes in the hypothalamus-pituitary-adrenal axis.

The liver is the predominant site of steroid inactivation, which occurs through several enzymatic steps. The liver also conjugates 95% of active and inactive steroids with glucuronide or sulfate so that they can be excreted more readily by the kidney (see Chapter 1). The circulating half-life of cortisol is about 70 minutes.

Cortisol is reversibly inactivated by conversion to cortisone (see Fig. 7.14). This is catalyzed by the enzyme, 11β-hydroxysteroid dehydrogenase type 2 (11β-HSD2). Inactivation of cortisol protects the mineralocorticoid receptor (MR) in aldosterone-responsive cells (e.g., distal convoluted tubule cells of the kidney) because cortisol binds to the MR with high affinity. The inactivation of cortisol by 11β-HSD2 is reversible in that another enzyme, 11β-HSD1, converts cortisone back to cortisol. This activation of cortisol occurs in tissues expressing the glucocorticoid receptor (GR), including liver, adipose, skin, and CNS (Fig. 7.14).

Mechanism of Action of Cortisol

Cortisol acts primarily through the GR, which regulates gene transcription (see Fig. 1.22 in Chapter 1). In the absence of hormone, the GR resides in the cytoplasm in a stable complex with several molecular chaperones, including heat-shock protein 90 and cyclophilins. Cortisol-GR binding promotes dissociation of the chaperone proteins, followed by the following elements:

1. Rapid translocation of the cortisol-GR complex into the nucleus.
2. Dimerization and binding to the glucocorticoid-response elements (GREs) near the basal promoters of cortisol-regulated genes.
3. Recruitment of coactivator or corepressor proteins, followed by covalent modification of chromatin

(e.g., histone acetylation for activation; histone deacetylation for inactivation).
4. A change (increase or decrease) in the assembly of the general transcription factors, leading to changes in the transcription rate of the targeted genes.
5. Phosphorylation, followed by nuclear export and/or degradation of the GR, thereby terminating the signal.

Physiologic Actions of Cortisol

Cortisol has a broad range of actions on several organ systems (see Box 7.2). Several of the actions of cortisol were put forth as an integrated response to stress by Hans Selye in the 1930s, and cortisol is often characterized as a stress hormone. In general, cortisol contributes to the maintenance of blood glucose, CNS function, and cardiovascular function during fasting, and it increases blood glucose by hepatic gluconeogenesis during stress at the expense of muscle protein. Cortisol protects the body against the self-injurious effects of unbridled inflammatory and immune responses. Cortisol also partitions energy to cope with stress by inhibiting reproductive function. As stated subsequently, cortisol has several other effects on bone, skin, connective tissue, the GI tract, and the developing fetus that are independent of its stress-related functions.

Metabolic actions. As the term glucocorticoid implies, cortisol is a steroid hormone from the adrenal cortex that regulates blood glucose. Cortisol increases blood glucose by stimulating gluconeogenesis. Cortisol enhances the gene expression of the hepatic gluconeogenic enzymes, phosphoenolpyruvate carboxykinase (PEPCK) and glucose-6-phosphatase, through direct actions and by increasing responsiveness to glucagon and catecholamines. Cortisol also decreases GLUT4-mediated glucose uptake in skeletal muscle and adipose tissue. During a fast (low insulin-to-glucagon ratio), cortisol promotes glucose sparing by potentiating the effects of catecholamines on lipolysis, thereby making FFAs available as an energy source and glycerol available for gluconeogenesis. Cortisol inhibits protein synthesis and significantly increases proteolysis, especially in skeletal muscle, thereby providing a rich source of carbon for hepatic gluconeogenesis. Excessive cortisol causes muscle wasting.

During the digestive phase, when the insulin-to-glucagon ratio is high, cortisol synergizes with insulin in promoting hepatic glycogen synthesis. This ensures that glycogen stores are replete at a time of stress or fasting. Cortisol also synergizes with insulin to promote preadipocyte differentiation into adipocytes, an effect that is dependent on PPARγ. Again, this ensures storage of excess calories during the fed state that can be mobilized at a time of stress or fasting. The effect on adipose tissue is region specific: cortisol specifically increases abdominal and interscapular adipose tissue.

Cardiovascular actions. Cortisol reinforces the enhancement of the delivery of blood glucose to the brain by its positive effects on the cardiovascular system. Cortisol is permissive on the actions of catecholamines and thereby increases cardiac output and blood pressure. Cortisol stimulates erythropoietin synthesis and, hence, increases red blood cell production. Anemia occurs when cortisol is deficient, and polycythemia occurs when cortisol levels are excessive.

Antiinflammatory and immunosuppressive actions. Inflammation and immune responses are often part of a response to stress. However, inflammation and immune responses have the potential of doing significant harm, even to the extent of causing death, to the organism they are designed to protect if they are not held in homeostatic balance. As a stress hormone, cortisol plays an important role in maintaining immune homeostasis. Cortisol, along with epinephrine and norepinephrine, represses the production of proinflammatory cytokines and stimulates the production of antiinflammatory cytokines.

The inflammatory response to injury consists of local dilation of capillaries and increased capillary permeability with a resultant local edema and accumulation of white blood cells. These steps are mediated in part by prostaglandins, thromboxanes, and leukotrienes. Cortisol inhibits phospholipase A2, a key enzyme in prostaglandin, leukotriene, and thromboxane synthesis. Cortisol also stabilizes lysosomal membranes, thereby decreasing the release of the proteolytic enzymes that augment local swelling. In response to injury, leukocytes normally leave the vascular system and migrate to the site of injury. These changes are inhibited by cortisol, as is the phagocytic activity of the neutrophils, although bone marrow release of neutrophils is stimulated. Cortisol decreases the number of circulating eosinophils. The proliferation of connective tissue fibroblasts involved in inflammation and tissue repair is also inhibited. This latter response is important in the formation of barriers to the spread of certain infectious agents. Analogs of glucocorticoid are frequently used pharmacologically because of their antiinflammatory properties. When cortisol levels are high, many of the body's defense mechanisms against infection are inhibited.

Cortisol inhibits the immune response and, for this reason, glucocorticoid analogs have been used as immunosuppressants in organ transplantations. High cortisol levels decrease the number of circulating T lymphocytes (particularly helper T lymphocytes) and decrease their ability to migrate to the site of antigenic stimulation. Glucocorticoids promote atrophy of the thymus and other lymphoid tissue. Although corticosteroids inhibit cell-mediated immunity, antibody production by B lymphocytes does not appear to be impaired.

Fig. 7.9 contrasts the normal role of cortisol in response to a stress and the effects of chronically elevated cortisol due to a pathologic condition. There are important differences in the overall metabolic effects of cortisol between these two states, particularly with respect to lipid metabolism. During stress, cortisol synergizes with catecholamines and glucagon to promote a lipolytic and gluconeogenic metabolic response, while synergizing with catecholamines to promote an appropriate cardiovascular response. During chronically elevated levels of cortisol owing to a pathologic overproduction, cortisol synergizes with insulin in the context of elevated levels of glucose (because of an increased appetite) and hyperinsulinemia (because of elevated glucose and increased glucose intolerance) to promote truncal (abdominal, visceral) and interscapular adiposity.

Action on reproductive systems. Reproduction exacts a considerable energy cost on the organism. In humans, reproductive behavior and function are dampened in response to stress. Cortisol decreases the function of the reproductive axis at the hypothalamic, pituitary, and gonadal levels.

Actions on bone. Glucocorticoids increase bone resorption. They have multiple actions that alter bone metabolism. Glucocorticoids decrease intestinal calcium absorption and decrease renal calcium reabsorption. Both mechanisms lower serum calcium concentrations. As the serum calcium level drops, the secretion of parathyroid hormone (PTH) increases, and PTH mobilizes calcium from bone both by stimulating resorption of bone. In addition to this action, glucocorticoids directly inhibit osteoblast bone-forming functions (see Chapter 4). Although glucocorticoids are useful for treating the inflammation associated with arthritis, excessive use will result in bone loss (osteoporosis).

Actions on connective tissue. Cortisol inhibits fibroblast proliferation and collagen formation. In the presence of excessive amounts of cortisol, the skin thins and is more readily damaged. The connective tissue support of capillaries is impaired, and capillary injury (bruising) is increased.

Actions on kidney. Cortisol inhibits antidiuretic hormone (ADH) secretion and action, so it is an ADH antagonist. In the absence of cortisol, the action of ADH is potentiated, making it difficult to increase the free-water clearance in response to a water load and increasing the likelihood of water intoxication. As discussed earlier, cortisol binds to the MR with high affinity, but this action is normally blocked by the inactivation of cortisol to cortisone by the enzyme 11β-HSD2. However, the mineralocorticoid activity (i.e., Na^+ and water retention, K^+ and H^+ excretion) of cortisol depends on the relative amount of cortisol (or synthetic glucocorticoids) and the activity of

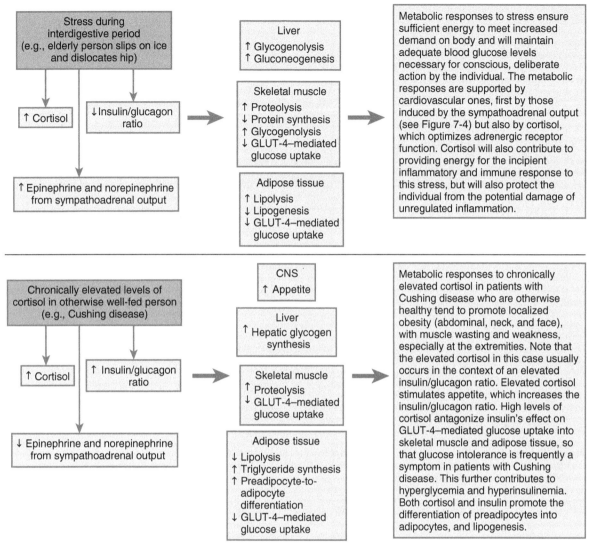

Fig. 7.9 Metabolic actions of cortisol (integrated with catecholamines and glucagon) in response to stress *(upper panel)* and contrasted to actions of chronically elevated cortisol (integrated with insulin) in an otherwise healthy individual *(lower panel)*.

11β-HSD2. Certain agents (such as compounds in black licorice) inhibit 11β-HSD2 and thereby increase the mineralocorticoid activity of cortisol. Cortisol increases the glomerular filtration rate by increasing cardiac output and acting directly on the kidney.

Actions on Muscle

Cortisol actions on muscle are complex. When cortisol levels are excessive, muscle weakness and pain are common symptoms. The weakness has multiple origins. In part it is a result of the **excessive proteolysis** (muscle wasting) that cortisol produces. High cortisol levels can result in hypokalemia (through the mineralocorticoid actions), which can produce muscle weakness because it hyperpolarizes and stabilizes the muscle cell membrane, thereby making stimulation more difficult.

Gastrointestinal actions. Cortisol exerts a trophic effect on the GI mucosa. In the absence of cortisol, GI motility decreases, GI mucosa degenerates, and GI acid and enzyme production decrease. Because cortisol stimulates appetite, hypercortisolism is frequently associated with weight gain. The cortisol-mediated stimulation of gastric acid and pepsin secretion increases the risk for ulcer development.

Psychological actions. The normal range of daily cortisol levels maintains optimal psychological function in humans. Psychiatric disturbances are associated with either excessive or deficient levels of corticosteroids. Excessive corticosteroids can initially produce a feeling of well-being, but continued excessive exposure eventually leads to emotional lability and depression. Frank psychosis can occur with either excess or deficient hormone. Cortisol has been shown to increase the tendency for insomnia and decrease rapid eye movement (REM) sleep. People who are deficient in corticosteroids tend to be depressed, apathetic, and irritable.

Actions of cortisol during fetal development. Cortisol is required for normal development of the CNS, retina, skin, GI tract, and lungs. The best-studied system is the lungs, in which cortisol induces differentiation and maturation of **type 2 alveolar cells**. These cells produce **surfactant** during late gestation that reduces surface tension in the lungs and thus allows for the onset of breathing at birth.

Regulation of Cortisol Production

Cortisol production by the zona fasciculata is regulated by the hypothalamus-pituitary-adrenal axis involving corticotropin-releasing hormone (CRH), ACTH, and **cortisol** (see Chapter 5). The hypothalamus and pituitary stimulate cortisol production and cortisol negatively feeds back on the hypothalamus and pituitary to maintain its setpoint.

A subset of the hypophysiotropic parvicellular neurons secrete CRH, which binds to the Gs-coupled CRH receptor on proopiomelanocortin (POMC) cells (also called *corticotropes*) in the pars distalis (see Chapter 5). Both **neurogenic** (e.g., fear) and **systemic** (e.g., hypoglycemia, hemorrhage, cytokines) forms of stress stimulate CRH release (Box 7.3). CRH is also under **strong diurnal rhythmic** regulation emerging from the suprachiasmatic nucleus so that cortisol levels surge during early predawn and morning hours and then continually decline throughout the day and evening (refer to Fig. 5.14 in Chapter 5, which shows diurnal variation for ACTH). CRH acutely stimulates ACTH release and chronically increases *POMC* gene expression and corticotrope hypertrophy and proliferation. Some parvicellular neurons coexpress CRH and **vasopressin** (also called **ADH**). Vasopressin that reaches the anterior pituitary binds to the Gq-coupled vasopressin-3 receptor (V3 receptor) on corticotropes and potentiates the actions of CRH.

ACTH binds to the **melanocortin-2 receptor (MC2R)** located on cells in the zona fasciculata. The MC2R is

BOX 7.3   Stimuli for Corticotropin-Releasing Hormone Secretion

- Diurnal input from suprachiasmatic nucleus
- Proinflammatory cytokines/infection
- Hypoglycemia
- Hemorrhage
- Neurogenic stress (e.g., fear)
- Physical stress (e.g., surgery)

coupled primarily to a Gs-cAMP-PKA signaling pathway. The effects of ACTH can be subdivided into three phases:

1. **Acute effects of ACTH** occur within minutes. Cholesterol is rapidly mobilized from lipid droplets by posttranslational activation of HSL and transported to the outer mitochondrial membrane. ACTH both rapidly increases StAR protein gene expression and activates StAR protein through PKA-dependent phosphorylation. Collectively, these acute actions of ACTH increase pregnenolone levels.
2. **Chronic effects of ACTH** occur over a period of several hours. These involve increasing the transcription of the genes encoding the steroidogenic enzymes and their coenzymes. ACTH also increases the expression of the LDL receptor.
3. **Trophic actions of ACTH** on the zona fasciculata and reticularis occur over a period of weeks and months. This last effect is exemplified by atrophy of the zona fasciculata in patients receiving therapeutic (i.e., supraphysiologic) levels of glucocorticoid analogs for at least 3 weeks. Under these conditions, the exogenous corticosteroids completely repress CRH and ACTH production, resulting in the **atrophy of the zona fasciculata** and decline in endogenous cortisol production (Fig. 7.10). At the end of therapy, such patients need to be gradually weaned from exogenous glucocorticoids to allow the hypothalamus-pituitary-adrenal axis to reestablish itself and the zona fasciculata to enlarge and produce adequate amounts of cortisol.

Cortisol inhibits both ***POMC* gene expression** at the corticotropes and **pro-*CRH*** gene expression at the hypothalamus. However, intense stress can override the negative feedback effects of cortisol at the hypothalamus, thereby resetting the setpoint at a higher level.

Zona Reticularis

The innermost zone, the **zona reticularis**, begins to appear after birth at about age 5 years. **Adrenal androgens**, especially **DHEAS**, the main product of the zona reticularis, become detectable in the circulation at about 6 years of

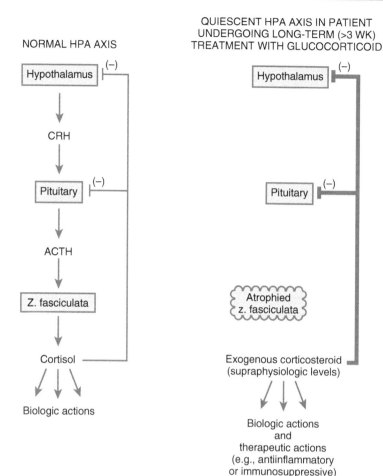

NORMAL HPA AXIS

QUIESCENT HPA AXIS IN PATIENT
UNDERGOING LONG-TERM (>3 WK)
TREATMENT WITH GLUCOCORTICOID

Fig. 7.10 Comparison of normal hypothalamus-pituitary-adrenal *(HPA)* axis to quiescent HPA in an individual receiving exogenous glucocorticoid therapy. The latter causes the zona fasciculata to atrophy after 3 weeks, requiring a careful withdrawal regimen that allows rebuilding of the adrenal tissue before total cessation of exogenous corticosteroid administration.

age. This onset of adrenal androgen production is called **adrenarche** and contributes to appearance of axillary and pubic hair at about age 8 years. DHEAS levels continue to increase, peak during the mid-20s, and then progressively decline with age.

The Zona Reticularis Makes Adrenal Androgens

The zona reticularis differs from the zona fasciculata in several important ways with respect to steroidogenic enzyme activity. First, 3β-HSD is expressed at a much lower level in the zona reticularis than in the zona fasciculata, so the **Δ5 pathway** predominates in the zona reticularis.

Second, the zona reticularis expresses cofactors or conditions that enhance the **17,20-lyase function of CYP17**, thereby generating the 19-carbon androgen precursor

molecule, **dehydroepiandrosterone (DHEA)**, from 17-hydroxypregnenolone. Additionally, the zona reticularis expresses **DHEA-sulfotransferase (SULT2A1 gene)**, which converts DHEA into **DHEAS** (Fig. 7.11). A limited amount of the Δ4 androgen, **androstenedione**, is also made in the zona reticularis. Small amounts of potent androgens (e.g., testosterone) or 18-carbon estrogens are normally produced by the human adrenal cortex (see Fig. 7.5 for summary).

Metabolism and Fate: DHEAS and DHEA

DHEAS can be converted back to DHEA by peripheral **sulfatases**. Importantly, several peripheral tissues (e.g., hair follicle, breast) express steroidogenic enzymes that can convert DHEA and androstenedione to the potent androgens, **testosterone** and **dihydrotestosterone** (see Chapter 9),

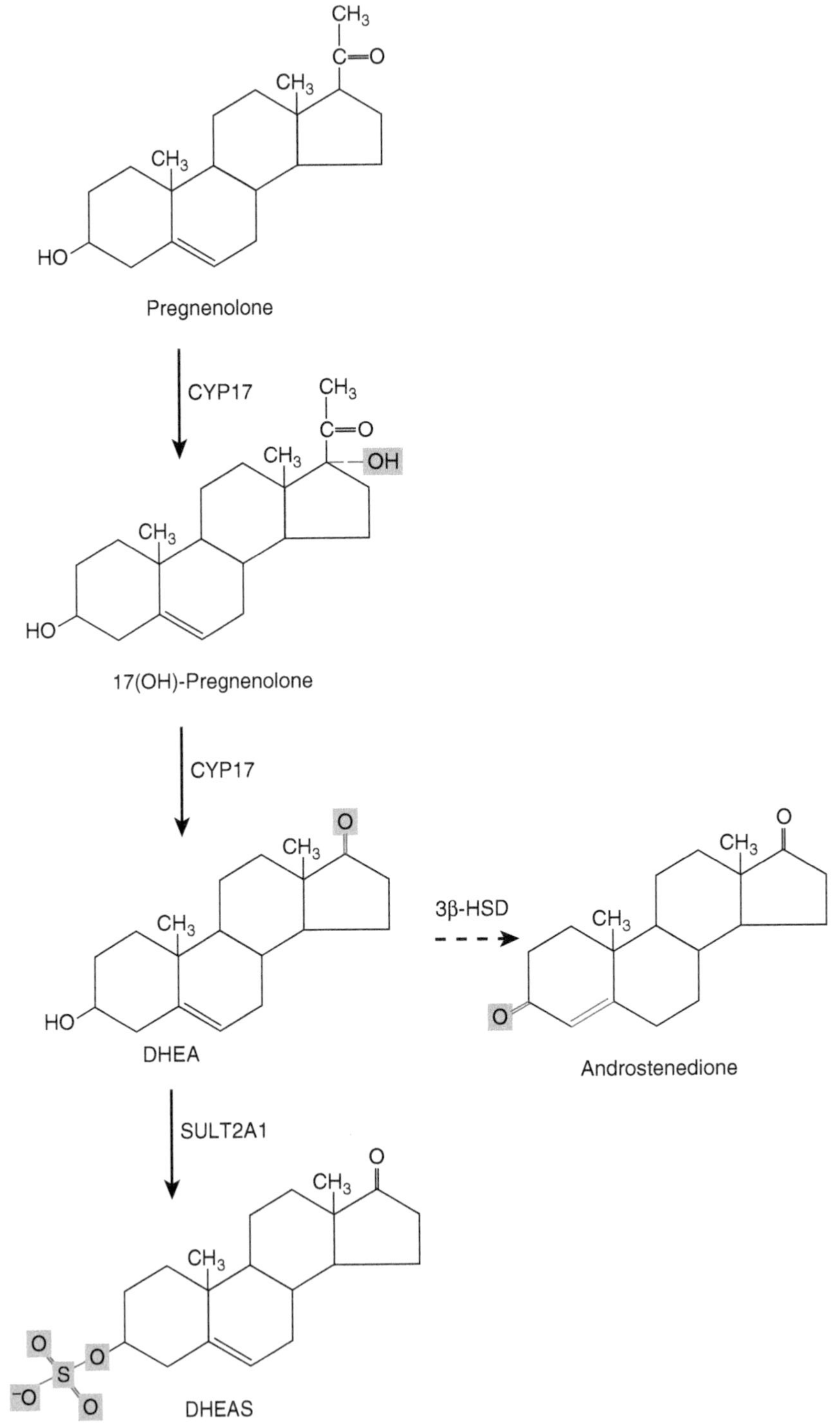

Fig. 7.11 Steroidogenic pathways in the zona reticularis. The first common reaction in the pathway, conversion of cholesterol to pregnenolone by CYP11A1, is not shown. The expression of 3β-hydroxysteroid dehydrogenase (3β-HSD) is relatively low in the zona reticularis, so androstenedione is a minor product compared with DHEA and DHEAS. The zona reticularis also makes a small amount of testosterone and estrogens (not shown).

or to the potent estrogen, estradiol (see Chapter 10). This peripheral conversion of DHEA, DHEAS, and androstenedione is the basis for masculinization of a female fetus or an adult woman by excessive adrenal androgen production.

DHEA binds to albumin and other transport globulins with low affinity and so is excreted efficiently by the kidney. The half-life of DHEA is 15 to 30 minutes. In contrast, DHEAS binds to albumin with very high affinity and has a half-life of 7 to 10 hours.

Physiologic Actions of Adrenal Androgens

In men, the peripheral conversion of adrenal androgens to active androgens is much lower than testicular production of active androgens. However, in women, the adrenal gland contributes to about 50% of circulating active androgens, which are required for axillary and pubic hair growth as well as libido. Under conditions of adrenal androgen excess (adrenal tumor, Cushing syndrome, congenital adrenal hyperplasia), masculinization of women can occur. This involves masculinization of external genitalia (e.g., enlarged clitoris) in utero and excessive facial and body hair (called hirsutism) and acne in adult women. Excessive adrenal androgens also appear to play a role in ovarian dysovulation (i.e., polycystic ovary syndrome). The ability of the breast to convert adrenal androgens into the active estrogen, estradiol, is a complicating factor in estrogen receptor–positive forms of breast cancer.

Apart from providing androgen precursors, it is not clear what other roles, if any, the zona reticularis plays in the adult human. DHEAS is the most abundant circulating hormone in young adults. DHEAS increases steadily until it peaks in the mid-20s and then steadily declines thereafter. Thus there has been considerable interest in the possible role of DHEAS in the aging process. However, the function of this abundant steroid in young adults and the potential impact of its gradual disappearance on aging are still poorly understood. It should be noted that the age-related decline in DHEA and DHEAS has been associated with the popular use of these steroids as dietary supplements, even though there are few (if any) studies to support the efficacy or safety of this practice.

Regulation of Zona Reticularis Function

ACTH promotes hormone production by the zona reticularis. Both DHEA and androstenedione display the same diurnal rhythm as cortisol (DHEAS does not because of its long circulating half-life). The zona reticularis shows the same atrophic changes as the zona fasciculata under conditions of little or no ACTH. However, other factors must regulate adrenal androgen function. Adrenarche occurs in the face of constant ACTH and cortisol levels, and the rise and decline of DHEAS is not associated with a similar

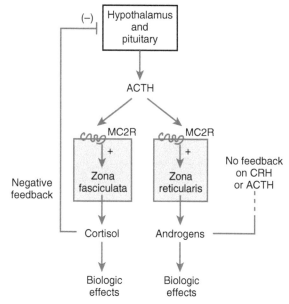

Fig. 7.12 The *loophole* in the hypothalamus-pituitary-adrenal axis. ACTH stimulates the production of both cortisol and adrenal androgens but only cortisol negatively feeds back on ACTH and CRH. Thus, if cortisol production is blocked (i.e., CYP11B1 deficiency), ACTH levels increase, along with adrenal androgens.

pattern of ACTH or cortisol production. However, the other factors, whether extraadrenal or intraadrenal, remain unknown.

A crucial clinical aspect of the regulation of the zona reticularis is that, although ACTH stimulates production of adrenal androgens, neither adrenal androgens nor their more potent metabolites (e.g., testosterone, dihydrotestosterone, estradiol-17β) negatively feed back on ACTH or CRH (Fig. 7.12). This means that an enzymatic defect associated with the synthesis of cortisol (e.g., CYP21 deficiency) is associated with a dramatic increase in both ACTH (no negative feedback from cortisol) and adrenal androgens (because of the elevated ACTH). It is this "loophole" in the hypothalamus-pituitary-adrenal axis that gives rise to congenital adrenal hyperplasia (discussed further later).

ZONA GLOMERULOSA

The thin, outermost zone is called the zona glomerulosa. This zone produces the mineralocorticoid, aldosterone, which regulates salt and volume homeostasis. The zona glomerulosa is only weakly influenced by ACTH. Rather, it is regulated primarily by the renin-angiotensin system, extracellular K⁺, and atrial natriuretic peptide (ANP).

The Zona Glomerulosa Makes Aldosterone

An important feature in the steroidogenic capacity of the zona glomerulosa is that it does not express CYP17. Therefore zona glomerulosa cells never make cortisol—nor do they make adrenal androgens in any form. Pregnenolone is converted to progesterone and DOC by 3β-HSD and CYP21, respectively (Fig. 7.13).

A completely unique feature of the zona glomerulosa among the steroidogenic glands is the expression of CYP11B2. The CYP11B2 gene lies close to CYP11B1 gene, which encodes the enzyme that catalyzes the 11-hydroxylation of 11-deoxycortisol in the zona fasciculata to form cortisol (see Fig. 7.5) on the same chromosome in humans. However, CYP11B2 has a different promoter that is regulated by different signaling pathways. The enzyme itself, called aldosterone synthase, catalyzes the last three reactions from DOC to aldosterone within the zona glomerulosa. These reactions are 11-hydroxylation of DOC to form corticosterone, 18-hydroxylation to form 18-hydroxycorticosterone, and 18-oxidation to form aldosterone (see Fig. 7.13).

Transport and Metabolism of Aldosterone

Aldosterone binds to transport proteins (albumin, corticosteroid-binding protein) with low affinity and therefore has a short biologic half-life of about 20 minutes. Almost all of aldosterone is inactivated by the liver in one pass, conjugated to a glucuronide group, and excreted by the kidney.

Mechanism of Aldosterone Action

Aldosterone acts much like cortisol (and other steroid hormones) in that its primary mechanism of action is through binding to a specific intracellular receptor, the MR. After dissociation of chaperone proteins, nuclear translocation, dimerization, and binding to mineralocorticoid-response element, the aldosterone-MR complex regulates the expression of specific genes.

Cortisol binds equally well to the MR and activates the same genes as does aldosterone. However, as discussed earlier, these cells also express 11β-HSD2, which converts cortisol to the inactive steroid, cortisone (Fig. 7.14). Cortisone can be converted back to cortisol by 11β-HSD1, which is expressed in several glucocorticoid-responsive tissues, including the liver and skin.

Physiologic Actions of Aldosterone*

Actions on Kidney. For more information on this subject, see Koeppen BM, Stanton BA: *Renal Physiology*, 6th ed., St. Louis, 2001, Mosby.

The primary action of aldosterone is to increase the reabsorption of Na$^+$, followed by H$_2$O, by the distal nephron. About 95% of Na$^+$ reabsorption in the nephron occurs before the distal nephron, independently of aldosterone regulation. However, the amount of Na$^+$ reabsorbed by the distal nephron can be regulated by a few percentages to match changes in dietary Na$^+$ intake. Na$^+$ uptake at the distal nephron is accompanied by Cl$^-$ and H$_2$O. As emphasized in the *Mosby Renal Physiology* monograph, "a 2% change in the fractional excretion of Na$^+$ would produce more than a 3 liter change in the volume of the extracellular fluid." Salt wasting and dehydration occur in patients with aldosterone insufficiency.

Aldosterone increases Na$^+$ reabsorption at the distal nephron (the latter portion of the distal convoluted tubule and the cortical collecting duct) primarily by increasing the expression of the α-subunit of the epithelial Na$^+$ channel (ENaC). Aldosterone also increases the stability of ENaC in the apical (luminal) membrane (Fig. 7.15). This action of aldosterone is mediated by the aldosterone-inducible serine/threonine kinase, SGK1. SGK1 gene expression is rapidly and profoundly increased by aldosterone. SGK1 prevents the ability of a protein, called *Nedd 4 to 2*, from targeting ENaC for degradation.

CLINICAL BOX 7.3

The importance of ENaC in the actions of aldosterone is made apparent by forms of **aldosterone resistance (type 1 pseudohypoaldosteronism; PHA1)**. PHA1 is characterized by symptoms related to lack of aldosterone (salt wasting, dehydration, hyperkalemia, hypotension, with very high levels of renin, angiotensin, and aldosterone; see later in the text). Some cases of PHA1 are due to inactivating mutations in one of the subunits of the ENaC. In the presence of these mutations, aldosterone cannot efficiently increase Na$^+$ reabsorption.

In contrast to PHA1, **Liddle syndrome** is characterized by hypertension, hypokalemia, and low renin and aldosterone levels. In these patients, ENaC subunits have mutations that prevent Nedd 4 to 2 from interacting with them and targeting them for degradation. Therefore in Liddle syndrome, the ENaCs reside in the apical membrane much longer and transport more Na$^+$ independently of aldosterone.

Aldosterone also promotes Na$^+$ reabsorption by increasing the activity of the basolateral Na$^+$/K$^+$ ATPase in the distal nephron, although the hormone does not acutely increase gene expression of this transporter.

Aldosterone also stimulates K$^+$ and H$^+$ excretion. Aldosterone increases gene expression of the renal outer medullary K$^+$(ROMK) channel and the density of this channel in the apical membrane of the distal nephron

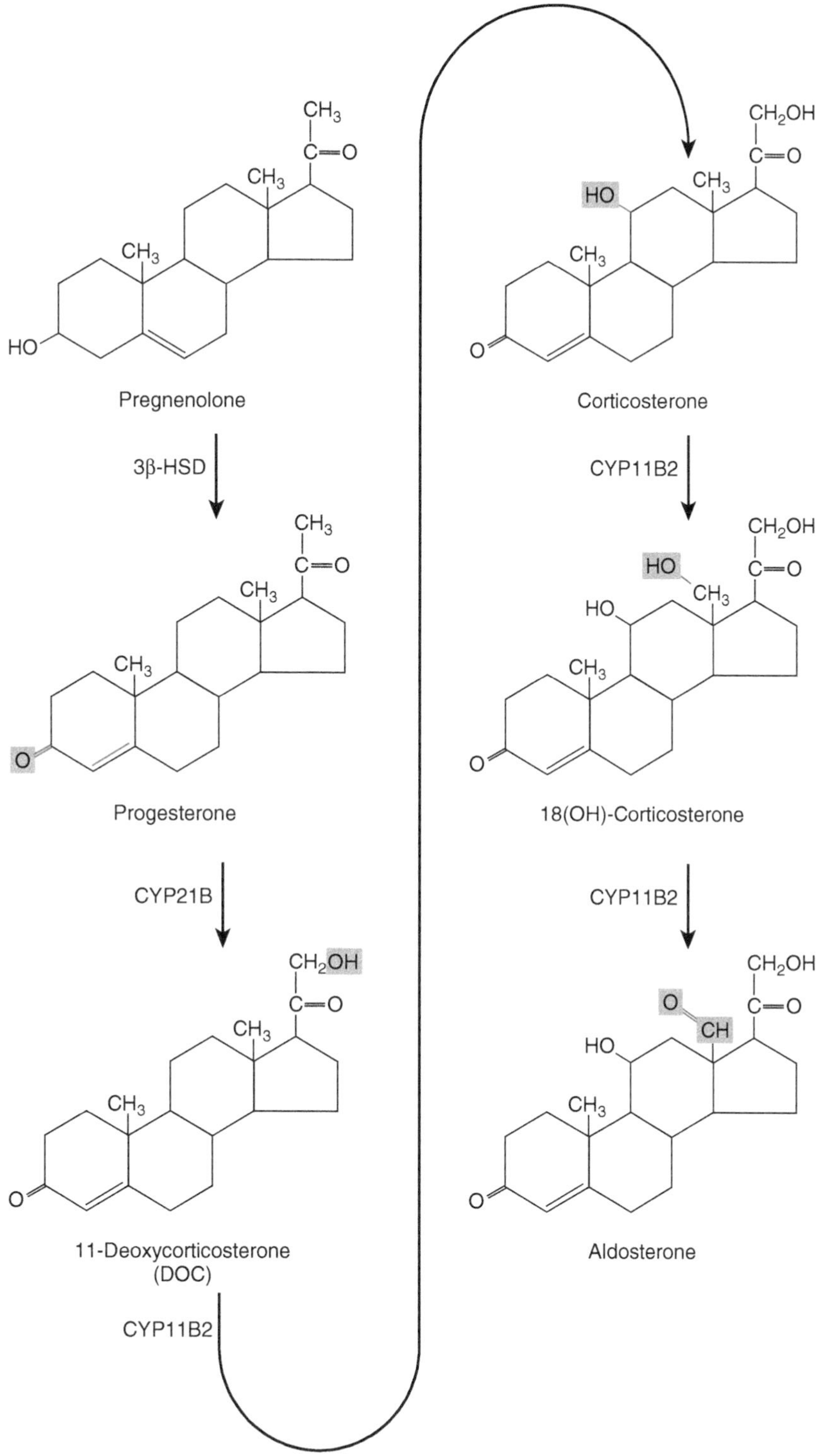

Fig. 7.13 Steroidogenic pathways in the zona glomerulosa. The first common reaction in the pathway, conversion of cholesterol to pregnenolone by CYP11A1, is not shown. Note that the last three reactions are catalyzed by CYP11B2.

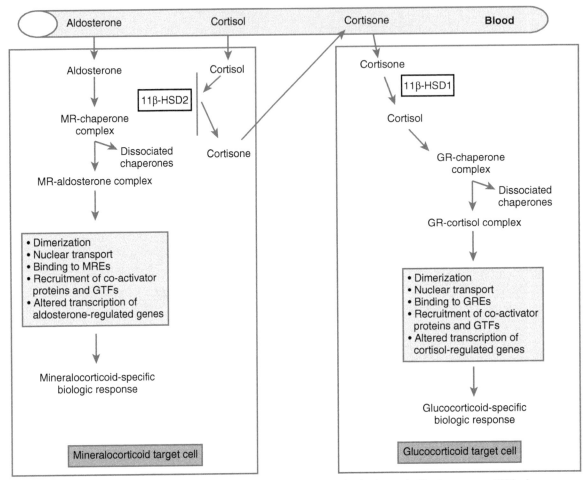

Fig. 7.14 The mineralocorticoid receptor *(MR)* is protected from activation by cortisol by the enzyme, 11β-hydroxysteroid dehydrogenase type 2 (11β-HSD2), which converts cortisol to inactive cortisone. Cortisone can be converted back to cortisol in glucocorticoid target cells by the enzyme, 11β-HSD1. Cortisol binds to the glucocorticoid receptor *(GR)* in cortisol target cell. *MRE*, mineralocorticoid receptor-response element; *GTF*, gene transcription factor.

(see Fig. 7.15). The excretion of K⁺ is linked to the reabsorption of Na⁺, in that the ENaC and the Na⁺, K⁺-ATPase establish the electrochemical conditions for apical secretion of K⁺. In this sense, SGK1 indirectly promotes K⁺ secretion. Additionally, SGK1 increases ROMK channel insertion into the apical membrane and increases its transporting activity. The importance of aldosterone on K⁺ and H⁺ homeostasis is emphasized by the findings that **hyperaldosteronism** leads to **hypokalemia** and **metabolic alkalosis**.

Continuous aldosterone administration results in aldosterone *escape* in 2 to 3 days. Initially, sodium retention and volume expansion are promoted, but the volume expansion does not continue indefinitely. As extracellular volume and therefore vascular volume increases, the glomerular filtration rate increases. This increases the rate of sodium delivery to the nephron and therefore the rate of renal sodium excretion, which limits the ability of aldosterone to continue expanding extracellular volume. The increase in vascular volume will stimulate the release of ANP, which promotes renal Na⁺ excretion. However, escape from the effects of aldosterone on potassium and hydrogen ion excretion does not occur, and potassium depletion and metabolic alkalosis can persist. Further, some forms of congenital adrenal hyperplasia that lead to increased mineralocorticoids are associated with long-term hypertension.

Actions on Other Epithelia

The colon is an important extrarenal site in terms of aldosterone regulation of salt and water homeostasis. As in the distal nephron, aldosterone increases sodium and water reabsorption and increases K⁺ excretion in the colon.

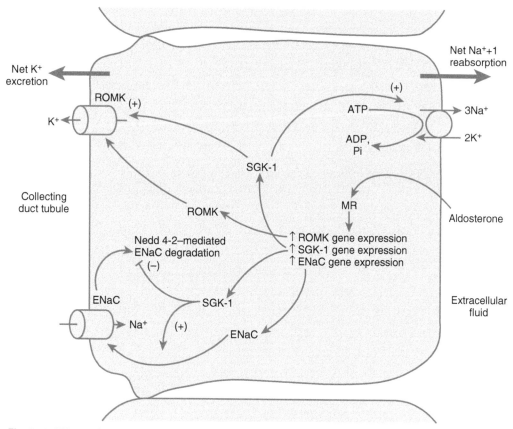

Fig. 7.15 Effects of aldosterone on collecting duct. Aldosterone increases gene expression of the kinase SGK1, the epithelial sodium channel ENaC, and the renal outer medullary potassium channel ROMK. SGK1 kinase activity reinforces aldosterone actions by increasing ENaC insertion into the membrane and inhibiting Nedd 4 to 2–dependent degradation of ENaC. SGK1 also increases the activity of ROMK and the basolateral sodium-potassium ATPase.

Aldosterone has similar effects on epithelia of salivary glands, sweat glands, and gastric glands.

Actions on Heart Muscle

Clinical studies in humans have revealed a deleterious effect of aldosterone on cardiovascular function independent of its effects on renal sodium and water reabsorption. Aldosterone has a proinflammatory, profibrotic effect on the cardiovascular system and promotes left ventricular hypertrophy and remodeling. This effect of aldosterone is associated with increased morbidity and mortality in patients with essential hypertension.

Regulation of Aldosterone Secretion

Given that Na^+ reabsorption and water uptake represent major actions of aldosterone, it would make sense that Na^+ levels and volume would feed back on aldosterone

> **BOX 7.4   Regulation of Aldosterone Production by Zona Glomerulosa Cells**
>
> **Stimulators**
> - Angiotensin II
> - Extracellular K^+
> - Acute elevated adrenocorticotropic hormone (ACTH)
>
> **Inhibitors**
> - Atrial natriuretic peptide (ANP)
> - Chronic elevated ACTH

production (Box 7.4). This occurs through the renin-angiotensin system (RAS). In the kidney, the vascular smooth muscle cells of the afferent arteriole adjacent to the glomerulus, called juxtaglomerular (JG) cells, are specialized to secrete a proteolytic enzyme called renin. JG cells release renin in response to a decrease in blood pressure in the afferent arteriole—as detected by baroreceptors in the wall of the afferent arteriole (Fig. 7.16). JG cells also release renin in response to decreased systemic blood pressure—as detected by baroreceptors. Decreased systemic blood pressure also leads to activation of sympathetic fibers that directly innervate JG cells through β1-adrenergic receptors. In addition to stimulation by decreased blood pressure, decreased delivery of Na$^+$ to specialized cells of the ascending loop of Henle, collectively called the macula densa, causes these cells to signal to the JG cells to release renin.

Once secreted, renin acts on circulating angiotensinogen (renin substrate) to produce the decapeptide, angiotensin I. Angiotensin I is converted to angiotensin II (8 amino acids) by angiotensin-converting enzyme (ACE) in the lungs (see Fig. 7.16). Angiotensin II binds to the Gq-coupled angiotensin I receptor on zona glomerulosa cells and most vascular smooth muscle cells. Angiotensin II is a potent stimulus for aldosterone production. Angiotensin II increases StAR and CYP11B2 (aldosterone synthase) expression. As the name suggests, angiotensin II

is also a potent vasoconstrictor and plays a direct role in compensation for vascular volume depletion.

Two other regulators of aldosterone production are extracellular K$^+$ and ANP. Rising serum K$^+$ levels depolarize the glomerulosa cell membrane, thereby stimulating voltage-sensitive calcium channels to open. The resultant calcium influx stimulates aldosterone production. In contrast to angiotensin II and extracellular K$^+$, ANP is a signal of too much aldosterone causing an expanded extracellular fluid volume and increased blood pressure. ANP is secreted by the heart and acts directly on zona glomerulosa cells to inhibit aldosterone production. Note that ANP also inhibits aldosterone indirectly by inhibiting renin release and plays an important role in the aldosterone escape response (see earlier in the text).

PATHOLOGIC CONDITIONS INVOLVING THE ADRENAL CORTEX

Adrenocortical Insufficiency (Addison Disease)

Addison disease is a primary adrenal insufficiency in which the levels of both mineralocorticoids and glucocorticoids

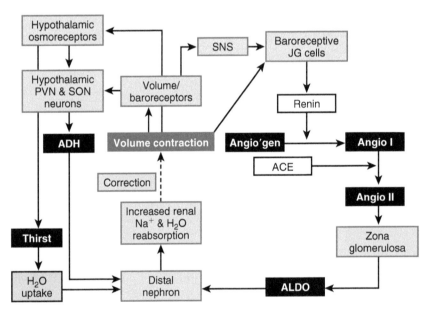

Fig. 7.16 Integrated response to volume contraction. Volume change and increased osmolarity will activate specific receptors that lead to the release of ADH and an increase in thirst. ADH promotes water reabsorption by the distal nephron (see Chapter 5). Volume contraction will also activate the juxtaglomerular cells directly through decreased blood pressure in the afferent arteriole of the glomerulus and through activation of the sympathetic nervous system *(SNS)*. Renin converts angiotensinogen *(Angio'gen)* to angiotensin I *(Angio I)*. Angiotensin I–converting enzyme *(ACE)* in the lung then generates angiotensin II (Angio II). Angiotensin II directly stimulates aldosterone *(ALDO)* production at the zona glomerulosa. Aldosterone acts on the distal nephron to increase Na$^+$ reabsorption, which results in an increase in water reabsorption due to osmotic drag.

are usually extremely low. In North America and Europe, the most prevalent cause of Addison disease is autoimmune destruction of the adrenal cortex. Because of the cortisol deficiency, ACTH secretion increases. Elevated levels of ACTH can compete for the MC1R in melanocytes, causing an increase in skin pigmentation, particularly in skin creases, scars, and gums (Fig. 7.17; also see Chapter 5). The loss of the mineralocorticoids results in contraction of extracellular volume, producing circulatory hypovolemia and therefore a drop in blood pressure. Because the loss of cortisol decreases the vasopressive response to catecholamines, peripheral resistance drops, adding to the tendency toward hypotension. Hypotension predisposes people to circulatory shock. These people are also prone to have hypoglycemia when stressed or fasting. The hyperglycemic actions of other hormones, such as glucagon, epinephrine, and growth hormone, generally will prevent hypoglycemia at other times. Although volume depletion occurs because of the loss of mineralocorticoids, water intoxication can develop if a water load is given. The loss of cortisol impairs the ability to increase free-water clearance in response to a water load and hence rid the body of the excess water. Patients with Addison disease exhibit hyperkalemic acidosis. Because cortisol is important for muscle function, muscle weakness occurs in cortisol deficiency. The loss of cortisol results in anemia, decreased GI motility and secretion, and decreased iron and vitamin B$_{12}$ absorption. The appetite decreases because of the cortisol deficiency, and this decreased appetite, coupled with the GI dysfunction, will predispose these persons to weight loss. These patients often show disturbances in mood and behavior and are more susceptible to depression (Box 7.5). Treatment involves replacement therapy with glucocorticoid and mineralocorticoid analogs.

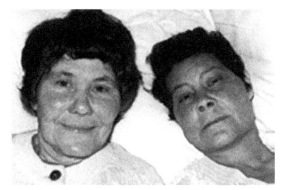

Fig. 7.17 Woman on the *right* has Addison disease. Note her increased pigmentation relative to her healthy twin sister on the *left*. (From Hall R, Evered DC: *Color Atlas of Endocrinology*, 2nd ed., London, 1990, Mosby-Wolfe.)

Adrenocortical Excess
Cushing Syndrome

Hypercortisolism is termed Cushing syndrome. Pharmacologic use of exogenous corticosteroids is now the most common cause of Cushing syndrome. The next most prevalent cause is ACTH-secreting tumors (pituitary or extrapituitary). The form of Cushing syndrome caused by a functional pituitary adenoma is called Cushing disease. A fourth cause is primary hypercortisolism resulting from a functional adrenal tumor. If the disorder is primary or a result of corticosteroid treatment, ACTH secretion

---

BOX 7.5   Manifestations of Primary Adrenocortical Insufficiency

Cortisol Deficiency
- Gastrointestinal disturbances
  - Anorexia
  - Nausea
  - Vomiting
  - Diarrhea
  - Abdominal pain
  - Weight loss
- Mental disturbances
  - Apathy
  - Psychosis
  - Confusion
- Metabolic disturbances
  - Hypoglycemia, especially under stress or fasting
  - Impaired gluconeogenesis
  - Increased insulin sensitivity
  - Cardiovascular/renal disorders
  - Impaired free-water clearance
  - Impaired pressor response to catecholamines
  - Hypotension
- Pituitary
  - Increased adrenocorticotropic hormone secretion
  - Hyperpigmentation

Aldosterone Deficiency
- Inability to conserve sodium
- Decreased extracellular fluid volume
- Decreased blood volume
- Weight loss
- Decreased cardiac output
- Increased renin production
- Hypotension
- Shock
- Impaired renal secretion of potassium and hydrogen
- Hyperkalemia
- Metabolic acidosis

will be suppressed, and increased skin pigmentation will not occur. However, if the hypersecretion of the adrenal is a result of an ACTH-secreting nonpituitary tumor, ACTH levels sometimes become high enough to increase skin pigmentation even in the presence of hypercortisolism.

Increased cortisol secretion causes a tendency to gain weight, with a characteristic **abdominal and interscapular (buffalo hump) fat distribution** (Table 7.2). The face appears round (**moon face**), and the cheeks may be reddened (**plethora**), in part because of the **polycythemia** and in part due to thinning of the skin (Fig. 7.18A). The limbs will be thin as a result of **skeletal muscle wasting** (from increased proteolysis), and **muscle weakness** will be evident (from muscle proteolysis and hypokalemia). Proximal muscle weakness is apparent, so the patient may have difficulty with stair climbing or rising from a sitting position. The abdominal fat accumulation, coupled with atrophy of the abdominal muscles and thinning of the skin, will produce a large, protruding abdomen. Purple abdominal **striae** are seen as a result of the damage to the skin by the prolonged proteolysis, increased intraabdominal fat, and loss of abdominal muscle tone (see Fig. 7.18B).

Capillary fragility is seen as a result of damage to the connective tissue supporting the capillaries. Patients are likely to show signs of **osteoporosis and poor wound healing**. They have metabolic disturbances that include **glucose intolerance, hyperglycemia, and insulin resistance**. Prolonged hypercortisolism can lead to manifestations of **diabetes mellitus**. However, the lipolytic effect of cortisol

by itself is so minor that if high insulin levels are present, lipogenesis, rather than lipolysis, predominates.

Insulin probably plays an important role in the increased adipose tissue mass typically seen with hypercortisolism.

TABLE 7.2 Clinical Manifestations of Hypercortisolism

Symptom	Metabolic Results
Weight gain	Centripetal fat distribution, increased appetite
Protein wasting	Thin skin, abdominal striae
Capillary fragility (ecchymoses)	
Muscle wasting, muscle weakness	
Osteoporosis	
Poor wound healing	
Growth retardation	
Carbohydrate intolerance	Impaired glucose use, hyperglycemia
Insulin resistance	
Mineralocorticoid effects of cortisol	Hypertension, hypokalemia
Immunologic suppression	Increased susceptibility to infections
Other manifestations	Hirsutism, oligomenorrhea, polycythemia, personality changes

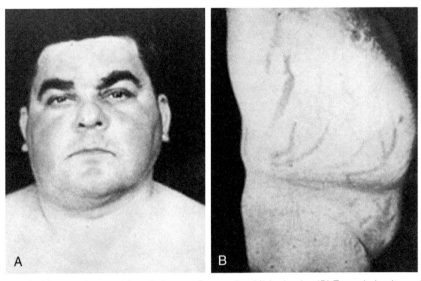

Fig. 7.18 (A) Cushing syndrome with typical moon face and reddish cheeks. (B) Truncal obesity and abdominal striae. (From Wilson JD, Foster DW: *Williams' Textbook of Endocrinology,* 8th ed., Philadelphia, 1992, Saunders.)

Cortisol interacts with insulin to promote the differentiation of preadipocytes into adipocytes. For reasons not fully understood, hypercortisolism is associated with a peculiar pattern of fat deposition, which is called *centripetal fat distribution* because the adipose tissue is concentrated in the trunk, whereas wasting is seen in the arms and legs. Adipose tissue tends to accumulate in the abdomen. Visceral adipose tissue expresses a high level of 11β-HSD1, thereby efficiently converting cortisone to cortisol and increasing differentiation of preadipocytes to adipocytes. However, other mechanisms are likely to contribute. Also, hypercortisolism increases the size of interclavicular fat pads, producing the buffalo hump characteristic of this endocrine imbalance (see Table 7.2).

Because there are many hyperglycemic hormones, a cortisol deficiency is not likely to produce hypoglycemia unless fasting occurs or the person is stressed. However, cortisol is essential for proper mobilization of proteins for glucose production. Changes in the serum after cortisol administration include increased blood urea nitrogen; decreased serum alanine (because it is used in gluconeogenesis); the increased branched-chain amino acids leucine, isoleucine, and valine; and increased serum fatty acid levels. The change in branched-chain amino acid levels is indicative of decreased muscle protein synthesis and increased proteolysis, whereas the increase in fatty acids reflects adipose tissue lipolysis. Because of the suppression of the immune system caused by the glucocorticoids, patients are more susceptible to infection. Mineralocorticoid activities of the glucocorticoids and the possible elevation of aldosterone secretion produce salt retention and subsequent water retention, resulting in hypertension.

Because ACTH also regulates the zona reticularis, Cushing disease is associated with excessive adrenal androgen secretion. In women, this can produce hirsutism, male pattern baldness, and clitoral enlargement (adrenogenital syndrome).

Conn Syndrome

Primary hyperaldosteronism is called Conn syndrome. It frequently occurs as a result of aldosterone-secreting tumors. Excessive mineralocorticoid secretion results in potassium depletion, sodium retention, muscle weakness, hypertension, and hypokalemic alkalosis. Although extracellular fluid volume increases, edema is not common because of hypervolemia-induced ANP release that results in natriuresis.

Congenital Adrenal Hyperplasia

Any enzyme blockage that decreases cortisol synthesis will increase ACTH secretion and produce adrenal hyperplasia. The most common form of congenital adrenal hyperplasia occurs as a result of a deficiency of the enzyme 21-hydroxylase (CYP21). These individuals cannot produce normal quantities of cortisol, deoxycortisol, DOC, corticosterone, or aldosterone. Because of impaired cortisol production, ACTH will be elevated. High ACTH will drive adrenal androgen production by the zona reticularis. As shown in Fig. 7.12, androgens do not feed back on ACTH or CRH and thus stay elevated. A female fetus will be masculinized. Conversely, conversion of adrenal androgens to estrogen can cause feminization (e.g., breast development, called gynecomastia) in males.

Because patients with Addison disease are unable to produce the mineralocorticoids, aldosterone, DOC, and corticosterone, they have difficulty retaining salt and maintaining extracellular volume. Consequently, they are likely to be hypotensive. If the blockage is at the next step, 11β-hydroxylase (CYP11B1), DOC will be formed, and the levels of DOC will accumulate. Because DOC has significant mineralocorticoid activity and the levels become high, these individuals tend to retain salt and water at an excessive rate and become hypertensive. If there is a deficiency of CYP17, neither cortisol nor sex hormones are produced. The inability of the gonads to produce normal androgen levels during fetal development can result in a female phenotype for both males and females. A complete deficiency of 3β-HSD2 is embryonic lethal. An incomplete deficiency results in the inability to produce adequate quantities of mineralocorticoids, glucocorticoids, androgens, and estrogens. The adrenal produces large quantities of the weak androgen DHEA, which can lead to masculinization of females because of the expression of 3β-HSD1 in some nonendocrine tissues.

SUMMARY

1. The adrenal gland is composed of a cortex, which is of mesodermal origin, and a medulla, which is of neuroectodermal origin. The cortex produces steroid hormones (cortisol, aldosterone, and inactive adrenal androgens), and the medulla produces catecholamines (epinephrine and, to a lesser extent, norepinephrine).

2. Regulated enzymes in medullary catecholamine synthesis are tyrosine hydroxylase and β-dopamine hydroxylase, which are induced by sympathetic stimulation, and phenylethanolamine-N-methyltransferase, which is induced by cortisol.

3. Catecholamines increase serum glucose and fatty acid levels. They stimulate gluconeogenesis, glycogenolysis,

and lipolysis. Catecholamines increase cardiac output and bronchiolar dilation but have selective effects on blood flow to different organs.

4. A pheochromocytoma is a tumor of chromaffin tissue from the adrenal medulla that produces excessive quantities of catecholamines. Symptoms of pheochromocytoma are often sporadic and include hypertension, headaches, sweating, anxiety, palpitations, chest pain, and orthostatic hypotension.

5. The adrenal cortex displays clear structural and functional zonation: the zona glomerulosa produces the mineralocorticoid, aldosterone; the zona fasciculata produces the glucocorticoid, cortisol; and the zona reticularis produces the androgen precursors, DHEAS, DHEA, and, to a much lesser extent, androstenedione.

6. Cortisol acts by binding to the glucocorticoid receptor. During stress, cortisol increases blood glucose by increasing gluconeogenic gene expression in the liver and breaking down muscle protein to supply gluconeogenic precursors. Cortisol also decreases glucose uptake by muscle and adipose tissue and has permissive actions on glucagon and catecholamines. Cortisol has multiple effects on other tissue. From a pharmacologic point of view, the immunosuppressive and antiinflammatory effects are the most important.

7. Cortisol is regulated by the CRH-ACTH-cortisol axis. Cortisol negatively feeds back at the hypothalamus on CRH-producing neurons and on the pituitary corticotropes. CRH is regulated by several forms of stress, including proinflammatory cytokines, hypoglycemia, neurogenic stress, and hemorrhage, and by diurnal inputs.

8. Adrenal androgens—DHEA, DHEAS, and androstenedione—are androgen precursors. They can be converted to active androgens peripherally and provide about 50% of circulating androgens in women. In adult men, the role of adrenal androgens, if any, remain obscure. In women, adrenal androgens promote pubic and axillary hair growth and libido. Excessive adrenal androgens in women can lead to various degrees of virilization and ovarian dysfunction.

9. The zona glomerulosa of the adrenal cortex is the site of aldosterone production. Aldosterone is the strongest naturally occurring mineralocorticoid in humans. Aldosterone promotes Na^+ and water uptake by the distal nephron, while promoting renal K^+ and H^+ excretion. Aldosterone promotes Na^+ and water uptake in the colon and salivary glands. Aldosterone has a proinflammatory, profibrotic effect on the cardiovascular system and causes left ventricular hypertrophy and remodeling.

10. Major actions of angiotensin II on the adrenal cortex are increased growth and vascularity of the zona glomerulosa, increased StAR and CYP11B2 enzyme activity, and increased aldosterone synthesis.

11. Major stimuli for aldosterone production are a rise in angiotensin II and a rise in serum potassium concentration. The major inhibitory signal is ANP.

12. Addison disease is adrenocortical insufficiency. Common symptoms include hypotension, hyperpigmentation, muscle weakness, anorexia, hypoglycemia, and hyperkalemic acidosis.

13. Cushing syndrome results from hypercortisolemia. If the basis of the disorder is increased pituitary adrenocorticotropin secretion, the disorder is called *Cushing disease*. Common symptoms of Cushing syndrome include centripetal fat distribution, muscle wasting, proximal muscle weakness, thin skin with abdominal striae, capillary fragility, insulin resistance, and polycythemia.

14. Congenital adrenal hyperplasia results from a congenital enzyme deficiency that blocks production of cortisol. The enzyme blockage results in elevated ACTH secretion, which stimulates adrenal cortical growth and secretion of precursors produced before the block. A 21-hydroxylase (CYP21B) deficiency is the most common form.

SELF-STUDY PROBLEMS

1. How does epinephrine influence metabolic pathways in the liver? Adipose tissue?

2. Explain how catecholamines can cause vasoconstriction in some blood vessels, while causing vasodilation in others.

3. Why does the adrenal cortex undergo atrophy in response to prolonged administration of synthetic glucocorticoids?

4. Why does masculinization of women (adrenogenital syndrome) often occur in patients with Cushing disease?

5. Explain the interaction of ENaC and SGK1 in the actions of aldosterone.

6. Explain the differences between the causes of orthostatic hypotension in patients with pheochromocytoma and those with Addison disease.

KEYWORDS AND CONCEPTS

3β-hydroxysteroid dehydrogenase (3β-HSD)
11β-HSD1
11β-Hydroxylase (CYP11B1)
11β-Hydroxysteroid dehydrogenase type 2 (11β-HSD2)
17,20-Lyase function
17-Hydroxylase function
21-Hydroxylase (CYP21)
α- and β-Adrenergic receptors
Δ4 pathway
Δ5 pathway
Addison disease
Adrenal androgens
Adrenal cortex
Adrenal glands
Adrenal medulla
Adrenarche
Adrenocortical insufficiency
Adrenogenital syndrome
Aldosterone
Aldosterone escape
Aldosterone synthase
Androstenedione
Angiotensin II
Angiotensin-converting enzyme (ACE)
Angiotensinogen (renin substrate)
Antiinflammatory and immunosuppressive actions
Angiotensin II receptor
Atrial natriuretic peptide (ANP)
Cardiac output
Chromaffin cells
Congenital adrenal hyperplasia
Conn syndrome
Corticosteroid-binding globulin (CBG; transcortin)
Corticosterone
Cortisol
Cortisone
Cushing disease
Cushing syndrome

CYP11A1
CYP11B1
CYP11B2
CYP21
Dehydroepiandrosterone sulfate (DHEAS)
Deoxycorticosterone (DOC)
Epinephrine
Fight-or-flight response
Glucocorticoid
Glucocorticoid receptor (GR)
Glucocorticoid-response elements (GREs)
Hirsutism
Hypokalemia and metabolic alkalosis
Juxtaglomerular cells
Liddle syndrome
Macula densa
Masculinization
Melanocortin-2 receptor (MC2R)
Mineralocorticoid
Mineralocorticoid receptor (MR)
Norepinephrine
Phenylethanolamine-N-methyl transferase (PNMT)
Pheochromocytoma Progesterone (P4)
Renal outer medullary K+ (ROMK) channel
Renin
Renin-angiotensin system (RAS)
Salt wasting and dehydration
Scavenger receptor-BI (SR-BI; the HDL receptor)
Steroidogenic acute regulatory protein (StAR protein)
Suprarenal glands
Type 1 pseudohypoaldosteronism
PHA1
Tyrosine hydroxylase
Vasopressin (ADH)
Zona fasciculate
Zona glomerulosa
Zona reticularis

Life Cycle of the Male and Female Reproductive Systems

OBJECTIVES

1. Map out an overview of meiosis.
2. Describe the general anatomic components of the male and female reproductive systems.
3. Describe the development of the male and female reproductive systems in utero.
4. Describe the regulation of puberty.
5. Describe the changes in adolescent boys and girls that occur during puberty (Tanner stages).
6. Explain the causes and physiologic changes that occur during menopause.
7. Explain the decline of androgens in men (andropause).

Many of the functional deficiencies and clinical syndromes associated with reproduction are linked to the following elements in some way (as a cause or as a consequence):

- **Embryonic development** of the male and female systems
- Onset of reproductive maturity and activity at **puberty**
- Age-related changes that lead to a decline in reproductive function with aging (**menopause and andropause**)

Thus before discussing the male and female reproductive systems in detail, it is useful to familiarize oneself with the general components of each system and their changes in development and function during life.

GENERAL COMPONENTS OF A REPRODUCTIVE SYSTEM

The two anatomic components of the reproductive system are the **gonads** and the **reproductive tracts**. The gonads (**testes** in men, **ovaries** in women) have both endocrine and exocrine functions, because they produce hormones and gametes (sperm and eggs). The major hormone product of the testes is **testosterone**. The major hormone products of the ovaries are **estrogen** before ovulation and **progesterone plus estrogen** after ovulation. Like the thyroid and adrenal glands, adult gonadal endocrine function is regulated within a **hypothalamus-pituitary-gonadal axis**. The female reproductive axis is remarkable in that it involves both negative and positive feedback. The testes produce **sperm** essentially in a

continuous manner, whereas the ovaries produce **eggs** in a discontinuous manner at a rate of about one egg per month.

The **reproductive tracts** (also referred to as *internal and external genitalia*) serve to transport gametes and, in women, allow for fertilization, implantation, gestation, and labor. Because natural fertilization in humans involves internal insemination of the female tract by the male, the male tract includes an intromittent organ, the **penis**, and the female tract includes the copulatory organ (and birth canal), the **vagina**. The external portions of the tracts, called the **external genitalia**, receive innervation that is associated with sexual excitement and orgasm, thereby reinforcing human sex drive. The **mammary glands** are an adjunct to the female reproductive system, providing nourishment and immune protection to the newborn and infant. Normal gametogenesis in the gonads, the development and physiology of the male and female reproductive tracts, and postpubertal development of the breasts are absolutely dependent on the endocrine function of the gonads.

OVERVIEW OF MEIOSIS

Sexual reproduction in humans requires the production of specialized **haploid cells** (called **gametes**) through the process of **meiosis** (Fig. 8.1). The male gametes are called sperm and are produced in the testes. The female gametes are called **eggs** (or ova) and are produced in the ovaries. **Sexual reproduction** has the advantage of generating

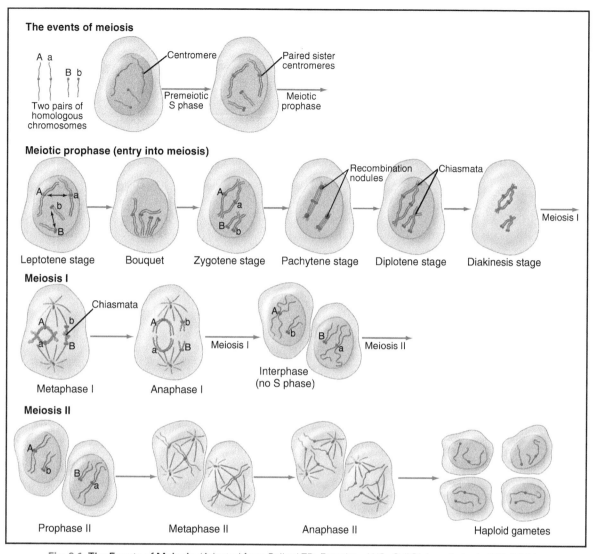

The events of meiosis

A a
B b
Two pairs of homologous chromosomes

Centromere
Premeiotic S phase

Paired sister centromeres
Meiotic prophase

Meiotic prophase (entry into meiosis)

Recombination nodules
Chiasmata

A   a
b
B

Leptotene stage   Bouquet   Zygotene stage   Pachytene stage   Diplotene stage   Diakinesis stage

Meiosis I

Meiosis I

Chiasmata

A   b
a   B

Metaphase I   Anaphase I

A   b
a   B

Meiosis I

A
b
B
a

Interphase (no S phase)

Meiosis II

Meiosis II

A
b
B
a

Prophase II   Metaphase II   Anaphase II   Haploid gametes

Fig. 8.1 **The Events of Meiosis.** (Adapted from Pollard TD, Earnshaw WC: *Cell Biology,* 2nd ed., Philadelphia, 2008, Saunders.)

new genotypes within the progeny, thereby increasing the **genetic diversity** of a species. Genetic diversity in humans is advantageous primarily because it dilutes out the dosage and effects of deleterious mutations, although it also has adaptive value. The diversification of genetic material occurs during sexual reproduction at three levels:

1. In humans, the 23 chromosomes from the father are complemented by 23 homologous chromosomes from the mother after fertilization. This generates 46,XX or 46,XY individuals with DNA from two unrelated individuals.

2. Meiosis promotes the random recombination of chromosomes. During production of gametes, the 23 pairs of chromosomal homologs undergo **independent assortment** during meiosis so that the possible combinations of chromosomes in a haploid gamete equals 2^{23}, or 8,400,000 genetically distinct gametes.

3. Before entry into meiosis, chromosomes are replicated, generating **sister chromatids** that closely adhere to each other along their length. During the first meiotic prophase, homologous chromosomes (now as

sister chromatids) **pair**, forming a **bivalent**. Before or during pairing, double-stranded breaks are induced in a chromatid, followed by the complex process of **crossing-over** between homologous chromosomes. This process occurs at two or three sites in each chromosome and introduces **genetic recombination**, thereby further scrambling the DNA that will reside in a gamete.

As shown in Fig. 8.1, meiosis consists of two phases. During the premeiotic prophase, chromosomes are replicated and consist of **sister chromatids** that are tightly adhered to each other at the centromeres and along their entire length. **Prophase I** involves the complex process of **crossing-over**, followed by **alignment and disjunction** (separation) of the homologous chromosomes. Because of crossing-over, points of chromosomal adhesion, called **chiasmata**, occur. Chiasmata resist separation of homologous chromosomes and thereby help to guide the alignment of chromosomes along the metaphase plate. Chiasmata are disassembled during **anaphase I,** allowing the disjunction (separation) of homologous chromosomes.

A **kinetochore** is a large protein complex associated with the **centromere** of a chromosome and connects to **microtubule spindles** that pull the chromatids to opposite poles. Importantly, in meiosis I, the kinetochores of the sister chromatids rotate and fuse to each other. This results in the movement of sister chromatids to the same pole at anaphase I. Consequently, homologous chromosomes are separated during meiosis I, but chromatids are not (see Fig. 8.1). After meiosis I, cells enter a brief interphase, but do not replicate DNA (i.e., no S phase). During this time, sister chromatids become separated, except at their centromeres. **Meiosis II** proceeds much more rapidly and involves the separation of chromatids. This involves the loss of cohesion between sister centromeres at anaphase II so that kinetochores can become attached to spindles on opposite poles. The final product is haploid gametes.

As discussed later, there are striking sex-specific differences in the details of meiotic induction and progression, as well as in gamete maturation, interaction with somatic nurse cells, and release.

CLINICAL BOX 8.1

Although meiosis and sexual reproduction confer concrete advantages to humans, correct **disjunction** or separation of chromosomes must occur at both phases of meiosis to maintain the integrity of the genotype (i.e., maintenance of **euploidy**). Failure of correct separation in either meiosis I or meiosis II is called **nondisjunction** and results in the addition of genetic material at one pole and the deletion of genetic material at the opposite pole. Nondisjunction causes **aneuploidy** (one or more chromosomes are not diploid) or **polyploidy** (all chromosomes are not diploid). It is likely that the resulting gametes, if they participate in fertilization and embryogenesis, will result in spontaneous abortion. The mistake of nondisjunction occurs with alarming frequency, in that 50% of conceptions are estimated to result in spontaneous abortion, of which more than 60% are caused by aneuploidy. Overall, spontaneous abortion acts as a safeguard against mistakes in chromosome number. In rare cases, aneuploid individuals survive. For example, gain of an extra chromosome 21 (**trisomy 21**) is compatible with life and results in **Down syndrome**. These individuals suffer abnormal development of the CNS and a decreased life expectancy.

BASIC ANATOMY OF THE REPRODUCTIVE SYSTEMS

Overview of the Male Reproductive System

The **testes** are the male gonads. Each testis (right and left) resides outside of the abdominopelvic cavity within the scrotum (Fig. 8.2). The testis produces sperm within tubules (seminiferous tubules). The lumina of the tubules empty into the anastomosing network of tubules called the **rete testis**, which in turn empty into about 20 **efferent ductules**. Ultimately, efferent ductules converge into one lumen in the **epididymis**. The right and left **epididymides, vas deferens,** and **ejaculatory ducts** transport sperm from each testis to the midline **male urethra**.

The male tract also contains two large accessory sex glands, the **seminal vesicles** and the **prostate**. These glands produce most of the volume of the **semen**, which mixes with spermatozoa as they enter the urethra. Semen components largely provide a buffered, bacteriostatic, and nutrient-rich microenvironment for sperm after ejaculation into the vagina.

The male urethra becomes the distal portion of the male tract and consists of **prostatic** (intrapelvic), **membranous** (a short segment within the deep perineal space), and **penile** (extrapelvic in superficial perineal space) segments. The urethra receives lubricating and cleansing secretions from the paired bulbourethral glands and the paraurethral glands (glands of Littre). The penile segment courses through the length of the penis. The **penis** serves as an intromittent organ designed for internal

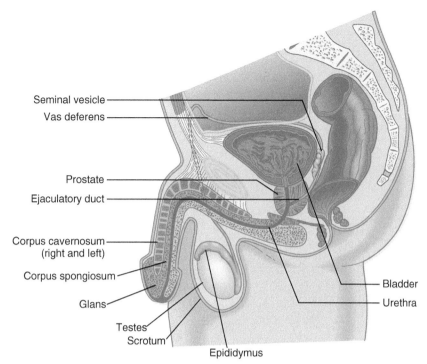

Fig. 8.2 The anatomy of the male reproductive tract. (Adapted from Koeppen BM, Stanton BA: *Berne and Levy Physiology,* 7th ed., updated edition, Philadelphia, 2017, Mosby.)

insemination within the vagina. Sensory (pudendal) innervation of the penis leads to **orgasm** during coitus, thereby reinforcing libido.

The Female Reproductive System

The **ovaries** are the female gonads. Each ovary (right and left) resides within the pelvic cavity (Fig. 8.3). There are no tubules in the ovary. Instead, the gametes (primary oocytes) become invested with epithelial and stromal cells that make up an **ovarian follicle; one follicle contains a single oocyte.** With growth, the follicle ultimately creates a fluid-filled lumen (called an **antrum**). At the time of gamete release, the gamete (now an egg arrested in meiotic metaphase II) and a thin covering of epithelial cells become free-floating within this lumen. Ovulation involves a complex set of events that essentially erode the follicular and ovarian walls at the point where the follicle is pushing against the ovarian surface, followed by the release of the egg.

Unlike the male tract, the egg is released into the pelvic cavity and has to be captured by the proximal segment of the female tract called the **oviduct** (see Fig. 8.3). The oviduct has an opening at its proximal, free end (the infundibulum), through which the captured egg is transported.

There is usually only one egg ovulated, either from the right or left side, depending on which side had the largest follicle at the beginning of the menstrual cycle. The oviduct transports the egg toward the midline **uterus** and allows for the movement of sperm from the uterus laterally toward the egg. Fertilization and early development (5 to 6 days) normally occur in the oviduct. The early embryo (blastocyst) eventually moves into the uterine lumen and implants into the uterine mucosa. The growing fetus is supported in part by the elastic and fibrous inferior end of the uterus called the **cervix**. At term, the newborn is expelled from the uterus through the cervix and vagina.

The **vagina** acts as both the copulatory organ and the birth canal. The female external genitalia surround the superficial opening of the vagina (called **introitus**). The **labia majora** are homologous to an unclosed scrotum. **Vestibular bulbs** (deep to the **labia minora**) and the **clitoris** represent structures homologous to the erectile tissue of the penis. However, unlike the penis, erection of these structures is not required for fertility. Sensory (pudendal) innervation of these structures and the vaginal wall may lead to **orgasm** during coitus, thereby providing reinforcement to libido.

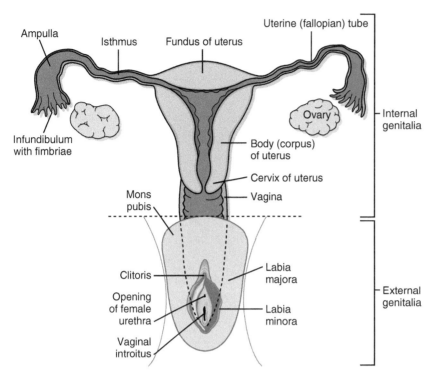

Fig. 8.3 The anatomy of the female reproductive tract. (Adapted from Koeppen BM, Stanton BA: *Berne and Levy Physiology*, 7th ed., updated edition, Philadelphia, 2017; Mosby.)

SEXUAL DEVELOPMENT IN UTERO

The **genetic sex** of a fetus depends on the nature of the sex chromosomes contributed by the egg and the sperm. Normally, there are 46 chromosomes, consisting of 22 pairs of autosomes and one pair of sex chromosomes. The sex chromosomes are called *X* and *Y* chromosomes; **46,XX** is the normal karyotype for the female, and **46,XY** is the normal karyotype for the male. **Genetic sex determines gonadal sex.** The gonads then either produce **hormones** (if male) or **no hormones** (if female). The hormonal environment determines the sex of the reproductive tract and external genitalia.

Male Development

During the first 6 weeks of development, mesodermal cells within the genital ridge develop into a **bipotential gonadal primordium** (Table 8.1). During this period, **primordial germ cells** migrate from the yolk sac endoderm into the gonadal tissue. By 6 weeks of gestation, the gonads contain germ cells, supporting cells, and stromal cells that will become androgen-producing steroidogenic cells in both sexes.

The short arm of the Y chromosome contains the *SRY* **gene** (sex-determining region on the Y chromosome) that encodes the transcription factor, **SRY**. SRY, along with other

TABLE 8.1   Time Frame for Fetal Development of Male Reproductive System

Gestational Age (wk)	Developmental Feature
6-8	Differentiation of testes
8	Retention of Wolffian ducts
	Regression of Müllerian ducts
9-12	Development of male-type external genitalia

transcription factors, plays a major role in the induction of differentiation of the bipotential gonad into a **testis** between weeks 6 and 7 of gestation (Fig. 8.4). With testicular development, the supportive epithelial cells differentiate into **Sertoli cells** and form the **seminiferous tubules.** Sertoli cells perform two critical functions in early embryogenesis: (1) they surround male germ cells (called **spermatogonia**) and produce an enzyme (CYP26B1; also produced by Leydig cells) that degrades locally produced **retinoic acid**, thereby preventing meiotic progression of spermatogonia; and (2) they express **antimüllerian hormone** (**AMH**, also referred to as **müllerian-inhibitory substance**), which causes the degeneration of the müllerian ducts (see later in the text).

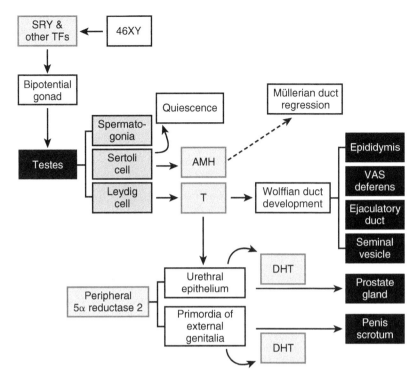

Fig. 8.4 Embryonic development of the male reproductive system. *AMH,* Antimüllerian hormone; *DHT,* dihydrotestosterone; *T,* testosterone; *TFs,* transcription factors.

Hormones mediate **phenotypic gender** expression. The fetus originally develops with bipotential internal and external genitalia (Figs. 8.5 and 8.6). Internally, there are two **Wolffian** (also called **mesonephric) ducts,** which have the potential for differentiating into the nonurethral segment of the male tract (epididymis, vas deferens, ejaculatory duct, and seminal vesicles), and two **Müllerian** (also called **paramesonephric) ducts,** which have the potential for differentiating into most of the female reproductive tract (the oviducts, uterus, cervix, and proximal third of the vagina). Whether male or female reproductive tracts develop depends on the presence or absence of two hormones produced by the fetal testis-**testosterone and AMH** (Box 8.1).

The persistence and differentiation of the **Wolffian ducts** into the proximal nonurethral male tract requires testosterone (see Fig. 8.4). By week 8, testosterone is produced by stromal cells that have differentiated into **Leydig cells.** Androgen production is first promoted by the placental, luteinizing hormone (LH)-like hormone, called **human chorionic gonadotropin (hCG),** and later by fetal pituitary LH. At this time, testosterone acts more like a paracrine factor than a true hormone, in that testosterone from each testis promotes the differentiation of the ipsilateral tract (Fig. 8.7).

The degeneration of the müllerian ducts requires production of AMH by the Sertoli cells of the testis (see Fig. 8.4). AMH is a glycoprotein homodimer belonging to the transforming growth factor-β (TGF-β) gene family. Accordingly, AMH binds to a coreceptor with serine-threonine kinase activity. AMH binds specifically to the **AMH receptor type II (AMHR-II),** which binds to and activates a type-I receptor. As described in Chapter 1, this activates a Smad-dependent signaling pathway.

CLINICAL BOX 8.2

Persistent müllerian duct syndrome (PMDS) can occur in 46,XY males. The persistence of müllerian derivatives (oviducts, uterus, cervix, vaginal tissue) frequently disrupts the descent of one or both testes, resulting in unilateral or bilateral **cryptorchidism.** Correction of cryptorchidism is performed by surgery. Mutations in both the *AMH* gene and AMH receptor II (AMHR-II) have been identified in families with PMDS. Most cases involve homozygous mutations that occur with a high frequency in certain Mediterranean and North African populations that have a high incidence of consanguinity.

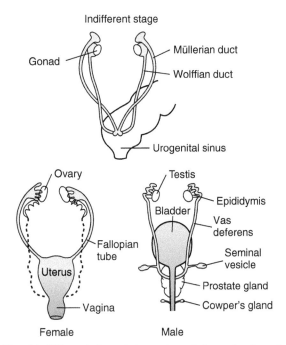

Fig. 8.5 Differentiation of internal genitalia and primordial ducts. (Redrawn from George FW, Wilson JD: Embryology of the genital tract. In Walsh PC, Retik AB, Stamey TA, Vaughan ED, editors: *Campbell's Urology*, 6th ed., Philadelphia, 1992, Saunders.)

The differentiation of the prostate gland and male external genitalia occurs between week 9 and week 11 (Box 8.2; see Figs. 8.5 and 8.6). This requires the expression of an enzyme, 5α-reductase-2, within the primordia of these structures (urogenital sinus, genital tubercle urethral folds, and labioscrotal swellings). 5α-reductase-2 catalyzes the peripheral conversion of testosterone to dihydrotestosterone (DHT). Testosterone and DHT bind to the same androgen receptor, but DHT is required in these tissues. The cell-specific actions of testosterone and DHT are not completely understood but may depend on cell-specific expression of coregulatory proteins, the chromatin context of cell-specific androgen-regulated genes, or cell-specific differences in the stability of the hormone-receptor complex. In any case, conversion of testosterone to DHT is absolutely required for the normal development of the prostate and external genitalia.

CLINICAL BOX 8.3

A **5α-reductase-2 deficiency** results in decreased DHT formation. Affected persons typically have a well-developed internal male tract (except for the prostate gland), but incompletely masculinized external genitalia (i.e., **ambiguous genitalia**) with microphallus and hypospadias. The testes are either inguinal or labial. Severely affected patients can be mistaken for females at birth. The testosterone production is normal, and at puberty, when testosterone production greatly increases, some masculinization of the external genitalia may occur. Also, **5α-reductase-1** activity in the skin appears at puberty, which may generate enough DHT to induce the pubertal changes. These include increased muscle mass, deepening of the voice, and descent of the testis into the labioscrotal folds. Patients who are diagnosed in infancy are assigned a male sex and treated with androgen therapy to induce growth of the penis and surgical repair of hypospadias. A male or female sexual identity may develop in patients who are diagnosed after puberty, and they may require some form of corrective surgery. It is not uncommon for patients to switch from a female sexual identity to a male one after puberty.

FEMALE DEVELOPMENT

In a normal 46,XX embryo, the absence of SRY allows for the expression of other transcription factors that induce the differentiation of the gonad into an ovary (Fig. 8.8). However, full ovarian differentiation does not occur until the end of the first trimester of pregnancy (Box 8.3). The germ cells differentiate into oogonia and divide mitotically. Starting at about 11 weeks of gestation, all oogonia enter meiosis and become primary oocytes arrested in first meiotic prophase. Oocytes become surrounded by a single layer of squamous supportive cells called granulosa cells and their basal lamina. These structures are called primordial follicles and appear in the second trimester. Although some follicular development (see Chapter 10) occurs during pregnancy, the ovary remains hormonally quiescent during gestation.

The absence of Sertoli cell–derived AMH allows for the persistence and development of the müllerian duct into oviducts, uterus, cervix, and the inner one-third of the vagina (see Figs. 8.5 and 8.8; see Box 8.1). In the absence of a testis and testosterone, the Wolffian duct degenerates. If high testosterone levels are present in a female fetus because of a congenital adrenal hyperplasia (see Chapter 7), or because of a maternal endocrine disorder, both sets of ducts can be retained (see Fig. 8.7).

In the absence of androgen exposure, the external genitalia develop into the labia majora, labia minora, clitoris, vestibular bulbs and glands, and outer two-thirds of the vagina (see Figs. 8.6 and 8.8; see Box 8.2).

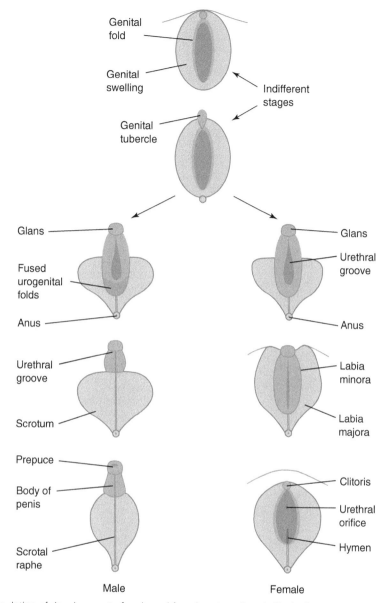

Fig. 8.6 Regulation of development of male and female external genitalia. In the presence of dihydrotestosterone (DHT) between 9 and 12 weeks of gestation, male external genitalia develop from the genital tubercle, genital fold, genital swelling, and urogenital sinus. In the absence of DHT, female external genitalia develop.

BOX 8.1 Regulation of Development of Internal Genitalia

- The Wolffian ducts, when stimulated with testosterone, become the epididymis, vas deferens, seminal vesicles, and ejaculatory ducts.
- The Müllerian ducts, in the absence of Sertoli cell Müllerian-inhibiting substance, become the fallopian tubes, uterus, cervix, and upper one-third of the vagina.

PUBERTY

Regulation of Timing of Puberty

The reproductive axis is driven by **gonadotropin-releasing hormone (GnRH) neurons** in the mediobasal hypothalamus that secrete GnRH in a pulsatile pattern. GnRH, in turn, stimulates production of pituitary LH and **follicle-stimulating hormone (FSH)** (see Chapter 5).

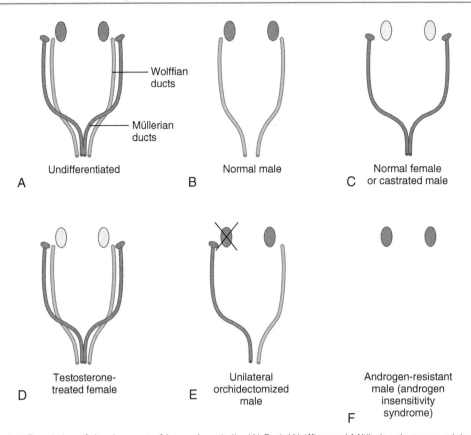

Fig. 8.7 Regulation of development of internal genitalia. (A) Both Wolffian and Müllerian ducts are originally present in both male and female fetuses (undifferentiated). (B) If functional testes are present, Wolffian ducts develop, and Müllerian ducts regress. (C) If no testes are present, Müllerian ducts develop, and Wolffian ducts are lost. (D) If a female fetus is exposed to testosterone, both ductile systems can remain. (E) If a testis is removed unilaterally (orchidectomized), the Müllerian duct will develop, and the Wolffian duct will regress on one side. (F) A male with functional testes but androgen insensitivity will show regression of both ductile systems.

BOX 8.2   Regulation of Development of External Genitalia

- *In the presence of dihydrotestosterone,* the genital tubercle, genital fold, genital swelling, and urogenital sinus become the penis, scrotum, and prostate.
- *In the absence of dihydrotestosterone,* the genital tubercle, genital fold, genital swelling, and urogenital sinus become the labia majora, labia minora, clitoris, and lower two-thirds of the vagina.

The GnRH neurons display activity during gestation, which decreases at parturition. GnRH neurons display a significant increase in activity in the first 2 years of infancy ("minipuberty of infancy"), followed by about a decade of very low activity of the reproductive axis

(Fig. 8.9). The resurgence in activity of the reproductive system during adolescence is called **puberty** and induces dramatic phenotypic and behavioral changes. These changes precede maturation of the personality and emotional stability.

The timing of puberty is variable among countries and among ethnic populations within countries. In the United States the average age of puberty in girls has declined over the past half-century, probably because of enhanced health and nutrition and, more recently, possibly because of increased rates of childhood obesity (although this has not been firmly established). African American girls typically reach pubertal milestones about 6 months earlier than Caucasian girls. The clinical significance of the timing of puberty relates to underlying disorders or diseases that induce the onset of puberty at an abnormally young age (called **precocious puberty**), or at an abnormally older age

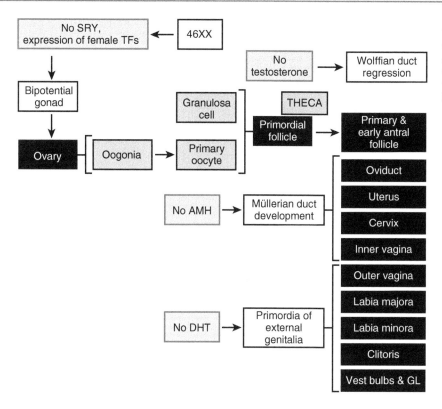

Fig. 8.8 Embryonic development of the female reproductive system. *AMH*, Antimüllerian hormone; *DHT*, dihydrotestosterone; *TFs*, transcription factors; *Vest bulbs & GL*, vestibular bulbs and gland.

BOX 8.3   Time Frame for Fetal Development of the Female Reproductive System

7 to 12 Weeks
- Meiosis of oogonia and arrest at first meiotic prophase
- Ovarian organogenesis
- Formation of primordial follicles

11 to 12 Weeks
- Oviducts, uterus, cervix, external genitalia, and vagina

20 to 25 Weeks
- Primary follicles in ovary

(**delayed puberty**), or not at all. The average age of breast development (first sign of puberty) in North American girls is about 10 years old. The average age of testicular enlargement (first sign of puberty) in North American boys is about 11.5 years old. The threshold for earliest onset of normal versus precocious puberty is 8 years in girls and 9 years in boys. These ages may be too high as the age of puberty declines.

After birth, the reproductive axes of both sexes show significant activity for 1 to 2 years (see Fig. 8.9). This is followed by the development of mechanisms that imposes a significant (but not absolute) suppression of GnRH neuronal activity. The exact nature of the inhibitory signals that result in the "nadir of childhood" reproductive activity remains poorly understood. The fact that some tumors that cause swelling or tissue destruction in the vicinity of the posterior hypothalamus can induce **gonadotropin-dependent precocious puberty** has led some to propose the existence of an inhibitory center within the central nervous system (CNS). There is also some evidence for an exquisite sensitivity of the hypothalamus and pituitary to negative feedback by steroid hormones (i.e., a low setpoint, or gonadostat). This is indicated by the findings that primary agonadal children typically have higher gonadotropin levels than normal children (although gonadotropin levels are low in both cases because of CNS inhibition). At puberty, these inhibitory mechanisms are presumably terminated.

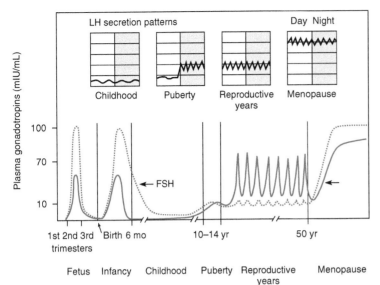

Fig. 8.9 Relative serum luteinizing hormone *(LH)* and follicle-stimulating hormone *(FSH)* levels across the life span in women. (Redrawn from Braunwald E, et al: *Harrison's Principles of Internal Medicine,* 4th ed., New York, 1987, McGraw-Hill.)

In addition to the release from CNS inhibition, there is also strong evidence for the activation of stimulatory centers in the CNS that induce pulsatile GnRH production at puberty. Recently much attention has been given to the role of the neurotransmitter **Kisspeptin (Kiss1)** as an inducer of GnRH pulsatile release at puberty. Kisspeptin is encoded by the **KISS1 gene.** Kiss1 is a 54-amino acid peptide that is expressed by neurons in the hypothalamus. Kiss1 acts through a G-protein–coupled receptor called **Kiss1R** (previously called GPR54), which is expressed by GnRH neurons. Kiss1 levels increase in the hypothalamus at puberty, and intracerebral infusion of Kiss1 in female monkeys induced precocious puberty. Null mutations in Kiss1R have been described in individuals with compromised pubertal changes, whereas gain-of-function mutations in human Kiss1 and Kiss1R cause gonadotropin-dependent precocious puberty.

During the **peripubertal period**, pulsatile sleep-associated surges in GnRH begin to occur (see Fig. 8.9). Gonadotrope sensitivity to GnRH increases, resulting in an increase in LH secretion. At puberty, the frequency and amplitude of the GnRH pulses increase. This change increases LH and FSH secretion throughout the day and ultimately gonadal steroid hormone production. The maturation of the positive feedback by estrogen on GnRH and gonadotropin secretion in women occurs late in puberty (see Fig. 8.9; spikes during reproductive years). The first menstrual period (**menarche**) occurs, average, 2.6 years after the onset of puberty.

CLINICAL BOX 8.4

Kallmann syndrome type 1 is a **tertiary** (i.e., hypothalamic) endocrine disorder and a form of isolated **hypogonatropic hypogonadism**. This genetic disorder is often associated with anosmia (absence of sense of smell) or hyposmia (poor sense of smell). It is due to loss of a functional protein, called *anosmin,* that is encoded by the X-linked *KAL1* gene. The syndrome is caused by the inability of all or some of the **GnRH neurons** to properly migrate to the mediobasal hypothalamus from the nasal placode (see Chapter 5). Anosmin is similar to adhesion molecules, and so may play a guiding role in GnRH migration. Males are more frequently affected than females. Men affected with this disorder have undescended testes (**cryptorchism**). Although there is normal embryonic differentiation of the Wolffian duct–derived structures, penis development is deficient, and microphallus often develops. These effects probably result from the fact that early fetal development of the internal genitalia is controlled by testicular androgens that are initially regulated by **placental hCG** (see Chapter 11), rather than fetal LH. Adult growth and function of Wolffian duct–derived structures and prostate gland are impaired. The inability of the fetus to secrete normal quantities of LH has an impact on testicular function later in development, when androgens regulate growth of the external genitalia. The severity of the impairment of LH secretion is variable, as is the severity of the reproductive problems associated with the disorder. Puberty is delayed.

TABLE 8.2   Tanner Pubertal Stages in Male

Stage	Genitals	Pubic Hair
1	Preadolescent	Preadolescent; no pubic hair
2	Scrotum and testes enlarge; change in scrotal skin texture	Sparse, long, downy pubic hair, chiefly at base of penis
3	Growth of penis in length and further growth of testes and scrotum	Hair darker and coarser
4	Growth of penis in length and breadth, darkening of scrotal skin	Adult-type hair, but area covered is less than that in adult
5	Adult-sized genitalia	Adult hair texture and quantity; hair is distributed in diamond-shaped escutcheon with hair extending up linea alba

Data from Marshall WA, Tanner JM: Variations in the pattern of pubertal changes in boys. *Arch Dis Child* 45:13, 1970.

TABLE 8.3   Tanner Pubertal Stages in Female

Stage	Breast	Pubic Hair
1	Prepubertal	Prepubertal; no pubic hair
2	Breast bud and papilla elevated; small mound present	Slight growth of fine, downy hair
3	Enlargement of breast mound; palpable glandular tissue	Hair darker, coiled, denser
4	Areola and nipple elevated	Adult-type hair, but area covered is less than in adult
5	Adult breast	Adult-type hair with triangular-shaped distribution

Data from Marshall WA, Tanner JM: Variations in pattern of pubertal changes in girls. *Arch Dis Child* 44:291, 1969.

Physiologic Changes Associated With Puberty

The developmental milestones associated with puberty in British boys and girls were objectively described by Marshall and Tanner and are referred to as **Tanner stages**. The progression of secondary sex characteristics was characterized as having five stages, ending in adults as stage 5. For boys, these changes include testicular size, penis size (Table 8.2), and pubic hair. For girls, these changes include breast development (Table 8.3) and pubic hair. Changes are driven by increasing sex steroids. Also, adrenal androgens increase (**adrenarche**) before gonadal gametogenesis and hormonogenesis (**gonadarche**), at about 6 to 7 years of age in girls and 7 to 8 years of age in boys. Adrenal androgens are converted to testosterone, DHT, and estradiol and therefore contribute to growth of pubic and axillary hair, particularly in girls.

Males

The first sign of puberty (Tanner stage 1) in males is an increase in **testicular volume** (Fig. 8.10). Before puberty, there are a few partially differentiated Leydig cells. During puberty, the steroid-producing Leydig cells differentiate from mesenchymal peritubular cells and divide to form

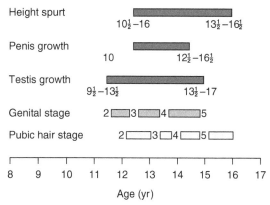

Fig. 8.10 Normal sequence of changes of male puberty. Numbers 2 to 5 refer to Tanner stages. (Data from Marshall WA, Tanner JM: Variations in the pattern of pubertal changes in boys. *Arch Dis Child* 45:13, 1970.)

the typical clusters seen in the adult testis. Within the seminiferous tubules, meiosis and spermatogenesis are initiated at puberty, and while testosterone and FSH levels increase, the rate of spermatogenesis reaches adult levels. The sperm-supporting Sertoli cells divide and become

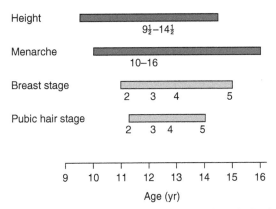

Fig. 8.11 Sequence of events during female puberty indicating ranges of ages at which each event normally occurs. Numbers 2 to 5 refer to Tanner stages. (Data from Marshall WA, Tanner JM: Variations in the pattern of pubertal changes in boys. *Arch Dis Child* 45:13, 1970.)

more active at puberty, forming the occluding junctions and performing other hormonally dependent functions, including secretion of fluid. **Spermarche** represents the age at first ejaculation as nocturnal emissions and sperm in the urine.

Puberty is associated with numerous primary and secondary sexual changes, including growth and onset of function of the prostate and seminal vesicles; increased growth of the penis; increased muscle mass; thickening of vocal cords; appearance of pubic (**pubarche**), facial, and body hair; and development of libido (see Table 8.2). Many of these changes are dependent on the conversion of testosterone to DHT.

Females

The timing of puberty in females is influenced by the level of body fat, as lean girls tend to enter puberty later than heavier girls, while female athletes with low body fat levels often have amenorrhea. This may be due in part to the fact that adipose tissue expresses significant levels of CYP19 (aromatase), which aromatizes androgens to estrogens (see Chapter 9). Growing evidence, however, suggests that leptin, which is also produced by adipose tissue, plays a permissive role in hypothalamic maturation at puberty. Several years before menarche (onset of menstrual cycles), adrenarche occurs. This is manifested by the development of pubic hair and axillary hair.

A hallmark of puberty in women is breast growth with some limited development (Fig. 8.11). At puberty, the increase in estrogen induces an enlargement and darkening of the areola, which is the pigmented, hairless circle surrounding the nipple, and some limited ductal growth beneath the areola and nipple. The onset of these mammary gland changes is referred to as **thelarche**. Once ovulatory cycles begin, progesterone stimulates further growth and maturation of the mammary glands. Progesterone also increases stromal edema and vacuolation of the epithelia, thereby inducing a sensation of fullness or tenderness during the late luteal phase (see Chapter 10). Table 8.3 shows the Tanner stages of pubertal development for women, and Fig. 8.11 shows the ages at which these changes occur.

The pubertal growth spurt refers to a significant increase in growth velocity. The growth spurt occurs early in puberty in girls, but toward the end of puberty in boys. The growth spurt is under complex hormonal regulation, involving triiodothyronine (T_3), growth hormone and its target, insulin-like growth factor-I (IGF-I), and sex steroids. Estradiol promotes normal bone density in both sexes. Also, estradiol promotes the cessation of long bone growth by inducing the closure of the epiphyseal plates in both sexes. Men who either have a null mutation in the estrogen receptor (ERα) or are deficient in CYP19-aromatase continue long-bone growth well beyond their second decade.

MENOPAUSE AND ANDROPAUSE

Menopause

As discussed earlier, all ovarian oogonia commit to meiosis, so no stem cell population exists (as it does in the testis). Menopause generally is thought to result from primary ovarian deficiency due to depletion of a sufficient number of functional follicles. Menopause typically occurs between 46 and 55 years of age. It extends over several years. Initially, the cycles become irregular and are periodically anovulatory. This is referred to as the **menopausal transition**. The cycles tend to shorten, primarily in the follicular phase. Eventually, the woman ceases to cycle altogether. The final menstrual period is determined retrospectively after 1 year of amenorrhea, and the stage of life from this final period to death is termed **postmenopause**.

The observation that some morphologically normal oocytes can be present in the postmenopausal ovary, however, suggests that oocyte depletion is not the sole cause of menopause. These remaining follicles are hypothesized to be less sensitive to gonadotropins. It has been proposed recently that age-related changes in the CNS, including critical patterns of GnRH secretion, precede follicular depletion and may play an important role in menopause. Because follicles do not develop in response to LH and FSH secretion, estrogen and progesterone levels drop. Loss of the negative feedback inhibition of estrogen on GnRH, LH, and FSH results in a marked rise in serum LH and FSH. FSH levels rise more than LH levels. This may result from ovarian inhibin loss.

The serum estradiol levels drop to about one-sixth the mean levels in younger cycling women, and progesterone levels drop to about one-third those in the follicular phase in younger women. Production of these hormones does not cease entirely, but the primary source of estradiol and active androgens (testosterone, DHT) in the postmenopausal woman becomes the peripheral conversion of adrenal androgens. Because estrone is the primary estrogen produced in adipose tissue, it becomes the predominant circulating form of estrogen in postmenopausal women. The decrease in circulating levels of sex steroids and inhibin results in an increase in gonadotropins, especially FSH. FSH levels increase even before the menopausal transition.

Most of the signs and symptoms associated with menopause result from estrogen deficiency. Some of the consequences of estrogen loss at menopause are the following:

1. The vaginal epithelium atrophies, becomes dry, and with loss of vaginal flora, increases in pH. These changes often result in increased incidence of vaginal and urinary tract infections, as well as pain during intercourse.
2. Bone loss is accelerated, potentially leading to osteoporosis. The effect of menopause on osteoporosis is staggering: greater than 1 million fractures per year occur in the United States due to menopausal osteoporosis. A significant fraction of these fractures are hip fractures, which greatly increase morbidity and mortality and increase the loss of independence.
3. Hot flashes result from periodic increases in core temperature, which produce peripheral vasodilation, sweating, and a feeling of malaise. Hot flashes are also correlated with sleep disturbances, which can significantly affect a woman's daily productivity and quality of life. Hot flashes are correlated with LH pulses, and current thinking proposes that a CNS mechanism leads to both events. Hot flashes typically subside within 1 to 5 years of the onset of menopausal symptoms.
4. The incidence of cardiovascular disease increases markedly after menopause. This is due, in part, to the reversal of the beneficial effect of estrogen on high-density lipoprotein levels. However, lifestyle plays an important role, and menopause can affect lifestyle—if a woman is losing sleep because of hot flashes, she is less likely to exercise during the day. There are other psychosocial effects of menopause, including fatigue and depression.

Most of the menopausal sequelae respond well to estrogen replacement therapy (ERT), or estrogen and progesterone replacement therapy (hormone replacement therapy, or HRT). Results from the Women's Health Initiative and other studies, however, have provided conflicting findings on the safety of estrogens and progestins (which were not in the form of bioidentical estradiol-17β and progesterone) for HRT in postmenopausal women, emphasizing the need for physicians to fully consider each woman's individual medical and family history before deciding on the course of therapy for the alleviation of postmenopausal symptoms. In general, use of the lowest effective dose and for the shortest effective duration is standard. New analysis from the Women's Health Initiative indicates that ERT given before the age of 60 years (i.e., short-term ERT) was not associated with an increased risk for thromboembolic events, stroke, or breast cancer.

Andropause

There is no distinct andropause in men. As men age, however, gonadal sensitivity to LH decreases and androgen production drops. While this occurs, serum LH and FSH levels rise. Although sperm production typically begins to decline after age 50 years, many men can maintain reproductive function and spermatogenesis throughout life.

SUMMARY

1. The male and female reproductive systems are composed of a gonad (testis and ovary) and a reproductive tract.
2. The gonads perform an endocrine function, which is regulated within a hypothalamic-pituitary-gonad axis.
3. The gonads perform an exocrine function by the production of gametes. This function is absolutely dependent on gonadal hormones.
4. Meiosis is central to sexual reproduction. Meiosis generates haploid gametes through two divisions, meiosis I and meiosis II, with no DNA synthesis in between. The major advantage of sexual reproduction is the recombination of genetic material. This occurs by independent segregation of chromosomes, combining the haploid genome of eggs with the haploid genome of sperm, and through crossing-over.
5. The process of crossing-over involves synapsis of homologous chromosomes (each with two sister chromatids) to form a bivalent, followed by a complex process that exchanges DNA sequence information between homologous strands. Chiasmata form at

these sites, which help organize chromosomes at the metaphase plate.

6. Chromosomes must undergo accurate disjunction (separation) in both divisions. Defects in disjunction lead to nondisjunction, resulting in aneuploidy or polyploidy.

7. The male reproductive system includes the testis, in which the seminiferous tubules generate spermatozoa. These are guided out of the testis by the rete testis and efferent ductules. Sperm then enter the epididymis, vas deferens, ejaculatory duct, and male urethra. Sperm receive seminal fluid (semen) from the seminal vesicles and the prostate. The tract ends in the penis, which is an intromittent organ designed for internal semination.

8. The female reproductive system includes the ovaries, oviducts, uterus, cervix, vagina, and external genitalia. The female tract does not join with the female urethra.

9. The gamete within the ovary is a primary oocyte arrested in prophase of meiosis I. Just before ovulation, the oocyte completes meiosis I and becomes arrested at metaphase of meiosis II (now called an *egg*).

10. Release of an egg involves a complex process that includes the focal breakdown of the follicular and ovarian walls.

11. Early embryos have a bipotential gonad, into which primordial germ cells have migrated from the yolk sac. Genetic sex (46,XY or 46,XX) determines gonadal sex. Gonadal sex will create a hormonal environment that determines the development of the reproductive tract and external genitalia.

12. SRY is a major factor involved in male development (formation of a testis) at 6 to 7 weeks of gestation.

13. Formation of a testis involves the organization of seminiferous tubules lined by spermatogonia and Sertoli cells. Leydig cells develop in the peritubular compartment.

14. Meiosis is blocked in the male by the production of CYP26B1, which breaks down and inactivates retinoic acid.

15. Sertoli cells secrete AMH, thereby inducing the regression of the female Müllerian tract.

16. Leydig cells, under stimulation by hCG and, later, fetal LH, produce testosterone. Testosterone promotes the differentiation of the Wolffian tract into the epididymis, vas deferens, ejaculatory duct, and seminal vesicle.

17. Testosterone also induces descent of the testis into the scrotum.

18. Testosterone is peripherally converted to DHT by 5α-reductase-2. DHT induces the differentiation of the urogenital sinus into the proximal male urethra and the prostate gland. DHT induces the primordia of the external genitalia to form the penis and scrotum.

19. A deficiency of 5α-reductase-2 may lead to female or ambiguous external genitalia in a 46,XY fetus. The female phenotype changes to a male phenotype at puberty, requiring reassessment of sexual identity, followed by appropriate surgery and hormonal replacement.

20. Lack of SRY in a 46,XX female embryo allows female-specific transcription factors to drive ovarian differentiation. This is completed much later than testicular differentiation.

21. Oogonia develop from primordial germ cells and divide mitotically to generate about 1 million oogonia per ovary. All oogonia enter meiosis and become oocytes arrested at the prophase of meiosis I. Oocytes become surrounded by epithelial cells and their basal lamina, generating a structure called the primordial follicle.

22. Absence of AMH allows the female Müllerian duct to develop into the oviducts, uterus, cervix, and the inner one-third of the vagina. Absence of testosterone causes the male Wolffian duct to regress. Absence of DHT allows the external genitalia to form female structures (labia majora, labia minora, clitoris, vestibular bulbs and glands) and the outer two-thirds of the vagina.

23. The human reproductive axis involves hypothalamic pulsatile GnRH neurons and pituitary gonadotropes that secrete LH and FSH. After significant activity in early infancy, the reproductive axis diminishes to very low activity for about a decade. This may be due to both active inhibition from the CNS and exquisite sensitivity to negative feedback.

24. Puberty involves a significant activation of the reproductive axes and the reproductive system. This probably involves cessation of CNS inhibition, along with stimulation by other CNS centers.

25. Kisspeptin (Kiss1) is produced in the hypothalamus and binds to its receptor, Kiss1R, on GnRH neurons. Null mutation in Kiss1R cause deficient GnRH-dependent pubertal changes. Gain-of-function mutations in both Kiss1 and Kiss1R have been linked to precocious puberty.

26. The progression of puberty is semiquantified by the five Tanner stages. In boys, these involve assessment of testicular size (volume), penile growth, and pubic hair growth. In girls, Tanner staging involves assessment of breast development and pubic hair growth.

27. The pubertal growth spurt begins in early puberty in girls and in late puberty in boys. This involves an

increase in the growth velocity, which is dependent on increased growth hormone, IGF-I, T_3, and sex steroids.

28. Menopause involves the great diminution of ovarian steroid and inhibin output, probably owing to insufficient number of gonadotropin-responsive follicles. LH and FSH levels increase.

29. Menopause may be accompanied by thinning of the vagina, vasomotor instability (hot flashes), sleep disturbances, personality changes, osteoporosis, and an increased risk for cardiovascular disease.

30. Men do not experience an abrupt cessation in the reproductive axis. Some men are fertile at advanced ages. Some men experience a decrease in androgen production (an incomplete andropause), along with symptoms such as low libido and erectile dysfunction.

SELF-STUDY PROBLEMS

1. How does sexual reproduction increase genetic diversity?

2. Explain how a 46,XX embryo would develop in the presence of an SRY-autosome translocation (i.e., gain of SRY).

3. Explain the gonadal, internal tract, and external genitalia in a 46,XY individual with a null mutation in the AMH receptor.

4. Compare the adult male and adult female reproductive systems in terms of onset and progression of meiosis.

5. Explain why Wolffian duct derivatives develop in embryos with Kallmann syndrome type 1.

6. How do gain-of-function mutations in Kiss1R affect the timing of puberty?

7. Why do women become infertile at menopause, whereas men may remain fertile into their ninth decade?

8. List the consequences of menopause.

KEYWORDS AND CONCEPTS

Adrenarche, menopause
Andropause, precocious puberty
Anatomy of male and female reproductive tracts
Embryonic development: male and female reproductive systems
Differentiation of internal and external genitalia
Testosterone
5α-reductase
Antimüllerian hormone (AMH)
Dihydrotestosterone (DHT)

Müllerian and Wolffian ducts
Estrogen
Gametes: GnRH neurons
Kisspeptin (Kiss1)
Leydig cells
Follicle stimulating hormone (FSH) and luteinizing hormone (LH)
Meiosis
SRY gene
Tanner stages

The Male Reproductive System

OBJECTIVES

1. Describe the organization of the male gonad, the testis, and the process of spermatogenesis, and discuss how this process is supported by Sertoli cells.
2. Describe the steroidogenic pathway of Leydig cells that produces testosterone, the peripheral conversion of testosterone to estradiol-17β or dihydrotestosterone, and the actions of these steroids in men.
3. Explain the regulation of testicular function by the hypothalamic-pituitary-testicular axis.
4. Describe the role of the proximal male reproductive tract, especially the epididymis, in the further development of sperm.
5. Explain the more distal segments of the male reproductive tract, including the accessory sex glands, in the context of emission and ejaculation.
6. Describe the neurovascular events in the penis that are involved in erection.
7. Explain the following pathologic conditions of the male reproductive system: Klinefelter syndrome and androgen insensitivity that is coupled to testicular feminization.

In men, the reproductive system has evolved for continuous, lifelong gametogenesis, coupled to occasional internal insemination with a high density of sperm (greater than 60×10^6/mL in 3 to 5 mL of semen). This means that in adult men, the basic roles of gonadal hormones are as follows:

- Support of gametogenesis (spermatogenesis)
- Maintenance of the male reproductive tract and production of semen
- Maintenance of secondary sex characteristics and libido. There is no overall cyclicity of this activity in men.

HISTOPHYSIOLOGY OF THE TESTIS

A major difference between the testes and the ovaries is that the testes reside in the **scrotum** outside of the abdominopelvic cavity and are connected to the abdominopelvic male tract by the spermatic cord (see Fig. 8.2 in Chapter 8). Various mechanisms, including the cremasteric reflex, a venous countercurrent exchanger in the spermatic cord (pampiniform plexus), folding of scrotal skin, and sweat glands within the scrotal skin, cooperate to maintain a testicular temperature at about 35°C, which is crucial for sperm development. Failure of the testes to descend

through the inguinal canal into the scrotum during development results in depressed spermatogenesis and an increased risk of testicular cancer.

The human testis is covered by a connective tissue capsule and is divided into about 300 **lobules** by fibrous septa. Within each lobule are two to four loops of **seminiferous tubules** (Fig. 9.1). Each loop empties into an anastomosing network of tubules called the **rete testis**. The rete testis is continuous with small ducts, the **efferent ductules** that lead the sperm out of the testis into the head of the **epididymis** on the superior pole of the testis (see Fig. 9.8). Once in the epididymis, the sperm pass from the head, to the body, to the tail of the epididymis and then to the vas (ductus) deferens. Spermatozoa are stored in the tail of the epididymis and the vas deferens for several months as viable sperm.

The presence of the seminiferous tubules in the lobules of the testis creates two compartments within each lobule: an **intratubular compartment**, which is composed of the **seminiferous epithelium** of the seminiferous tubule; and a **peritubular compartment**, which is composed of neurovascular elements, connective tissue cells, immune cells, and the **interstitial cells of Leydig**, whose main function is to produce **testosterone** (Fig. 9.1D).

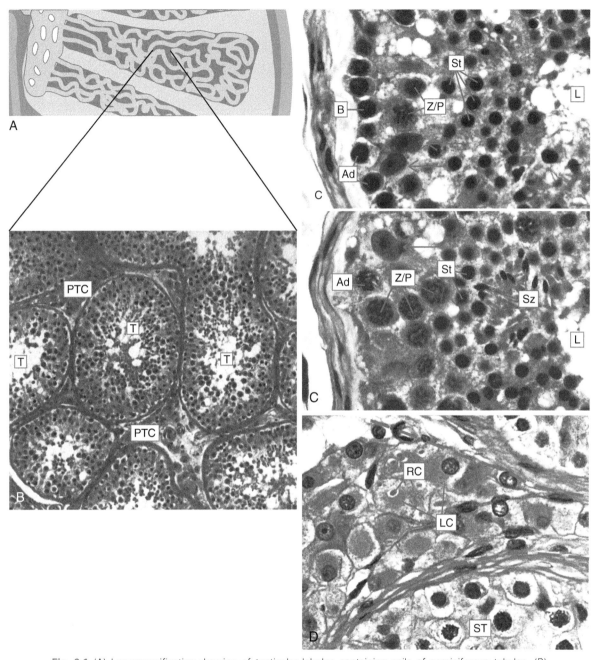

Fig. 9.1 (A) Low-magnification drawing of testicular lobules containing coils of seminiferous tubules. (B) Higher magnification of histologic organization of a section from the testicular lobule (as drawn in A), showing several seminiferous tubules *(T),* which collectively make up the intratubular compartment, and the peritubular compartment *(PTC).* (C) Higher magnification of histologic organization of two seminiferous tubules, showing Sertoli cells *(arrows),* spermatogonia *(Ad* and *B),* primary spermatocytes *(Z/P),* spermatids *(St),* and spermatozoa *(Sz). L,* Lumen of tubule. Note that the association of sperm cells differs in two adjacent tubules as a result of the difference in their stage of the spermatogenic cycle. (D) Higher magnification of histologic organization of the peritubular compartment (between *dashed lines*) showing a cluster of Leydig cells *(LC).* (A, From Porterfield SP: *Endocrine Physiology,* 2nd ed., St. Louis, 2001, Mosby. B to D, From Stevens A, Lowe J: *Human Histology,* 3rd ed., Philadelphia, 2005, Mosby.)

The Intratubular Compartment

The seminiferous tubule is lined by a complex seminiferous epithelium (Fig. 9.2) composed of two cell types:
- Sperm cells in various stages of spermatogenesis
- The Sertoli cell, which is a nurse cell in intimate contact with all sperm cells and which regulates many aspects of spermatogenesis

Developing Sperm Cells

The entire developmental process by which spermatogonia give rise to spermatozoa is called spermatogenesis. Spermatogenesis begins at puberty and involves the processes of mitosis and meiosis (Fig. 9.2). Stem spermatogonia (also called prespermatogonia) reside at the basal level of the seminiferous epithelium. Stem spermatogonia divide mitotically to generate daughter spermatogonia (spermatocytogenesis). These mitotic divisions are initially asymmetric, in that one daughter cell remains a *stem* spermatogonium (thereby undergoing self-renewal throughout life), whereas the second daughter cell will divide several times to amplify its population. After several mitotic divisions, the daughter spermatogonia complete S phase (DNA replication) and commit to meiotic division. Of note, these amplifying divisions are accompanied by incomplete cytokinesis, so all spermatogonia daughter cells and subsequent sperm cells (at different stages) remain interconnected by a cytoplasmic bridge. This configuration contributes to the synchrony of development of a clonal population of sperm cells.

Spermatogonia migrate apically away from the basal lamina as they enter the first meiotic prophase (see Fig. 9.2). At this time, they are called primary spermatocytes. During the first meiotic prophase, the hallmark processes of sexual reproduction involving synapsis, crossing-over, formation of chiasmata, and the first disjunction occur (see Chapter 8). Completion of the first meiotic division gives rise to secondary spermatocytes, which quickly (within 20 min) complete the second meiotic division.

The initial products of meiosis are haploid spermatids, which reside apically within the seminiferous epithelium, close to the lumen of the seminiferous tubule (see Fig. 9.2). Spermatids are small, round cells with a round nucleus. Spermatids undergo a remarkable metamorphosis called spermiogenesis that results in a spermatozoon (Fig. 9.3). The spermatozoon contains the following parts:
1. A head. The head consists of two major components:
   a. A condensed and streamlined nucleus. The chromatin of the nucleus is highly heterochromatic (i.e., condensed), and the nucleosomal histones are replaced by protamines. The DNA of a spermatozoan is transcriptionally silent.
   b. An acrosomal vesicle. The acrosomal vesicle contains hydrolytic enzymes transported to it from the Golgi. These enzymes will play an important role in fertilization and the prevention of polyspermy (see Chapter 11). The acrosomal vesicle attaches to the forward pole of the nucleus and descends along the side of the nucleus so that it partially covers the nucleus.
2. The neck. This contains two centrioles (proximal and distal). The proximal centriole attaches to the nucleus, and the distal centriole will generate a "9 + 2" configuration of microtubules that is called the axoneme.
3. The tail (also called the flagellum). The tail has a continuous axonemal core but is composed of structurally distinct regions called the middle piece, principal piece, and end piece. The middle piece is the thickest and contains a collar of mitochondria that will deliver adenosine triphosphate (ATP) for flagellar beating and motility. The outer circumference of the middle piece contains dense fibers. The principal piece and the end piece lack the mitochondrial sheath, and the end piece lacks the outer dense fibers.

The process of spermatogenesis takes about 72 days. A cohort of adjacent spermatogonia enters the process every 16 days, so the process is staggered along the length of a seminiferous tubule. Consequently, spermatogonia do not enter the process of spermatogenesis at the same time along the entire length of the tubule, or in synchrony with every other tubule (there are about 500 seminiferous tubules per testis). Because the seminiferous tubules within one testis total about 400 m in length, spermatozoa are continually being generated at many sites within the testis at any given time. Histologic examination of the seminiferous tubules reveals that there are specific associations, called spermatogenic stages, of sperm cells at any one point in time. In humans, there are six different stages that progress and repeat as a cycle at one point within the seminiferous tubule. This is referred to as the spermatogenic cycle. The stages are staggered spatially along the length of the seminiferous tubule, before repeating themselves. This spatial configuration of cycles is called a spermatogenic wave.

The final release of sperm, called spermiation, is an active process involving dissolution of adhesive junctions between Sertoli cells and spermatozoa. It is important to note that testicular spermatozoa after spermiation are not fully mature. Testicular spermatozoa are barely motile, and leave the seminiferous tubule passively within fluid produced by the Sertoli cells.

The Sertoli Cell

The Sertoli cell represents the true epithelial cell of the seminiferous epithelium and extends from the basal lamina to the lumen (Box 9.1; see Fig. 9.2). Sertoli cells surround sperm cells,

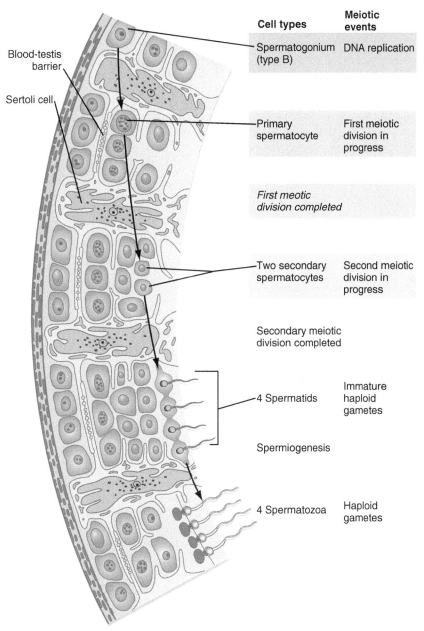

Cell types	Meiotic events
Spermatogonium (type B)	DNA replication
Primary spermatocyte	First meiotic division in progress
	First meotic division completed
Two secondary spermatocytes	Second meiotic division in progress
	Secondary meiotic division completed
4 Spermatids	Immature haploid gametes
	Spermiogenesis
4 Spermatozoa	Haploid gametes

Blood-testis barrier

Sertoli cell

Fig. 9.2 Seminiferous epithelium. Spermatogonia undergo mitosis (spermatocytogenesis) to produce both a reservoir of spermatogonia and maturing spermatogonia that differentiate into primary spermatocytes. These spermatocytes remain joined by cytoplasmic bridges (not shown). Primary spermatocytes undergo the complex process of the first meiotic division to become secondary spermatocytes, and then a rapid second meiotic division (reduction-division) to become haploid spermatids. Spermatids mature into spermatozoa by the process of spermiogenesis. Sertoli cells extend from the basal to the apical sides of the epithelium and create the blood-testis barrier between spermatogonia and primary spermatocytes. (From Koeppen B, Stanton B: *Berne and Levy Physiology,* updated 6th ed., Philadelphia, 2010, Mosby.)

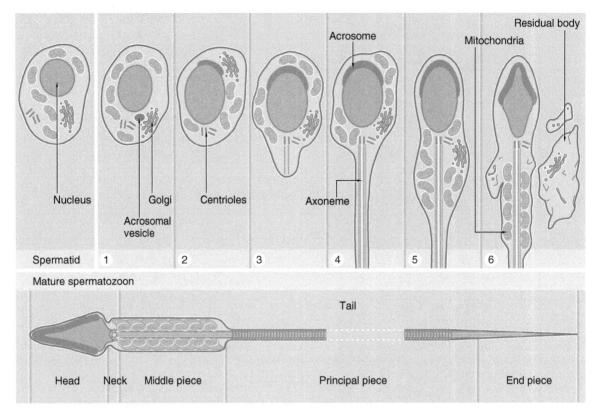

Fig. 9.3 Spermiogenesis and structure of a spermatozoon. The residual body is phagocytized by Sertoli cells. (From Young B, Lowe J, Stevens A, et al: *Wheater's Functional Histology*, 5th ed., Edinburgh, 2007, Churchill Livingstone.)

providing structural support within the epithelium, and form adherens-type junctions and gap junctions with all stages of sperm cells (see Fig. 9.2). Through the formation and breakdown of these junctions, Sertoli cells guide sperm cells toward the lumen as they advance to later stages in spermatogenesis. Accordingly, major secretory products of Sertoli cells include proteases and protease inhibitors. Spermiation requires the final breakdown of Sertoli cell–sperm cell junctions.

Another important structural feature of Sertoli cells is the formation of tight junctions among adjacent Sertoli cells (see Fig. 9.2). These occluding junctions divide the seminiferous epithelium into a **basal compartment**, containing the spermatogonia and early-stage primary spermatocytes, and an **adluminal** (i.e., toward the lumen) **compartment**, containing later-stage primary spermatocytes and all subsequent stages of sperm cells. Because early primary spermatocytes move apically from the basal compartment to the adluminal one, the tight junctions need to be disassembled and reassembled. These tight junctions form the physical basis for the **blood-testis barrier**, which creates a specialized, immunologically safe microenvironment for developing sperm. By blocking

paracellular diffusion, the tight junctions restrict movement of substances between the blood and the developing germ cells through a trans-Sertoli cell transport pathway and in this manner allow the Sertoli cell to control nutrient availability to germ cells. Accordingly, Sertoli cells also have the responsibility for providing nutrients to this environment, such as transferrin, iron, and lactate. For example, spermatogonia and released spermatozoa use fructose and glucose for energy. However, sperm undergoing meiosis cannot efficiently use glucose as an energy source. Sertoli cells acquire glucose by the GLUT1 transporter, metabolize it to lactate, and transfer it to developing sperm, which express a sperm-specific lactate transporter. This process is dependent on hormonal stimulation (follicle-stimulating hormone [FSH] and testosterone; see later in the text) but also appears to be optimized by local sperm cell–generated paracrine factors.

Thus healthy Sertoli cell function is essential for sperm cell viability and development. In this respect, it should be noted that spermatogenesis is absolutely dependent on testosterone produced by peritubular Leydig cells (see later), yet it is the Sertoli cells that express the **androgen receptor**, not the

---

BOX 9.1   Functions of Sertoli Cells

Supportive ("Nursing")

- Maintaining, breaking, and reforming multiple junctions with developing sperm
- Maintaining blood-testis barrier
- Phagocytosis
- Transfer of nutrients and other substances from blood to developing sperm cells
- Expression of paracrine factors and receptors for sperm-derived paracrine factors

Exocrine

- Production of fluid to move immobile sperm out of testis toward epididymis
- Production of androgen-binding protein
- Determination of release of spermatozoa (spermiation) from seminiferous tubule

Endocrine

- Expression of androgen receptor and follicle-stimulating hormone receptor
- Production of Müllerian-inhibiting substance, also called *anti-Müllerian hormone*
- Aromatization of testosterone to estradiol-17β (this has local effect, not strictly endocrine)

---

developing sperm cells. Similarly, the pituitary hormone FSH is also required for maximal sperm production, and again, it is the Sertoli cell that expresses the FSH receptor, not the developing sperm. Thus these hormones support spermatogenesis indirectly through stimulation of Sertoli cell function.

Sertoli cells have multiple additional functions. Sertoli cells express the enzyme CYP19 (also called aromatase), which converts Leydig cell–derived testosterone to the potent estrogen, estradiol-17β (see later in the text). This local production of estrogen may enhance spermatogenesis in humans. Sertoli cells also produce androgen-binding protein (ABP). ABP is encoded by the same gene as for sex hormone–binding globulin (SHBG; Chapter 1; see later in the text) but has different carbohydrate groups and is specifically expressed intratesticularly. ABP maintains a high androgen level within the adluminal compartment, the lumina of the seminiferous tubules, and the proximal part of the male reproductive tract. Sertoli cells also produce a large amount of fluid. This fluid provides an appropriate bathing medium for the sperm and assists in moving the immotile spermatozoa from the seminiferous tubule into the epididymis. Sertoli cells perform an important phagocytic function. This allows Sertoli cells to engulf residual bodies, which represent cytoplasm that is shed by spermatozoa during spermiogenesis, as well as dead sperm cells.

Finally, the Sertoli cell has an important endocrine role. During development, Sertoli cells produce anti-Müllerian hormone (AMH), also called Müllerian-inhibiting substance (MIS), which induces regression of the embryonic Müllerian duct that is programmed to give rise to the female reproductive tract (see Chapter 8). The Sertoli cells also produce the hormone inhibin. Inhibin is a heterodimer protein hormone related to the transforming growth factor-β (TGF-β) family. FSH stimulates inhibin production, which then exerts negative feedback on gonadotropes to inhibit FSH production. Thus inhibin keeps FSH levels within a specific range (see later in the text).

The Peritubular Compartment

The peritubular compartment (see Fig. 9.1) contains the primary endocrine cell of the testis, the Leydig cell. This compartment also contains common cell types of loose connective tissue and an extremely rich peritubular capillary network that must provide nutrients to the seminiferous tubules (by way of Sertoli cells) while conveying testosterone away from the testes to the peripheral circulation.

The Leydig Cell

Leydig cells are steroidogenic stromal cells. These cells synthesize cholesterol de novo, as well as acquiring it through low-density lipoprotein (LDL) receptors and, to a lesser extent, high-density lipoprotein (HDL) receptors (the HDL receptor is also called scavenger receptor-B1 [SR-B1]), and store cholesterol as cholesterol esters, as described for adrenocortical cells (see Chapter 7). Free cholesterol is generated by a cholesterol hormone-sensitive lipase (HSL) and transferred to the outer mitochondrial membrane, and then to the inner mitochondrial membrane in a steroidogenic acute regulatory protein (StAR)-dependent manner (refer to Fig. 7.6 in Chapter 7). As in all steroidogenic cells, cholesterol is converted to pregnenolone by CYP11A1. Pregnenolone is then processed to progesterone, 17α-hydroxyprogesterone, and androstenedione by 3β-hydroxysteroid dehydrogenase type 2 (3β-HSD2) and CYP17 (Fig. 9.4). Recall from Chapter 7 that CYP17 is a bifunctional enzyme, with a 17-hydroxylase activity and a 17, 20-lyase activity. CYP17 displays a robust level of both activities in the Leydig cell. In this respect, the Leydig cell is similar to the zona reticularis cell, except that it expresses a higher level of 3β-HSD, so that the Δ4 pathway is ultimately favored. Another major difference is that the Leydig cell expresses a Leydig cell–specific isoform of 17β-hydroxysteroid dehydrogenase (17β-HSD3), which converts androstenedione to testosterone (see Fig. 9.4). Mutation of this specific gene in men results in a form of disorders of sexual development (DSD; see later in the text).

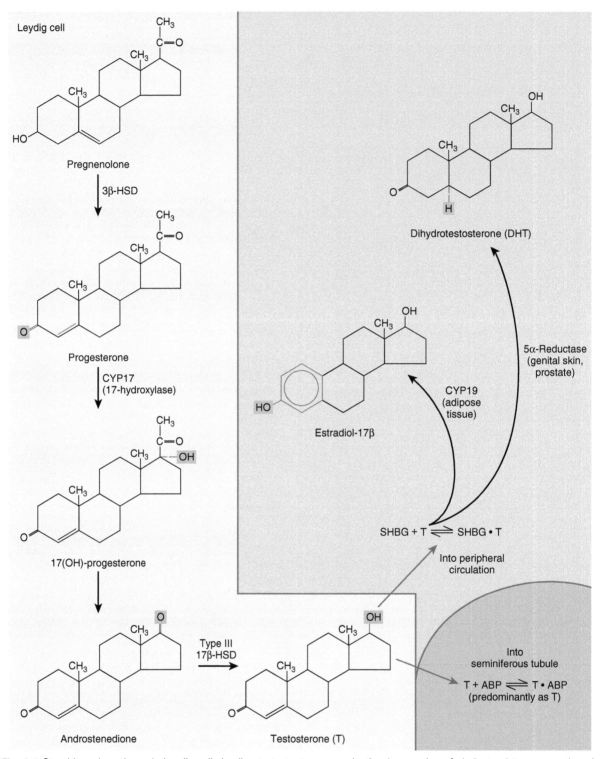

Fig. 9.4 Steroidogenic pathway in Leydig cells leading to testosterone production (conversion of cholesterol to pregnenolone is not shown). Testosterone (*T*) diffuses both into the neighboring seminiferous tubules and into the peritubular capillary network to be carried into the peripheral circulation. In the lumina of seminiferous tubules, T is concentrated by binding to androgen-binding protein *(ABP)*. T is carried in the peripheral circulation by sex hormone–binding globulin *(SHBG)* and albumin. The Leydig cell makes limited amounts of DHT and estradiol-17β, but considerably more of these two steroids is made by peripheral conversion.

TRANSPORT, ACTIONS, AND METABOLISM OF ANDROGENS

Intratesticular Androgen

The testosterone produced by Leydig cells has several metabolic fates and multiple actions (Box 9.2; Table 9.1). Because of the proximity of Leydig cells to the seminiferous tubules, significant amounts of testosterone diffuse into the seminiferous tubules and become concentrated within the adluminal compartment by ABP. Testosterone within the seminiferous tubules is maintained at a significantly higher level than the circulating testosterone level. This concentration of intratubular testosterone is absolutely required for normal spermatogenesis. As noted, Sertoli cells express the enzyme CYP19 (aromatase), which converts a small amount of testosterone into the highly potent estrogen estradiol-17β. Human sperm cells express at least one isoform of the estrogen receptor (ER), and there is some evidence from CYP19-aromatase–deficient men that this locally produced estrogen optimizes spermatogenesis in humans.

Peripheral Conversion to Estrogen

In several tissues (especially adipose tissue), testosterone is converted to estrogen (see Fig. 9.4) by the enzyme CYP19 (also called aromatase). This peripheral conversion is the primary source of estrogen production in men.

BOX 9.2 Actions of Androgens

- Regulation of differentiation of male internal and external genitalia in fetus
- Stimulation of growth, development, and function of male internal and external genitalia
- Stimulation of sexual hair development
- Stimulation of sebaceous gland secretion
- Stimulation of erythropoietin synthesis
- Control of protein anabolic effects
- Stimulation of bone growth
- Closure of epiphyses after conversion to estradiol
- Initiation and maintenance of spermatogenesis
- Stimulation of androgen-binding protein synthesis (synergizes with follicle-stimulating hormone)
- Maintenance of secretions of sex glands
- Regulation of behavioral effects, including libido

TABLE 9.1 Approximate Hormone Production Rates in Adult Man

Testosterone	5 mg/day
Estradiol	10-15 µg/day
Dihydrotestosterone	50-100 µg/day

CLINICAL BOX 9.1

Studies in men with **CYP19-aromatase deficiency** have shown that inability to produce estrogen results in tall stature, owing to lack of epiphyseal closure in long bones, and osteoporosis. Thus peripheral estrogen plays an important role in bone maturation and biology in men. These studies also implicated estrogen in promoting insulin sensitivity, improving lipoprotein profiles (i.e., increasing HDL, decreasing triglycerides and LDL), and exerting negative feedback on pituitary gonadotropins.

Peripheral Conversion to Dihydrotestosterone

Testosterone can also be converted into a potent, nonaromatizable androgen, 5α-dihydrotestosterone (DHT), by the enzyme 5α-reductase (see Fig. 9.4). There are two isoforms of 5α-reductase: type 1 and type 2. Major sites of 5α-reductase-2 expression are the male urogenital tract, genital skin, hair follicles, and liver. 5α-reductase-2 generates DHT, which is required for masculinization of the external genitalia and development of the prostate gland in utero, and in many of the changes associated with puberty (see Chapter 8), including growth and activity of the prostate gland, growth of the penis, darkening and folding of the scrotum, growth of pubic and axillary hair, facial and body hair, and increased muscle mass (Fig. 9.5). Onset of 5α-reductase-1 expression occurs at puberty. This isozyme is expressed primarily in the skin and contributes to sebaceous gland activity and acne associated with puberty.

CLINICAL BOX 9.2

Because DHT has strong growth-promoting (i.e., trophic) effects on its target organs, the development of selective 5α-reductase-2 inhibitors has benefited the treatment of prostatic hypertrophy and prostatic cancer.

Peripheral Testosterone Actions

Individuals with 5α-reductase-2 deficiency are born with ambiguous or feminized external genitalia, thereby demonstrating the need for conversion of testosterone to DHT for an effect on some androgen-responsive tissues. However, testosterone can act as itself in several cell types (see Fig. 9.5). As mentioned previously, testosterone regulates Sertoli cell function. Testosterone induces the development of the portion of the male reproductive tract that originates from the mesonephric duct (see Chapter 8) in the absence of 5α-reductase. Testosterone has several metabolic effects, including increasing very-low-density lipoprotein (VLDL) and LDL while decreasing HDL, promoting the deposition of abdominal adipose tissue, increasing red blood cell production, promoting bone growth and health, and having a protein anabolic effect on muscle. Testosterone is sufficient to maintain erectile function and libido.

Mechanism of Androgen Action

Testosterone and DHT act through the same **androgen receptor (AR)**. As described for other steroid hormone receptors (see Chapter 1), the AR resides in the cytoplasm bound to chaperone proteins in the absence of ligand. Testosterone-AR binding or DHT-AR binding causes dissociation of chaperone proteins, followed by nuclear translocation of the androgen-AR complex, dimerization, binding to an androgen-response element (ARE), and recruitment of coregulatory proteins to the vicinity of a specific gene's promoter. It remains unclear how testosterone and DHT differ in

their ability to activate the AR in the context of different cell types.

Transport and Metabolism of Androgens

As testosterone enters the peripheral circulation, it quickly reaches equilibrium with serum proteins. About 60% of circulating testosterone is bound to **SHBG**, 38% is bound to albumin, and about 2% remains as *free* hormone (see Fig. 9.4). Testosterone and its metabolites are excreted primarily in the urine. About 50% of excreted androgens are found as **urinary 17-ketosteroids**, with most of the remainder being conjugated androgens or diol or triol derivatives. Only about 30% of the 17-ketosteroids in urine are from the testis; the rest are produced from adrenal androgens. Androgens are **conjugated** with glucuronate or sulfate in the liver, and these conjugated steroids are excreted in the urine.

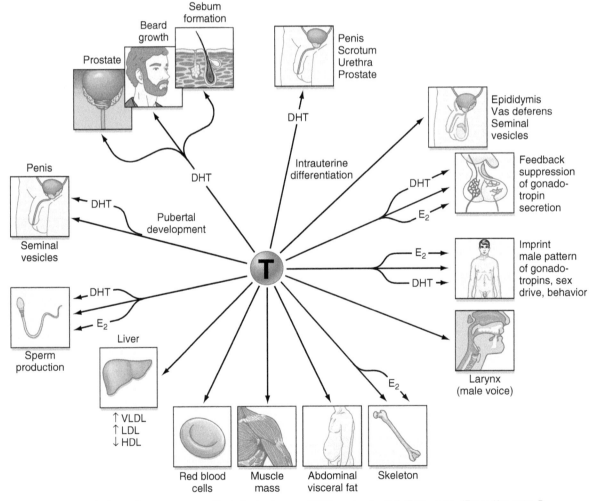

Fig. 9.5 Actions of testosterone, dihydrotestosterone *(DHT)*, and estradiol *(E₂)* in men. (From Koeppen B, Stanton B: *Berne and Levy Physiology,* updated 6th ed., Philadelphia, 2010, Mosby.)

Androgen analogs are administered orally, sublingually, by intramuscular injection, by transdermal patch, and by subdermal slow-release pellets.

HYPOTHALAMUS-PITUITARY-TESTIS AXIS

The testis is regulated by an endocrine axis involving parvicellular hypothalamic **gonadotropin-releasing hormone (GnRH)**–secreting neurons and pituitary gonadotropes that produce both **luteinizing hormone (LH)** and **FSH** (Fig. 9.6). In addition, the function of GnRH neurons is dependent on kisspeptin, a peptide produced by neighboring hypothalamic neurons. Recall from Chapter 5 that LH and FSH are pituitary glycoprotein hormones. They are heterodimers, composed of a common α-subunit—the α-glycoprotein subunit (αGSU)—and a specific β-subunit (either LH-β or FSH-β).

Regulation of Leydig Cell Function

The Leydig cell expresses the **LH receptor**. LH acts on Leydig cells much like adrenocorticotropic hormone (ACTH) does on zona fasciculata cells (see Chapter 7). The LH receptor is coupled to a Gs-cyclic adenosine monophosphate cAMP-PKA signaling pathway (see Chapter 1). **Rapid effects** include hydrolysis of cholesterol esters and new expression of StAR. **Less acute effects** include an increase in steroidogenic enzyme gene expression and in the expression of the LDL receptor and SR-BI. Over the **long term**, LH promotes Leydig cell growth and proliferation.

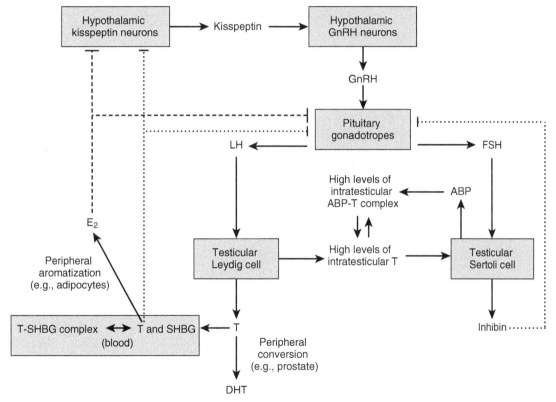

Fig. 9.6 Summary of regulation of testicular function. Gonadotropin-releasing hormone *(GnRH)* neurons are stimulated to release GnRH by kisspeptin. GnRH stimulates the pituitary gonadotropes to secrete luteinizing hormone *(LH)* and follicle-stimulating hormone *(FSH)*. LH acts on Leydig cell to produce testosterone *(T)*. FSH acts on Sertoli cells, and both T and FSH stimulate all functions of the Sertoli cells. In terms of regulatory loops, Sertoli cells produce inhibin, which negatively feeds back on the pituitary gonadotropes to selectively inhibit FSH production, and Sertoli cells produce androgen-binding protein *(ABP)*, which maintains very high levels of both free T and T complexed with ABP, within the testis. Testosterone enters the blood and is complexed with sex hormone binding globulin *(SHBG)*. Free T negatively feeds back on gonadotropes and kisspeptin neurons directly, but also after its peripheral aromatization to estradiol *(E₂)*. T can also be converted to dihydrotestosterone *(DHT)*, which does not contribute to regulation within the hypothalamus-pituitary-testis axis.

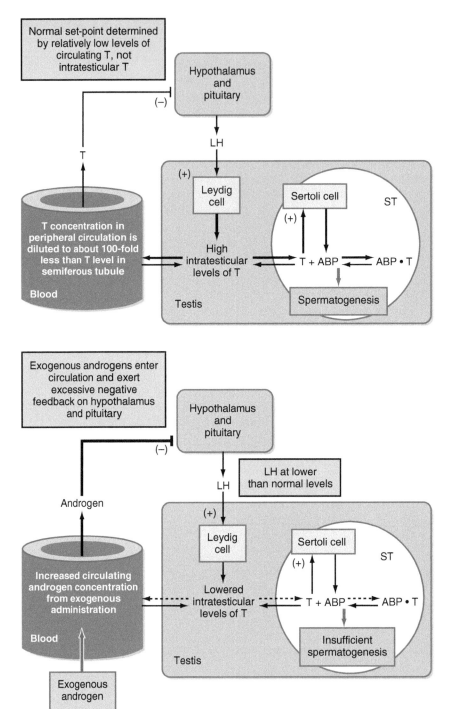

Fig 9.7 The difference in intratesticular testosterone versus circulating testosterone concentrations and its importance in the hypothalamus-pituitary-testis axis. *Upper panel,* Feedback loop in a normal adult man. *Lower panel,* Administration of testosterone (or an androgenic analog) increases circulating testosterone (androgen) levels, which in turn increases negative feedback on release of luteinizing hormone *(LH).* Decreased LH levels diminish Leydig cell activity and intratesticular production of androgen. Lowered intratesticular testosterone levels result in reduced sperm production and can cause infertility. Note that the inhibin feedback loop has been omitted from this diagram. (From Koeppen B, Stanton B: *Berne and Levy Physiology,* updated 6th ed., Philadelphia, 2010, Mosby.)

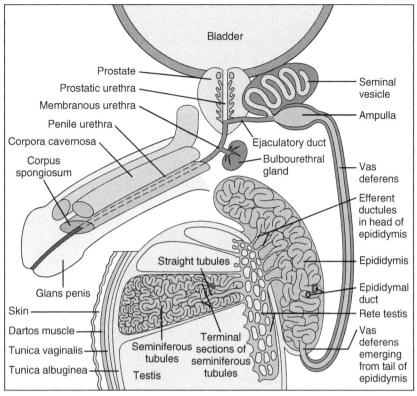

Fig. 9.8 Diagram of male reproductive tract, including the intratesticular portion of the tract. (Redrawn from Stevens A, Lowe J: *Human Histology,* 3rd ed., Philadelphia, 2005, Mosby.)

Testosterone negatively feeds back on LH and FSH production by the pituitary gonadotrope, both as testosterone and as estradiol-17β (see Fig. 9.6). Both steroid hormones inhibit the expression of LH-β, the GnRH receptor, and to a lesser extent, FSH-β. These steroids also indirectly inhibit the release of GnRH via their inhibition of hypothalamic kisspeptin neurons. DHT does not appear to be involved in negative feedback on the pituitary or hypothalamus.

Regulation of Sertoli Cell Function

Although testosterone and estrogen exert negative feedback on both LH and FSH, they selectively inhibit LH more effectively than FSH. From a historic standpoint, this finding raised the possibility that a Sertoli cell–derived factor might feed back on FSH production. The Sertoli cell is stimulated by both testosterone and FSH. The FSH receptor also is coupled primarily to a Gs-cAMP-PKA pathway. In addition to stimulating the synthesis of proteins involved in the *nurse cell* aspect of Sertoli cell function (e.g., ABP), FSH stimulates the synthesis of the dimeric protein **inhibin**. Inhibin has a common α-subunit, coupled with either a β$_A$-subunit, called **inhibin A**, or a β$_B$-subunit, called **inhibin B**. Only inhibin B

is expressed in men. Inhibin B expression is stimulated by FSH, and inhibin B exerts a negative feedback on the pituitary gonadotrope to selectively inhibit FSH production.

CLINICAL BOX 9.3

There exists an important *loophole* in the male reproductive axis, which is based on the fact the **intratesticular levels of testosterone** need to be greater than 100-fold higher than circulating levels of the hormone to maintain normal rates of spermatogenesis, but it is the **circulating levels of testosterone** that provide the negative feedback to the pituitary and hypothalamus. This means that exogenous administration of testosterone can raise circulating levels sufficient to inhibit LH but not sufficient to concentrate in the testis at the required concentration for normal spermatogenesis. The decreased LH levels, however, will diminish intratesticular production of testosterone by Leydig cells, which will result in reduced levels of spermatogenesis (Fig. 9.7). This *loophole* is currently being investigated as a possible strategy for developing a male oral contraceptive. It also is the basis for sterility in some cases of steroid abuse in men.

MALE REPRODUCTIVE TRACT

Once spermatozoa emerge from the efferent ductules, they leave the gonad and enter the extratesticular portion of the male reproductive tract (Fig. 9.8;). The segments of the tract are as follows: the epididymis (head, body, and tail), the vas deferens, the ejaculatory duct, the prostatic urethra, the membranous urethra, and the penile urethra. Unlike in the female tract:

- There is a continuous lumen from the seminiferous tubule to the end of the male tract (i.e., the tip of the penile urethra).
- The male tract connects to the distal urinary tract (i.e., male urethra).

In addition to conveying sperm, the primary functions of the male reproductive tract are as follows:

1. Sperm spend about a month in the epididymis, where they undergo further maturation. The epithelium of the epididymis is actively secretory and adds numerous proteins and glycolipids to the seminal fluid. Spermatozoa that enter the head of the epididymis are weakly motile but are strongly unidirectionally motile by the time they exit the tail. Spermatozoa also may undergo the process of decapacitation, which involves stabilization of their cell membranes to prevent spermatozoa from undergoing the acrosomal reaction before contact with an egg (see Chapter 11). Sperm become capacitated by the female reproductive tract within the oviduct (see Chapter 10). The function of the epididymis is dependent on luminal testosterone-ABP complexes that come from the seminiferous tubules and on testosterone from the blood. Of note, the epididymal epithelium is extremely tight, so a blood-epididymis barrier exists.

2. Sperm are stored in the tail of the epididymis and vas deferens. Sperm can be stored for several months without loss of viability. The primary function of the vas deferens, besides providing a storage site, is to propel sperm during sexual intercourse into the male urethra. The vas deferens has a very thick muscularis that is richly innervated by sympathetic nerves. Normally in response to repeated tactile stimulation of the penis during coitus, the muscularis of the vas deferens receives bursts of sympathetic stimulation, causing peristaltic contractions. The emptying of the contents of the vas deferens into the prostatic urethra is called emission. Emission immediately precedes ejaculation, which is the propulsion of semen out of the male urethra.

3. During emission, contraction of the vas deferens coincides with contraction of the muscular coats of the two accessory sex glands: the seminal vesicles (right and left) and the prostate gland (which surrounds the prostatic urethra). At this point, sperm become mixed with all the components of semen. The seminal vesicles secrete about 60% of the volume. These glands are the primary source of fructose, a critical nutrient for sperm. Seminal vesicles also secrete semenogelins, which induce partial coagulation of semen immediately after ejaculation. The alkaline secretions of the prostate, which make up about 30% of the volume, are high in citrate, zinc, spermine, and acid phosphatase. Prostate-specific antigen (PSA) is a serine protease that liquefies coagulated semen after a few minutes. PSA can be detected in the blood under conditions of prostatic infection, benign prostatic hypertrophy, and prostatic carcinoma and is currently used as one indicator of prostatic health. The predominant buffers in semen are phosphate and bicarbonate. The bulbourethral glands (also called Cowper glands) empty into the penile urethra in response to sexual excitement before emission and ejaculation. Paraurethral glands (glands of Littre) similarly secrete along the length of the male urethra. The mucous bulbourethral and paraurethral secretions lubricate, cleanse, and buffer the urethra. Average sperm counts are reported to be from 60 to 100 million/mL semen. Men with sperm counts below 20 million/mL, less than 50% motile sperm, or less than 60% normally formed sperm usually are infertile.

4. As noted, emission and ejaculation occur during coitus in response to a reflex arc that involves sensory stimulation from the penis (through the pudendal nerve) followed by sympathetic motor stimulation to the smooth muscle of the male tract and somatic motor stimulation (through the pudendal nerve) to the musculature associated with the base of the penis. However, for sexual intercourse to occur in the first place, the male partner has to achieve and maintain an erection of the penis. The penis has evolved as an intromittent organ designed to separate the walls of the vagina, pass through the potential space of the vaginal lumen, and deposit semen at the deep end of the vaginal lumen near the cervix. This process of internal insemination can be performed only if the penis is stiffened from the process of erection.

Erection is a neurovascular event (Fig. 9.9). The penis is composed of three erectile bodies: two corpora cavernosa and one corpus spongiosum. The penile urethra runs through the corpus spongiosum (and is also called the spongy urethra). These three bodies are composed of erectile tissue—an anastomosing network of potential cavernous vascular spaces lined with continuous endothelia within a loose connective tissue support. During the flaccid state, blood flow to the cavernous spaces is minimal (see Fig. 9.9A), because of vasoconstriction of vasculature that shunts blood flow away from the cavernous spaces. In response to sexual arousal, parasympathetic nerves innervating the vascular smooth muscle of the helicine arteries that supply blood to the cavernous spaces release

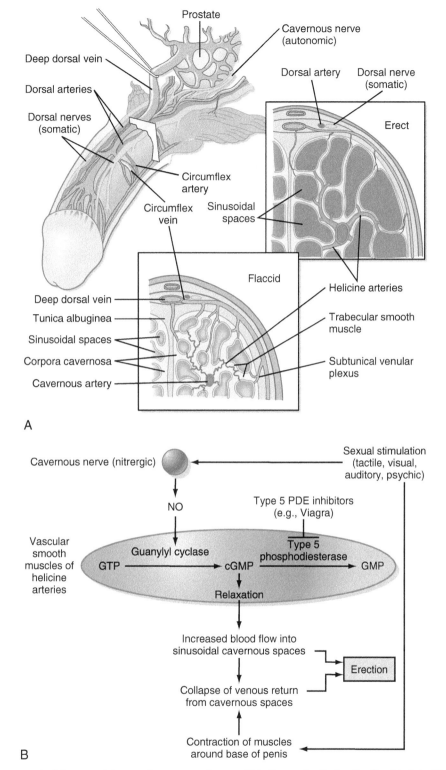

Fig. 9.9 (A) Arrangement of the vasculature and cavernous tissue within the penis. During the flaccid state, blood flow into the cavernous spaces is limited by contraction of the helicine arteries. (B) Outline of neurovascular events leading to penile erection. (From Bhasun S, et al. In Larsen P, Kronenberg H, Melmed S, et al, editors: *Williams Textbook of Endocrinology,* 10th ed., Philadelphia, 2003, Saunders.)

nitric oxide (NO). NO activates guanylyl cyclase, increasing cyclic guanosine monophosphate (cGMP), which decreases intracellular Ca^{2+} and causes relaxation of the vascular smooth muscle (see Fig. 9.9B). The vasodilation allows blood to flow into the spaces, causing engorgement and erection (see Fig. 9.9). The veins in the penis course to the circumference of the penis before emptying into the deep dorsal vein. During erection, the engorged tissue presses the veins against a noncompliant outer fascia, thereby reducing venous drainage. Finally, somatic stimulation increases contraction of muscles at the base of the penis, further promoting erection.

CLINICAL BOX 9.4

Inability to achieve or maintain an erection is termed **erectile dysfunction (ED)** and is one cause of **infertility**. Multiple factors can lead to ED, such as insufficient androgen production; neurovascular damage (e.g., from diabetes mellitus, spinal cord injury); structural damage to the penis, perineum, or pelvis; psychogenic factors (e.g., depression, performance anxiety); prescribed medications; and recreational drugs, including alcohol and tobacco. A major development in the treatment of some forms of ED is availability of selective cGMP phosphodiesterase inhibitors, which assist in the maintenance of an erection.

DISORDERS INVOLVING THE MALE REPRODUCTIVE SYSTEM

Klinefelter Syndrome (XXY Seminiferous Tubule Dysgenesis)

Men with an extra X chromosome have the genetic disorder called **Klinefelter syndrome** (also called **seminiferous tubular dysgenesis**). Although there are multiple permutations of the disorder, the most common form results in a 47,XXY karyotype. Affected persons are phenotypically male because of the presence of the Y chromosome, and they appear normal at birth. At puberty, increased levels of gonadotropins fail to induce normal testicular growth and spermatogenesis. Instead, the testis becomes fibrotic and hyalinized and remains small and firm. The seminiferous tubules are largely destroyed, resulting in infertility. However, some patches of tubules may exist, allowing for extraction of sperm to be used in intracytoplasmic sperm injection (ICSI) into an egg as part of an assisted reproductive procedure. Androgen production is usually low (but this is highly variable among patients), whereas the levels of gonadotropins are elevated, thereby indicating primary hypogonadism. A small penis and lack of body hair are two signs of reduced androgen production (Fig. 9.10). An elevated estradiol-to-testosterone ratio can lead to moderate feminization, including the potential for limited **gynecomastia** (inappropriate development of breasts). Klinefelter syndrome is associated with a compromised intellectual development, behavioral problems, alterations in bone growth and density, and several other comorbidities. Androgen replacement to induce virilization is the most common treatment.

Androgen Insensitivity Syndrome

Androgen insensitivity syndrome (AIS) results from a hereditary defect of the X chromosome gene controlling AR expression. Because the defect can range from partial to complete inability of the AR to respond to androgens, the degree of feminization of AIS is variable. Because the karyotype is 46,XY, the gonad develops into the testis, which produces testosterone and MIS in utero. The mesonephric (Wolffian) duct does not develop into male structures, however, because androgen action is deficient, and MIS causes the Müllerian duct to regress. Consequently, there are no functional internal genitalia.

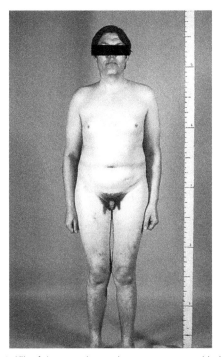

Fig. 9.10 Klinefelter syndrome in a young man. Limited gynecomastia is present, and body shape is somewhat feminine. (From Besser GM, Thorner MO: *Clinical Endocrinology*, 2nd ed., London, 1994, Mosby-Wolfe.)

The external genitalia typically develop as female, and the phenotype is female (Fig. 9.11). In severe AIS, the affected person has labia, a clitoris, and a short, blind vagina. Pubic and axillary hair is absent or sparse because the development of sexual hair is androgen dependent. Menstruation does not occur, and serum androgen levels are high or normal. When androgen production rises at puberty, estradiol production increases, both from the testes and from peripheral aromatization of androgens. LH levels remain elevated throughout adulthood because testosterone cannot exert negative feedback on the pituitary and hypothalamus because of a defective AR. The LH increase leads to dividing, hypertrophic Leydig cells that produce enhanced amounts of androstenedione, testosterone, and estradiol-17β. The androgens are peripherally converted to estrogens, which feminize the individual in a manner unopposed by androgenic actions. The phenotype that is derived from hyperstimulated Leydig cells secreting steroids that are converted into estrogens and lead to feminization is called **testicular feminization**. This is called a **disorder of sexual development (DSD)/androgen insensitivity syndrome**.

Note that the testes typically remain in the abdomen because androgen action is required for testicular descent. Because of gonadotropic hyperstimulation and exposure to elevated temperature, the gonads represent a probable site for cancerous growth and are surgically removed as a precaution.

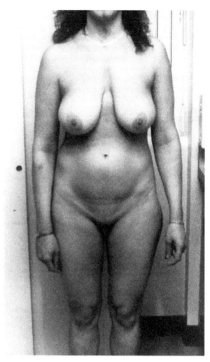

Fig. 9.11 A 46, XY patient with complete androgen insensitivity and female phenotype. Full breast development and female body form (e.g., widened pelvis) constitute evidence of testicular feminization. (From Quigley CA, De Bellis A, Marschke KB, et al: Androgen receptor defects: Historical, clinical, and molecular perspectives. *Endocr Rev* 16:271, 1995.)

▌ SUMMARY

1. Seminiferous tubules (the intratubular compartment) contain Sertoli cells and developing sperm. Sertoli cells have a *supportive* function, providing the proper microenvironment for sperm development. Tight junctions between adjacent Sertoli cells create the blood-testis barrier. Sertoli cells also have an important exocrine function, producing fluid and androgen-binding protein. In addition, Sertoli cells have an endocrine function, producing anti-Müllerian hormone and inhibin. Sertoli cells express the androgen receptor and the FSH receptor.

2. Spermatogenesis involves mitosis and meiosis. The final product is haploid spermatozoa. Normal spermatogenesis is dependent on FSH and high intratesticular levels of testosterone (T). High intratesticular levels of T are achieved by the secretion of androgen-binding protein by Sertoli cells. Sperm cells do not express the androgen receptor or the FSH receptor and are completely dependent on Sertoli cells for their development. FSH stimulates inhibin production, which selectively feeds back on FSH production by pituitary gonadotropes.

3. Leydig cells reside in the peritubular compartment. Leydig cells express the LH receptor and produce testosterone, as well as small amounts of DHT and estradiol-17β.

4. Testosterone can be converted peripherally to DHT (e.g., in the prostate gland) or estradiol-17β (e.g., in adipose tissue). Testosterone and DHT regulate secondary sex characteristics and are required for the normal development, growth, and function of the male reproductive tract. Estrogen is required for normal bone mineralization and epiphyseal plate closure in men, and for modulation of lipoprotein profile (lowered VLDL and LDL, increased HDL).

5. The endocrine function is regulated within a hypothalamus-pituitary-testis axis. GnRH is produced by hypothalamic neurons in response to stimulation by the peptide, kisspeptin. GnRH stimulates LH and FSH production by pituitary gonadotropes. Circulating levels of testosterone and estradiol-17β exert a negative feedback at both the pituitary and the hypothalamus.

6. The male reproductive tract includes the epididymis, the vas deferens, the ejaculatory duct, and the male urethra. The male tract also includes accessory sex glands, the seminal vesicles, and the prostate gland. The secretions of these glands produce most of the volume of semen. Semen serves to provide bulk to sperm, maintain an alkaline environment for sperm, provide nutrients to sperm, prevent sperm capacitation, and inhibit sperm motility in the male reproductive tract. Emission and ejaculation are achieved through primarily sympathetic stimulation of the muscularis of the male tract and somatic stimulation of pelvic muscles.

7. The male tract also includes a copulatory organ, the penis. Erection of the penis is required for internal insemination of the female tract. Erection of the penis is a neurovascular process, involving parasympathetic stimulation of erectile tissue arterioles leading to vasodilation and engorgement of the cavernous spaces. Multiple factors can lead to erectile dysfunction.

8. Klinefelter syndrome (gonadal dysgenesis) results when men have an extra X chromosome. Fibrotic changes in the testis destroy most of the seminiferous tubules.

9. Androgen insensitivity syndrome results from a hereditary defect in the gene controlling androgen receptor expression. As a result of diminished feedback, LH levels are elevated, as are testosterone levels. More testis-derived testosterone is converted to estrogens, resulting in a female phenotype (enhanced breast development, female pelvis). This process is called *testicular feminization*. The overall condition (high estrogen levels in the absence of androgen effects) gives rise to a disorder of sexual development.

SELF-STUDY PROBLEMS

1. What is the relationship of Sertoli cells to the basal and adluminal compartments of the seminiferous tubules?
2. Name two endocrine products of Sertoli cells and their function.
3. Describe the structure of a spermatozoon. What is the process from spermatid to spermatozoon called?
4. Explain how the congenital loss of 17β-hydroxysteroid dehydrogenase (type 3) would affect the following elements: spermatogenesis, external genitalia, breast development.
5. How does abuse of androgens cause low sperm count?
6. Name one event that occurs in developing sperm cells during the following processes: spermatocytogenesis, spermiogenesis, passage through the epididymis, emission.
7. What is the role of the seminal vesicles and prostate? What is PSA?
8. How does cGMP control erection?

KEYWORDS AND CONCEPTS

5α-Dihydrotestosterone (DHT)
5α-Reductase
17β-HSD3
Acrosomal vesicle
Adluminal compartment
Androgen insensitivity syndrome
Androgen receptor (AR)
Androgen-binding protein (ABP)
Anti-Müllerian hormone (AMH)
Aromatase
Axoneme
Basal compartment
Blood-epididymis barrier
Blood-testis barrier
Bulbourethral glands
Circulating levels of testosterone
Corpora cavernosa
Corpus spongiosum
Disorder of sexual development (DSD)
Efferent ductules

Ejaculation; emission
Epididymis
Erectile dysfunction (ED)
Erectile tissue
Flagellum
Fructose
Gynecomastia
Incomplete cytokinesis
Inhibin
Interstitial cells of Leydig
Intratesticular levels of testosterone
Intratubular compartment
Klinefelter syndrome
Leydig cell
Luminal testosterone-ABP complexes
Male pseudohermaphroditism
Penile urethra
Peritubular compartment
Primary spermatocytes
Prostate gland

Prostate-specific antigen (PSA)
Prostatic urethra
Pudendal nerve
Residual bodies
Rete testis
Scrotum
Secondary spermatocytes
Seminal vesicles
Seminiferous epithelium
Seminiferous tubular dysgenesis
Seminiferous tubules
Sertoli cell
Sex hormone–binding globulin (SHBG)
Spermatids

Spermatocytogenesis
Spermatogenesis
Spermatogenic cycle
Spermatogenic stages
Spermatogenic wave
Spermiation
Spermiogenesis
Spongy urethra
Stem spermatogonia
Testicular feminization
Testosterone
Urinary 17-ketosteroids
Vas (ductus) deferens

10

The Female Reproductive System

OBJECTIVES

1. Describe the anatomy and histology of the ovary and the development of the ovarian follicle.
2. Describe the steroidogenic pathways in the ovarian follicle and the functions of the ovarian steroids, estradiol-17β and progesterone.
3. Diagram the hypothalamus-pituitary-ovarian axis in the context of the monthly menstrual cycle.
4. Explain the changes in the physiology of the female reproductive tract throughout the menstrual cycle.
5. Describe the anatomy and function of the female external genitalia during the female sexual response.
6. Explain pathophysiologic conditions of the female reproductive system, including Turner syndrome and polycystic ovarian syndrome.

The physiology of pregnancy and the development and functions of the placenta and mammary glands are discussed in Chapter 11.

The female reproductive system is composed of the gonads, called ovaries, and the female reproductive tract. The mammary glands (breasts) are also part of the female reproductive system. Like the male gonads, the ovaries perform an endocrine function and a gametogenic function. The endocrine function is regulated within a hypothalamic-pituitary-ovarian axis, and ovarian hormones are absolutely necessary for the health and normal function of the female tract. The female reproductive system differs from the male system in several important general aspects (Box 10.1).

ANATOMY AND HISTOLOGY OF THE OVARY

The ovary is located within a fold of peritoneum called the broad ligament, usually close to the lateral wall of the pelvic cavity (Fig. 10.1). The ovary extends into the peritoneal cavity, and ovulated eggs briefly reside within the peritoneal cavity before they are captured by the oviducts. Nerves and blood vessels enter and exit the ovary at both its lateral and medial poles.

The ovary can be roughly divided into an outer cortex and an inner medulla (Fig. 10.2). The neurovascular elements run into the medulla of the ovary. The cortex of the ovary is composed of a densely cellular stroma. Within this stroma reside the ovarian follicles, which contain a primary oocyte surrounded by follicle cells (see later in the text). The cortex is covered by a connective tissue capsule, called the *tunica albuginea*, and a layer of simple epithelium, called ovarian surface epithelial cells. There are no ducts emerging from the ovary to convey its gametes to the reproductive tract. Thus the process of ovulation involves an inflammatory event that erodes the wall of the ovary and follicle. After ovulation, the ovarian surface epithelial cells rapidly divide to repair the wall. It is this highly mitogenic population of cells, the ovarian surface epithelial cells, which gives rise to more than 80% of cases of ovarian cancer.

GROWTH, DEVELOPMENT, AND FUNCTION OF THE OVARIAN FOLLICLE

The ovarian follicle is the functional unit of the ovary, performing both gametogenic and endocrine functions. A histologic section of the ovary from a premenopausal cycling woman contains follicular structures at many different points of their development. The life history of a follicle can be divided into the following stages:
1. Resting primordial follicle
2. Growing preantral (primary and secondary) follicle
3. Growing antral (tertiary) follicle
4. Dominant (preovulatory, graafian) follicle
5. Dominant follicle within the periovulatory period
6. Corpus luteum (of menstruation or of pregnancy)
7. Atretic follicles

BOX 10.1 Major Differences Between Male and Female Reproductive Systems

Male Reproductive System	Female Reproductive System
Gonads (testes) reside outside of abdominal cavity, in scrotum	Gonads (ovaries) reside within abdominal cavity
Gonad is continuous with reproductive tract	Gonad is not continuous with reproductive tract
Release of gametes (sperm) from gonads is continuous	Release of gamete (egg) from gonads occurs once per month
Gametic reserve is replenished throughout life	Gametic reserve is finite and exhausted by menopause
Testosterone exerts negative feedback on secretion of pituitary luteinizing hormone (LH) and follicle-stimulating hormone (FSH)	Estrogen exerts both negative and positive feedback on secretion of pituitary LH and FSH
Male tract serves only male gamete transport and maturation and delivery	Female tract serves male and female gamete transport and maturation, fertilization, placentation, and gestation
Activity of male tract does not show rhythm	Activity of female tract is based on the monthly menstrual cycle, or on the length of a pregnancy (normally about 9 months)
Testosterone is always the primary gonadal steroid	Estrogen is the primary gonadal steroid in the first half of the monthly cycle, and progesterone in the second half
The male reproductive system does not prepare for newborn	The female reproductive system prepares for newborn with breast development and milk production and is involved in breastfeeding of the newborn

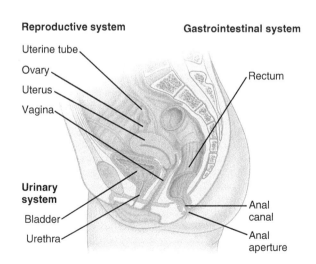

Reproductive system
- Uterine tube
- Ovary
- Uterus
- Vagina

Gastrointestinal system
- Rectum
- Anal canal
- Anal aperture

Urinary system
- Bladder
- Urethra

Fig. 10.1 Anatomy of the female pelvis and midsagittal section. (From Drake RL, Vogl W, Mitchell AWM: *Gray's Anatomy for Students,* Philadelphia, 2005, Churchill Livingstone.)

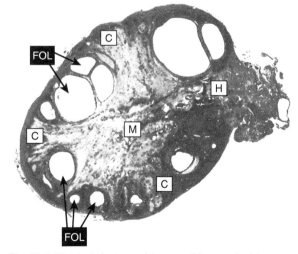

Fig. 10.2 Histologic features of the ovary. Micrograph of the ovary shows the hilum (*H*), medulla (*M*), and cortex (*C*). Follicular (*FOL*) formation and maturation occur in the cortex and are responsible for the cystic spaces seen here. (Modified from Stevens A, Lowe J: *Human Histology,* 3rd ed., Philadelphia, 2005, Mosby)

In this section, follicular biology is discussed in terms of the following elements:

- Growth and structure of the follicle
- State of the gamete
- Endocrine function of the follicle cells

Resting Primordial Follicle

Growth and Structure

Resting primordial follicles represent the earliest and simplest follicular structure in the ovary. Primordial follicles appear during midgestation through the interaction of gametes and somatic cells. The approximately 7 million oogonia enter the process of meiosis, thereby becoming primary oocytes (see Chapter 8). The primary oocytes arrest in prophase of meiosis I.

During this time, the primary oocytes become surrounded by a simple epithelium of somatic follicle cells, thereby creating primordial follicles (Fig. 10.3). The follicle cells (also called pregranulosa cells) establish gap junctions with each other and with the oocyte. The follicle cells themselves represent a true avascular epithelium, surrounded by a basal lamina. As in Sertoli cell–sperm interactions, the granulosa cells remain intimately attached to the oocyte throughout its development. Granulosa cells provide nutrients such as amino acids, nucleic acids, and pyruvate to support oocyte maturation.

Primordial follicles represent the ovarian reserve of follicles (Fig. 10.4). This is reduced from a starting number of about 7 million to fewer than 300,000 follicles at reproductive maturity. Of these, a woman will ovulate about 450 between menarche (first menstrual cycle) and menopause (cessation of menstrual cycles). At menopause, fewer than 1000 primordial follicles are left in the ovary. Primordial follicles are lost primarily from death due to follicular atresia. A small subset of primordial follicles, however, will enter follicular growth in waves. Because the ovarian follicular reserve represents a fixed, finite number, the rate at which resting primordial follicles die or begin to develop will determine the reproductive life span of a woman.

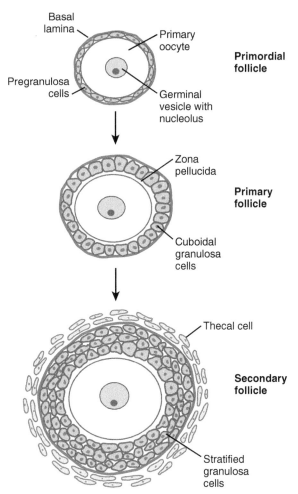

Fig. 10.3 Early follicular development from a primordial follicle to a secondary, preantral follicle.

Basal lamina — **Primary oocyte**
Pregranulosa cells — **Germinal vesicle with nucleolus**
Primordial follicle

Zona pellucida
Primary follicle
Cuboidal granulosa cells

Thecal cell
Secondary follicle
Stratified granulosa cells

The rate at which resting primordial follicles enter the growth process appears to be independent of pituitary gonadotropins. There is evidence in mice that follicle cells stimulate oocyte growth through paracrine factors. Reciprocal regulation of granulosa cell growth by the oocyte also probably occurs. Additional evidence indicates that factors from growing follicles provide restraint on the development of too many primordial follicles. One such factor appears to be anti-Müllerian hormone (AMH). AMH-knockout mice deplete their ovarian reserve more rapidly than do wild-type mice, as a result of a high rate of follicular development. In summary, whether a resting follicle enters the early growth phase is dependent primarily on intraovarian paracrine factors that are produced by both the follicle cells and oocytes.

CLINICAL BOX 10.1

Determination of the age at which a woman will reach menopause has a strong genetic component but also is influenced by environmental factors. For example, cigarette smoking significantly depletes the ovarian reserve. An overly rapid rate of atresia or development also depletes the reserve, giving rise to **premature ovarian failure,** defined as entering **menopause** before the age of 40 years. Premature ovarian failure can also be caused by severe infections or tumors of the pelvis, by chemotherapy and radiation, and by endocrine factors that disrupt the hypothalamus-pituitary-ovarian axis.

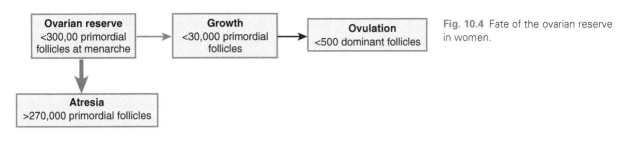

Fig. 10.4 Fate of the ovarian reserve in women.

The Gamete

As mentioned previously, the gamete in primordial follicles is derived from oogonia that have entered the first meiotic division and are now called **primary oocytes**. These primary oocytes progress through most of prophase of the first meiotic division (termed **prophase I**) over a 2-week period and then arrest in the diplotene stage. This stage is characterized by decondensation of chromatin, which supports transcription needed for oocyte maturation. Meiotic arrest at this stage, which may last up to 50 years, appears to be due to "maturational incompetence," or the lack of necessary cell cycle proteins to support the completion of meiosis. The nucleus of the oocyte, called the *germinal vesicle*, remains intact at this stage.

Endocrine Function

Although primordial follicles release paracrine factors, they do not produce ovarian steroid hormones.

Growing Preantral Follicles

Growth and Structure

One of the first visible signs of follicle growth is the appearance of **cuboidal granulosa cells** surrounding the oocyte. At this point, the follicle is referred to as a **primary follicle** (see Fig. 10.3). While granulosa cells proliferate, they form a multilayered (i.e., stratified) epithelium around the oocyte. At this stage, the follicle is referred to as a **secondary follicle** (see Fig. 10.3). Before the formation of a fluid-filled antral cavity, primary and secondary follicles are referred to as *preantral*. Once a secondary follicle acquires three to six layers of granulosa cells, it secretes paracrine factors that induce nearby stromal cells to differentiate into epithelioid **thecal cells.** Thecal cells form a flattened layer of cells around the follicle. Once a thecal layer forms, the follicle is referred to as a mature preantral follicle (see Fig. 10.3). In humans, it takes several months for a primary follicle to reach the mature preantral stage.

Follicular development is associated with an inward movement of the follicle from the outer cortex to the inner cortex, closer to the vasculature of the ovarian medulla.

Follicles release angiogenic factors that induce the development of one or two arterioles, which generate a vascular wreath around the follicle.

The Gamete

During the preantral stage, the oocyte begins to grow and produce cellular and secreted proteins. The oocyte initiates secretion of extracellular matrix glycoproteins, called *ZP proteins 1 to 4*, that form the **zona pellucida** (see Fig. 10.3). The zona pellucida ultimately increases to a thickness of 13 μm in humans and provides a species-specific binding site for sperm during fertilization (see Chapter 11). Of importance, granulosa cells and the oocyte project cellular extensions through the zona pellucida and maintain gap junctional contacts. The oocyte also continues to secrete paracrine factors that regulate follicle cell growth and differentiation.

Endocrine Function

The granulosa cells express the follicle-stimulating hormone (FSH) receptor during the preantral period but are dependent primarily on factors from the oocyte to grow. They do not produce ovarian hormones at this early stage of follicular development.

The newly acquired thecal cells are analogous to testicular Leydig cells (see Chapter 9), in that they reside outside of the epithelial *nurse cells,* express the luteinizing hormone (LH) receptor, and produce androgens. The main difference between Leydig cells and thecal cells is that thecal cells do not express high levels of a 17β-hydroxysteroid dehydrogenase (17β-HSD). Thus the major product of the thecal cells is androstenedione, as opposed to testosterone. Androstenedione production at this stage is absent or minimal.

Growing Antral Follicles

Growth and Structure

Mature preantral follicles develop into early **antral follicles** (Fig. 10.5) over a period of about 25 days, growing from a diameter of approximately 0.1 to 0.2 mm. Once the granulosa epithelium increases to six or seven layers, fluid-filled

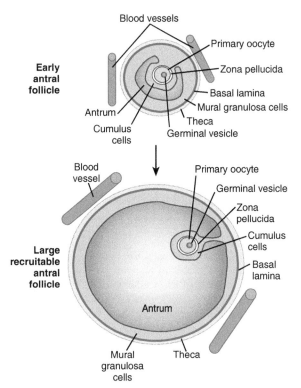

Fig. 10.5 Late follicular development from an early antral follicle to a large antral follicle.

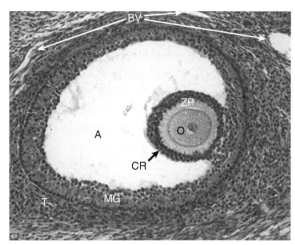

Fig. 10.6 Histologic features of ovarian graafian follicle. Ovum (*O*) is surrounded by zona pellucida (*ZP*). As a result of shrinkage artifacts, the zona pellucida appears larger than normal. Cumulus cells (*C*) are indicated, as is the large antrum (*A*). *BV*, Blood vessels in outer thecal stroma; *MG*, mural glomerulosa cell; *T*, thecal cells.

spaces appear between cells and coalesce into the antrum. Over a period of about 45 days, this wave of small antral follicles will continue to grow to **large, recruitable antral follicles** that are 2 to 5 mm in diameter. This period of growth is characterized by about a 100-fold increase in granulosa cells (from about 10,000 to 1,000,000 cells). It is also characterized by swelling of the antral cavity, which increasingly divides the granulosa cells into two discrete populations (Fig. 10.6; see Fig. 10.5):

1. The **mural granulosa cells** (also called **stratum granulosum**) are those that form the outer wall of the follicle. The basal layer is adhered to the basal lamina and in close proximity to the outer-lying thecal layers. Mural granulosa cells become highly steroidogenic and remain in the ovary after ovulation to differentiate into the corpus luteum.
2. The **cumulus cells** are the inner cells that surround the oocyte (they are also referred to as the **cumulus oophorus**). The layer of cumulus cells closest to the oocyte, the **corona radiata**, maintains gap and adhesion junctions with the oocyte. Cumulus cells are released from the ovary with the oocyte (collectively referred to as the **cumulus-oocyte complex**) during the process of **ovulation**. Cumulus cells are crucial for the ability of the fimbriated end of the oviduct to "capture" and move the oocyte by a ciliary transport mechanism along the length of the oviduct to the site of fertilization.

Early antral follicles are dependent on **pituitary FSH** for normal growth. Large antral follicles become **highly dependent** on pituitary FSH for their growth and sustained viability. As discussed later (under "Dominant Follicle"), 2- to 5-mm follicles are recruited to enter a rapid growth phase by a transient increase in FSH that occurs toward the end of a previous menstrual cycle.

The Gamete

The oocyte grows rapidly in the early stages of antral follicles; growth then slows in larger follicles. During the antral stage, the oocyte synthesizes cell-cycle proteins, such as **cyclin-dependent kinase-1 (CDK1)** and **cyclin B**, and the oocyte becomes competent to complete meiosis I at ovulation. Thus in preantral follicles, the oocyte fails to complete meiosis I because of a dearth of specific meiosis-associated proteins (i.e., they are incompetent to complete meiosis I). Larger antral follicles, however, gain **meiotic competence** but still maintain **meiotic arrest** until the midcycle LH surge. Meiotic arrest is achieved in the meiotically competent, prophase-arrested oocyte by the maintenance of elevated **cyclic adenosine monophosphate (cAMP)** levels. The oocyte expresses a constitutively active (i.e., active without a ligand) G-protein–coupled receptor, called **GPR3**, that maintains high cAMP levels (Figs. 10.7 and 10.8). Through a cAMP-PKA phosphorylation cascade, the **cyclin**

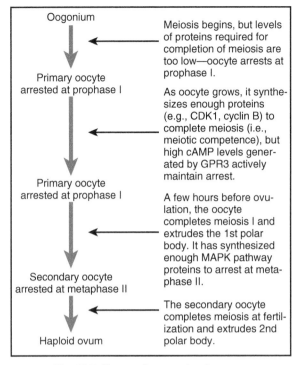

Fig. 10.7 Phases of oocyte development.

B–cyclin-dependent kinase, CDK1, complex (also called maturation-promoting factor, or MPF) is kept inactive. As discussed in Chapter 1, intracellular cAMP levels are determined by the activity of adenylyl cyclase, which generates cAMP, and by the activity of phosphodiesterases (PDEs), which metabolize cAMP to AMP. Cyclic guanosine monophosphate (cGMP) contributes to the maintenance-elevated cAMP levels in competent oocytes by inhibiting the oocyte-specific PDE, PDE3A. Cyclic GMP is made in the cumulus cells and mural granulosa cells and is transferred to the oocyte through gap junctions (see Fig. 10.8).

Endocrine Function

Thecal cells of large antral follicles produce significant amounts of androstenedione and, to a much lesser extent, testosterone (Fig. 10.9). This is due to high expression of CYP17 with both 17-hydroxylase and 17,20-lyase activities (Fig. 10.10A). Androgens are converted to estradiol-17β by the mural granulosa cells (see Fig. 10.9). At this stage, FSH stimulates proliferation of granulosa cells and induces the expression of CYP19-aromatase (Fig. 10.10B) required for estrogen synthesis. Additionally, the mural granulosa cells of the large antral follicles produce increasing amounts of inhibin B during the early follicular phase. Low levels of estrogen and inhibin exert a negative feedback effect on FSH secretion, thereby contributing to the selection of the follicle with the most FSH-responsive cells.

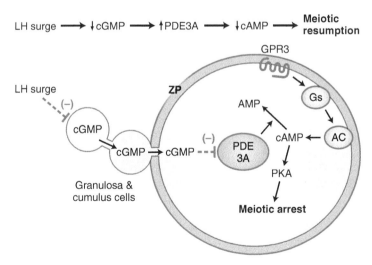

Fig. 10.8 Mechanisms involved in meiotic arrest of a meiotically competent primary oocyte. The smaller cells represent cumulus, stalk, and mural granulosa cells—all connected by gap junctions and all contributing to elevated cyclic guanosine monophosphate (cGMP) in the oocyte. AC, Adenylyl cyclase; PDE 3A, phosphodiesterase 3A; ZP, zona pellucida. (From Koeppen BM, Stanton BA, editors: Berne and Levy Physiology, 7th ed., Philadelphia, 2017, Mosby.)

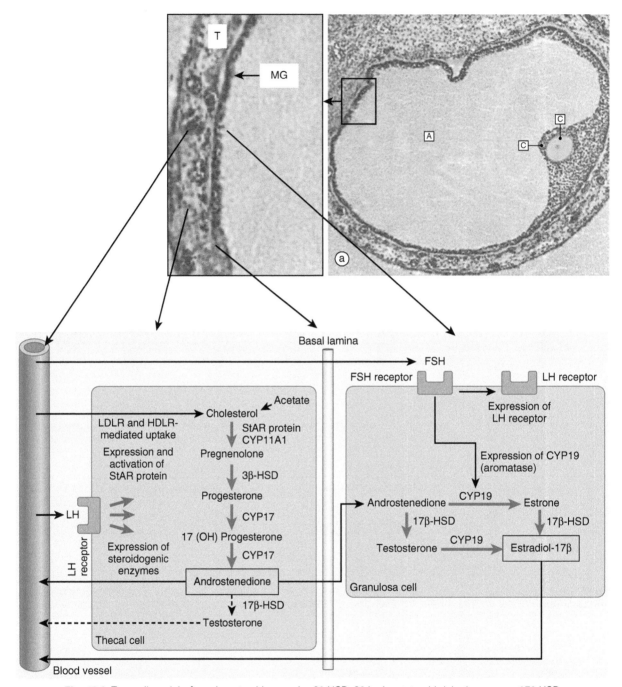

Fig. 10.9 Two-cell model of ovarian steroidogenesis. *3β-HSD*, 3β-hydroxysteroid dehydrogenase; *17β-HSD*, 17β-hydroxysteroid dehydrogenase; *FSH*, follicle-stimulating hormone; *HDLR*, high-density lipoprotein receptor; *LDLR*, low-density lipoprotein receptor; *LH*, luteinizing hormone; *StAR protein*, steroidogenic acute regulatory protein. (From Koeppen BM, Stanton BA, editors: *Berne and Levy Physiology*, 7th ed., Philadelphia, 2017, Mosby.)

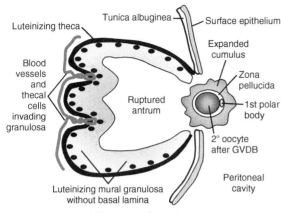

Fig. 10.10 Ovulation.

Dominant Follicle

Growth and Structure

At the end of a previous menstrual cycle, a crop of large (2- to 5-mm) antral follicles (see Fig. 10.4) is recruited to begin rapid, gonadotropin-dependent development. The total number of recruited follicles in both ovaries can be as high as 20 in a younger woman (<33 years of age), but rapidly declines at older ages. The number of recruited follicles is reduced to the ovulatory quota (which is one in humans) by the process of selection. While FSH levels decline, the rapidly growing follicles progressively undergo atresia, until one follicle is left. Generally, the largest follicle with the most FSH receptors of the recruited crop becomes the dominant follicle. Selection occurs during the early follicular phase. By midcycle, the dominant follicle becomes a large preovulatory follicle that is 20 mm in diameter and contains about 50 million granulosa cells by the midcycle gonadotropin surge.

The Gamete

The oocyte is competent to complete meiosis I but remains arrested in the dominant follicle through the mechanisms described earlier. Growth of the oocyte continues, but at a slower rate—the human oocyte reaches a diameter of about 140 μm by ovulation. The stalk by which cumulus cells are attached to the mural granulosa cells becomes increasingly attenuated.

Endocrine Function

The newly selected follicle emerges for the first time during its development as a significant steroidogenic *gland*. Ovarian steroidogenesis requires both theca and granulosa cells (see Fig. 10.9). As discussed earlier, theca cells express LH receptors and produce androgens. Basal levels of LH stimulate the expression of steroidogenic enzymes, as well

as the LDL receptor in the theca. Theca cells show robust expression of CYP11A1 (also called P-450 cholesterol side-chain cleavage), 3β-hydroxysteroid dehydrogenase (3β-HSD), and CYP17, with both 17-hydroxylase activity and 17,20-lyase activity. Androgens (primarily androstenedione but also some testosterone) released from the theca can diffuse into the mural granulosa cells or can enter the vasculature surrounding the follicle.

The mural granulosa cells of the selected follicle have a high number of FSH receptors and are very sensitive to FSH signaling. FSH strongly upregulates CYP19 (aromatase) gene expression and activity (see Fig. 10.9). CYP19 converts androstenedione to the weak estrogen, estrone, and converts testosterone to the potent estrogen, estradiol-17β. Granulosa cells express activating isoforms of 17β-HSD, which ultimately drives steroidogenesis toward the production of estradiol-17β (see later in the text). FSH also induces the expression of inhibin B during the follicular phase.

Of importance, FSH also induces the expression of LH receptors in the mural granulosa cells during the second half of the follicular phase (see Fig. 10.9). Thus mural granulosa cells become responsive to both gonadotropins, allowing these cells to maintain high levels of CYP19 in the face of declining FSH levels. Acquisition of LH receptors also ensures that mural granulosa cells will respond to the LH surge (see later).

The Dominant Follicle During the Periovulatory Period

The periovulatory period can be defined as the time from the onset of the LH surge to the expulsion of the cumulus-oocyte complex out of the ovary (i.e., ovulation). This process lasts 32 to 36 hours in women. Starting at the same time, and superimposed on the process of ovulation, is a change in the steroidogenic function of the theca and mural granulosa cells. This process is called luteinization and culminates in the formation of a corpus luteum that is capable of producing large amounts of progesterone, along with estrogen, within a few days after ovulation.

Growth and Structure

The LH surge induces dramatic structural changes in the dominant follicle that involve its rupture, ovulation of the cumulus-oocyte complex, and the biogenesis of a new structure called the corpus luteum from the remaining theca cells and mural granulosa cells. Major structural changes occur during this transition (see Fig. 10.10):

1. Before ovulation, the large preovulatory follicle presses against the ovarian surface, generating a poorly vascularized bulge of the ovarian wall called the stigma. The LH surge induces the release of

inflammatory cytokines and hydrolytic enzymes from the theca and granulosa cells. These secreted components lead to the breakdown of the follicle wall, tunica albuginea, and surface epithelium in the vicinity of the stigma. At the end of this process, the antral cavity becomes continuous with the peritoneal cavity.

2. The stalklike attachment of the cumulus cells to the mural granulosa cells detaches, and the cumulus-oocyte complex becomes free-floating within the antral cavity. As an indirect response to the LH surge (i.e., in response to LH-dependent paracrine factors), the oocyte releases the transforming growth factor-β (TGF-β)–related factor, GDF9. GDF9 (see earlier in the text) stimulates the cumulus cells to secrete hyaluronic acid and other extracellular matrix components. These secreted components enlarge the entire cumulus-oocyte complex, a process called cumulus expansion. This enlarged cumulus-oocyte complex is more easily captured and transported by the oviduct. The expanded cumulus also makes the cumulus-oocyte complex easier for spermatozoa to find. The cumulus-oocyte complex is released through the ruptured stigma in a slow, gentle process, indicating that the follicular fluid in the antrum is not under increased pressure. The specific forces that lead to expulsion of the cumulus-oocyte complex are unknown.

3. The basal lamina of the mural granulosa cells is enzymatically degraded, and blood vessels and outer-lying theca can push into the granulosa cells. Granulosa cells secrete angiogenic factors, such as vascular endothelial growth factor (VEGF), angiopoietin-2, and basic fibroblast growth factor (bFGF), which significantly increase the blood supply to the new corpus luteum.

The Gamete

Before ovulation, the primary oocyte is competent to complete meiosis but is arrested in prophase I as a result of high cAMP levels (see Fig. 10.8). The LH surge induces the oocyte to progress to metaphase of meiosis II. The oocyte subsequently arrests at metaphase II until fertilization. LH receptors are only present on the mural granulosa cells. The LH surge induces a series of events that ultimately lead to a decrease in cGMP in the oocyte. This decrease in cGMP removes the inhibition on the cAMP phosphodiesterase, PDE3A, which now becomes active and degrades cAMP in the oocyte.

The decrease in cAMP and protein kinase A (PKA) activity in the oocyte ultimately leads to activation of MPF, composed of CDK1 and cyclin B. MPF drives nuclear events that complete meiosis I with the extrusion of the first polar body. The secondary oocyte (called an egg) then arrests in metaphase of meiosis II. This is achieved by an increase in an activity called cytostatic factor (CSF). It is now known that CSF is composed of the kinase, c-Mos, its target mitogen-activated kinase kinase (MAPKK), also called MEK1 (see Chapter 1), and MAPK. Thus elevation of the MAPK signaling pathway is required for arrest at metaphase II, and fertilization leads to the rapid degradation of MAPK. It should be emphasized that our understanding of normal oocyte maturation has had a major impact on the ability to treat infertile couples through the process of in vitro fertilization (IVF). Normal oocyte biology dictates the type of hormonal treatment, the timing of egg retrieval, and the meiotic stage of eggs used for fertilization.

Endocrine Function

Both theca and mural granulosa cells express LH receptors at the time of the LH surge. The LH surge induces terminal differentiation (called luteinization) of the granulosa cells—a process that will continue for several days after ovulation. During the periovulatory period, the LH surge induces the following shifts in the steroidogenic activity of the mural granulosa cells (Fig. 10.11):

1. It transiently inhibits CYP19 expression and, consequently, estrogen production. The rapid decline in estrogen helps to turn off the positive feedback on LH secretion.

2. It causes the direct vascularization of the granulosa cells by inducing the breakdown of the basal lamina. This makes LDL and HDL cholesterol accessible to these cells for steroidogenesis. The LH surge also increases the expression of the LDL receptor and HDL receptor (SR-BI) in granulosa cells.

3. It increases the expression of StAR protein, CYP11A1 (side-chain cleavage enzyme), and 3β-HSD. Because CYP17 activity, especially the 17,20-lyase function, is largely absent in granulosa cells, these cells begin to secrete progesterone, and progesterone levels will gradually increase over the next week.

The Corpus Luteum

Growth and Structure

After ovulation, the remnant of the antral cavity fills with blood from damaged blood vessels in the vicinity of the stigma. This gives rise to a corpus hemorrhagicum with clotted blood within the former antral lumen (Fig. 10.12). Within a few days, red blood cells and debris are removed by macrophages, and fibroblasts fill in the antral cavity with a hyaline-like extracellular matrix. In the mature corpus luteum, the granulosa cells, now called granulosa

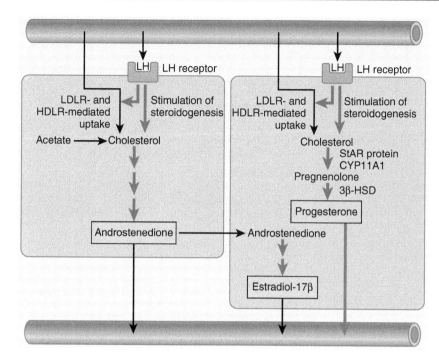

Fig. 10.11 Two-cell model of ovarian steroidogenesis during the luteal phase. *3β-HSD*, 3β-hydroxysteroid dehydrogenase; *HDLR*, high-density lipoprotein receptor; *LDLR*, low-density lipoprotein receptor; *LH*, luteinizing hormone; *StAR protein*, steroidogenic acute regulatory protein. Note the absence of a basal lamina. (From Koeppen BM, Stanton BA, editors: *Berne and Levy Physiology*, 7th ed., Philadelphia, 2017, Mosby.)

lutein cells, enlarge and become filled with lipid (cholesterol esters). The enlarged granulosa lutein cells collapse into and partially fill in the old antral cavity. Proliferation of these cells is very limited. The theca, along with blood vessels, mast cells, macrophages, leukocytes, and other resident connective tissue cells, infiltrates the granulosa layer at multiple sites.

The human corpus luteum is programmed to live for 14 ± 2 days (**corpus luteum of menstruation**), unless *rescued* by the LH-like hormone, human chorionic gonadotropin (hCG), that originates from an implanting embryo (hCG is the protein that is detected in pregnancy tests; see **Chapter 11**). If rescued, the **corpus luteum of pregnancy** will remain viable for as long as the pregnancy (usually about 9 months), and serves as the major source of progesterone that maintains pregnancy, until the placenta is developed enough to take over progesterone production (about 2 to 3 months). The mechanism by which the corpus luteum of menstruation regresses in 14 days is not fully understood, although the timing is very consistent. In response to paracrine factors and, perhaps, declining progesterone production, the corpus luteum becomes progressively unresponsive to pituitary LH and needs the extra amount of hCG to remain viable. The corpus luteum ultimately is turned into a scarlike body called the

corpus albicans (see Fig. 10.12), which sinks into the medulla of the ovary and is slowly absorbed.

The Gamete

The LH surge induces two parallel events, ovulation and luteinization. If ovulation occurs normally, the corpus luteum is devoid of a gamete.

Endocrine Function

Progesterone production by the corpus luteum (see Fig. 10.11) increases steadily from the onset of the LH surge and peaks during the midluteal phase. The main purpose of this timing is to transform the uterine lining into an adhesive and supportive structure for implantation and early pregnancy. As discussed in Chapter 11, the midluteal phase is synchronized with early embryogenesis, so the uterus is optimally primed when a blastocyst enters it around day 22 of the menstrual cycle. Estrogen production transiently decreases in response to the LH surge but then rebounds and also peaks at midluteal phase.

Luteal hormonal output is absolutely dependent on basal LH levels (see Fig. 10.11). In fact, progesterone output is closely correlated with the pulsatile pattern of LH release in women. Both FSH and LH are reduced to basal levels during the luteal phase by the negative feedback from progesterone and estrogen. Also, granulosa lutein

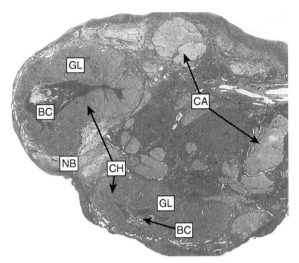

Fig. 10.12 Histologic features of the corpus hemorrhagicum. Micrograph of an ovary containing two corpora hemorrhagicum (*CH*). These arise from the coovulation of two dominant follicles, creating the potential for nonidentical twins. Each corpus luteum shows a central blood clot (*BC*) surrounded by a thick layer of lipid-rich granulosa lutein cells (*GL*). Degenerating corpora lutea are called corpora albicans (*CA*), which look like scar tissue and are eventually degraded. (Modified from Stevens A, Lowe J: *Human Histology,* 3rd ed., Philadelphia, 2005, Mosby.)

cells secrete **inhibin A**, which further represses FSH secretion. The elevated estrogen levels at midluteal phase may be responsible for the decrease in the sensitivity of the corpus luteum to LH, so progesterone and estrogen levels decline during the second half of the luteal phase unless an increase in circulating LH-like activity (i.e., in the form of hCG) compensates for the decreased sensitivity to LH.

CLINICAL BOX 10.2

The corpus luteum must generate large amounts of progesterone for an adequate number of days to support **implantation** and early **pregnancy**. Thus the duration of the life of the corpus luteum (14 days) is very regular, and a shortened luteal phase typically leads to **infertility**. The quality of the corpus luteum is largely dependent on the size and health of the dominant follicle from which the corpus luteum developed. Dominant follicle development, in turn, is dependent on normal hypothalamic and pituitary stimulation during the follicular phase. Numerous factors that perturb hypothalamic and pituitary output during the follicular phase, including **heavy exercise, starvation, high prolactin levels**, and **abnormal thyroid function**, can lead to **luteal phase deficiency (LPD)** and **infertility**.

The corpus luteum of other mammalian species also produces an insulin-like hormone called relaxin. The human corpus luteum produces very low levels of relaxin, however, and the physiologic role of circulating relaxin in humans has not been established.

Follicular Atresia

Follicular atresia refers to the demise of an ovarian follicle and represents by far the predominant process in the ovary. During atresia, the granulosa cells and oocytes undergo apoptosis. The theca cells typically persist and repopulate the cellular stroma of the ovary. The theca cells retain LH receptors and the ability to produce androgens and collectively are referred to as the **interstitial gland of the ovary**. Follicles can undergo atresia at any time during development.

Follicular Development and the Monthly Menstrual Cycle

The first half of the monthly menstrual cycle is referred to as the **follicular phase of the ovary** and is characterized by the recruitment and growth of 15 to 20 antral follicles (2 to 5 mm in diameter), selection of one of these follicles as the dominant follicle, and growth of the dominant follicle until ovulation. The dominant follicle must contain a fully developed, meiotically competent oocyte and somatic follicle cells that secrete high levels of estrogen. It takes several months for a primordial follicle to reach the size of an antral follicle that can be recruited (Fig. 10.13). Therefore it should be noted that much of follicular development occurs independently of the monthly menstrual cycle. The second half of the menstrual cycle is referred to as the **luteal phase of the ovary** and is dominated by the hormonal secretions of the corpus luteum. Nevertheless, small follicles continue to develop within the ovarian stroma during the luteal phase.

THE HUMAN MENSTRUAL CYCLE

As stated earlier, late follicular development and luteal function are absolutely dependent on normal hypothalamic and pituitary function. As in the male, hypothalamic neurons secrete **gonadotropin-releasing hormone (GnRH)** in a **pulsatile** manner. GnRH, in turn, stimulates LH and FSH production by pituitary gonadotropes. A high frequency of GnRH pulses (one pulse every 60 to 90 min) selectively promotes LH production, whereas a slow frequency (one pulse every 120 min) selectively promotes FSH production. A major difference between the male and the female reproductive axes is the **midcycle gonadotropin surge** in females, which is dependent on a high level of estrogen over a specific duration coming from the dominant follicle.

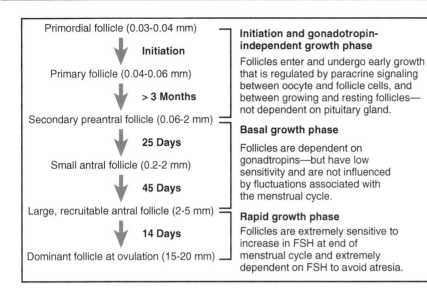

Primordial follicle (0.03-0.04 mm)

Initiation

Primary follicle (0.04-0.06 mm)

> 3 Months

Secondary preantral follicle (0.06-2 mm)

25 Days

Small antral follicle (0.2-2 mm)

45 Days

Large, recruitable antral follicle (2-5 mm)

14 Days

Dominant follicle at ovulation (15-20 mm)

Initiation and gonadotropin-independent growth phase

Follicles enter and undergo early growth that is regulated by paracrine signaling between oocyte and follicle cells, and between growing and resting follicles—not dependent on pituitary gland.

Basal growth phase

Follicles are dependent on gonadtropins—but have low sensitivity and are not influenced by fluctuations associated with the menstrual cycle.

Rapid growth phase

Follicles are extremely sensitive to increase in FSH at end of menstrual cycle and extremely dependent on FSH to avoid atresia.

Fig. 10.13 Timing and phases of follicular growth.

A highly dynamic *conversation* occurs among the ovary, pituitary, and hypothalamus, which orchestrates the events of the menstrual cycle (Fig. 10.14). This section outlines the main events involving the ovary and pituitary gonadotrope that regulate the menstrual cycle, with an overview of hypothalamic involvement. In the next section, the effects of the hormonal changes on the female reproductive tract, especially the uterus, are discussed.

The following outline of events, numbered as depicted in Fig. 10.14, begins with the ovary at the end of the luteal phase of a previous, nonfertile cycle:

Ovary—**event 1**: In the absence of fertilization and implantation, the corpus luteum regresses and dies (a phenomenon called **luteolysis**). This leads to a drastic decline in the levels of progesterone, estrogen, and inhibin A by day 24 of the menstrual cycle.

Pituitary gonadotrope—**event 2**: The gonadotrope perceives the end of luteal function as a release from negative feedback. This permits a rise in **FSH** that occurs about 2 days before the onset of menstruation. The basis for the selective increase in FSH is incompletely understood but may result from the **slow frequency of GnRH pulses** during the luteal phase, which is due to high progesterone levels.

Ovary—**event 3**: The rise in FSH levels recruits a crop of antral follicles (2 to 5 mm in diameter) to begin rapid, highly gonadotropin-dependent growth. These follicles produce low levels of **estrogen** and **inhibin B**.

Pituitary gonadotrope—**event 4**: The gonadotrope responds to the slowly rising levels of estrogen and inhibin B by decreasing FSH secretion. Loss of high levels of progesterone and estrogen causes an increase in the frequency of GnRH pulses, thereby selectively increasing **LH** synthesis and secretion by the gonadotrope. Thus the **LH/FSH ratio** slowly increases throughout the follicular phase.

Ovary—**event 5**: The ovary's response to declining FSH levels is **follicular atresia** of all the recruited follicles, except for one **dominant follicle**. Thus the process of selection is driven by an extreme dependency of follicles on FSH in the face of declining FSH secretion. Usually, only the largest follicle with the most FSH receptors and best blood supply (i.e., most angiogenic) survives. This follicle produces increasing amounts of estradiol-17β and inhibin B during the second half of the follicular phase. FSH also induces the expression of **LH receptors** in the mural granulosa cells of the dominant follicle.

Pituitary gonadotrope—**event 6**: Once the dominant follicle causes the circulating estrogen levels to exceed 200 pg/mL for about 50 hours in women, estrogen exerts a **positive feedback** on the gonadotrope, producing the midcycle LH surge. This is enhanced by the small amount of progesterone starting to be made at midcycle. The exact mechanism of the positive feedback is unknown, but it occurs largely at the level of the pituitary. **GnRH receptors** and the **sensitivity to GnRH signaling** increase dramatically in the gonadotropes. The hypothalamus contributes to the gonadotropin surge by increasing the frequency of GnRH pulses. There is some evidence that other neurons in the hypothalamus (e.g., kisspeptin neurons; see Chapter 8) respond to high levels of estrogen by increasing the frequency and amount of GnRH released.

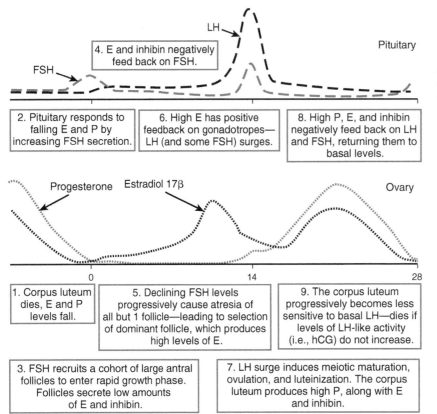

4. E and inhibin negatively feed back on FSH.

FSH

LH

Pituitary

2. Pituitary responds to falling E and P by increasing FSH secretion.

6. High E has positive feedback on gonadotropes— LH (and some FSH) surges.

8. High P, E, and inhibin negatively feed back on LH and FSH, returning them to basal levels.

Progesterone   Estradiol 17β

Ovary

0   14   28

1. Corpus luteum dies, E and P levels fall.

5. Declining FSH levels progressively cause atresia of all but 1 follicle—leading to selection of dominant follicle, which produces high levels of E.

9. The corpus luteum progressively becomes less sensitive to basal LH—dies if levels of LH-like activity (i.e., hCG) do not increase.

3. FSH recruits a cohort of large antral follicles to enter rapid growth phase. Follicles secrete low amounts of E and inhibin.

7. LH surge induces meiotic maturation, ovulation, and luteinization. The corpus luteum produces high P, along with E and inhibin.

Fig. 10.14 The human menstrual cycle—a conversation between the ovary and the pituitary, with the hypothalamus as a facilitator. See text for comments on the involvement of the hypothalamus. *E*, Estrogen; *FSH*, follicle-stimulating hormone; *hCG*, human chorionic gonadotropin; *LH*, luteinizing hormone; *P*, progesterone.

Ovary—event 7: The LH surge drives three general events in the ovary:

1. The primary oocyte completes meiosis I and arrests at metaphase of meiosis II. This is associated with **germinal vesicle breakdown (GVBD;** the germinal vesicle refers to the nucleus of the oocyte), which is the dissolution of the nuclear membrane and interphase nuclear structure, followed by the formation of a metaphase spindle and then the first oocyte cleavage. Development of a metaphase II-stage egg is complete by the time of ovulation.
2. The wall of the follicle and of the ovary at the stigma is broken down, and the free-floating cumulus-oocyte complex is extruded from the ovary (i.e., ovulation). This occurs about 32 to 36 hours after the onset of the LH surge.
3. The mural granulosa cells and theca cells are restructured to form the corpus luteum. This involves direct vascularization of the granulosa cells and their differentiation into progesterone- and

estrogen-producing cells. Note that estrogen production transiently drops for about 2 days after the onset of LH production, which may terminate the positive feedback. The granulosa cells also secrete inhibin A. The process of luteinization continues for several days after the onset of the LH surge. The small amount of progesterone secreted during the periovulatory period contributes to the magnitude of the LH surge.

Pituitary gonadotrope—event 8: Rising levels of progesterone, estrogen, and inhibin A by the mature corpus luteum negatively feed back on the pituitary gonadotrope. Even though estrogen levels exceed the 200 pg/mL threshold for positive feedback, the **high progesterone levels** block any positive feedback. Consequently, both FSH and LH levels decline to basal levels.

Ovary—event 9: Basal levels of LH (but not FSH) are absolutely required for normal corpus luteum function. The corpus luteum becomes progressively insensitive to LH signaling, however, and dies unless LH-like activity

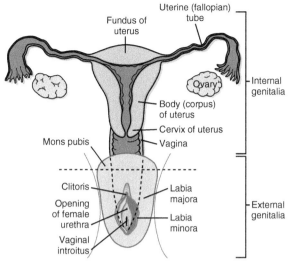

Fig. 10.15 The internal and external genitalia of the female reproductive tract. (Modified from Drake RL, Vogl W, Mitchell AWM: *Gray's Anatomy for Students,* Philadelphia, 2005, Churchill Livingstone.)

(i.e., hCG from an implanted embryo) increases. In a nonfertile cycle, the corpus luteum of menstruation will regress in 14 days, and progesterone and estrogen levels will start to decline by about 10 days.

Pituitary gonadotrope—event 10: Removal of negative feedback causes an increase in FSH at the end of the cycle, and the entire process begins again.

From this sequence of events, it is evident that the **ovary** is the primary clock for the menstrual cycle. The timing of the two main pituitary-based events—the transient rise in FSH that recruits large antral follicles and the LH surge that induces ovulation—is determined by two respective ovarian events:

- Highly regular life span of a corpus luteum and its demise after 14 days
- Growth of the dominant follicle to a point at which it can maintain a sustained high production of estrogen that induces a switch to positive feedback at the pituitary

The hypothalamic release of GnRH changes over the cycle. The frequency of GnRH pulses increases during the second half of the follicular phase and decreases during the luteal phase.

FEMALE REPRODUCTIVE TRACT

The female reproductive tract does not connect directly to the ovaries (Fig. 10.15). The internal portion of the tract consists of right and left oviducts and the following midline structures: uterus, cervix, and vagina. The external opening of the vagina is surrounded by the external genitalia.

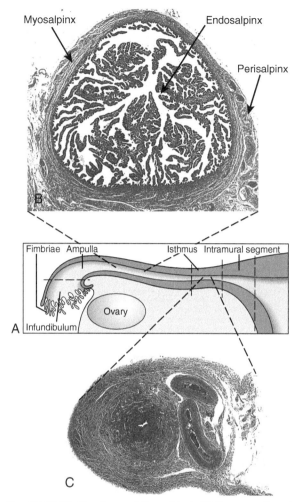

Fig. 10.16 (A) Structures of the oviduct. (B) Cross section of the oviduct at the ampulla, with a large lumen filled with mucosal (endosalpinx) folds. (C) Cross section of the oviduct at the isthmus, showing a much smaller lumen but a thicker muscularis (myosalpinx). (Modified from Stevens A, Lowe J: *Human Histology,* 3rd ed., Philadelphia, 2005, Mosby.)

The Oviduct

Structure and Function

The **oviducts** (also called the **uterine tubes** or **fallopian tubes**) are muscular tubes that are open at both ends. The end of the oviduct close to the surface of each ovary has finger-like projections, called **fimbriae**. The opposite end pierces the wall of the uterus and opens into the uterine lumen. The oviducts can be divided into four sections (Fig. 10.16). Going from ovary to uterus, these sections are named as follows:

1. **Infundibulum**, which includes the fimbriae
2. **Ampulla**, which has a relatively wide lumen and extensive folding of the mucosa

UTERINE LUMEN

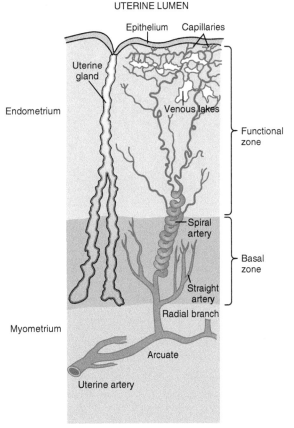

Fig. 10.17 Structure of the uterine endometrium. (Modified from Strauss J III, Coutifaris C: The endometrium and myometrium: Regulation and dysfunction. In Yen SSC, Jaffe RB, Barbieri RL, editors: *Reproductive Endocrinology*, 4th ed., Philadelphia, 1999, Saunders, pp 191-217.)

3. **Isthmus,** which has a relatively narrow lumen and less mucosal folding
4. **Intramural or uterine segment,** which extends through the uterine wall at the superior corners (horns) of the uterus

The wall of the oviduct is composed of a mucosa called the **endosalpinx,** a two-layered muscularis called the **myosalpinx,** and outer-lying connective tissue, the **perisalpinx, that contains numerous blood vessels** (Fig. 10.17). The endosalpinx is lined by a simple epithelium made up of two cell types: **ciliated cells and secretory cells.** The cilia are most numerous at the ovarian end (infundibulum and ampulla) and beat toward the uterus. The cilia on the fimbriae are the sole mechanism for transport of the ovulated cumulus-oocyte complex into the oviduct. Once the complex passes through the ostium of the oviduct and enters the ampulla, it is moved by both cilia and peristaltic contractions of the myosalpinx.

As shown in Fig. 10.17, the ovarian end of the oviduct (infundibulum and ampulla) has a wide lumen partially filled with a highly folded myosalpinx. This allows the cumulus-oocyte complex to be transported while in intimate contact with ciliated mucosal cells. The uterine end of the oviduct (isthmus and intramural segment) has a narrow lumen and a relatively thicker muscularis. This allows for slow transport of an early embryo to the uterus primarily by peristaltic waves of the muscularis.

The main functions of the oviducts are the following:

1. **Capture of the cumulus-oocyte complex** at ovulation and **transport** of the cumulus-oocyte complex to a midway point (the ampullary-isthmus junction), where fertilization takes place. Oviductal secretions coat and infuse the cumulus-oocyte complex and may be required for viability and fertilizability.
2. Providing a site for **sperm storage.** Women who ovulate up to 5 days after sexual intercourse can become pregnant. Sperm remain viable by adhering to the epithelial cells lining the isthmus. The secretions of the oviduct also induce **capacitation** and **hyperactivity of sperm** (see Chapter 11).
3. Providing nutritional support to the preimplantation embryo by the oviductal secretions. Also, the timing of the movement of the embryo into the uterus is critical because the human uterus has an implantation window of about 3 days. The oviduct needs to harbor the early embryo until it reaches the blastocyst stage (5 days after fertilization); then it allows the embryo to move into the uterine cavity (see Chapter 11).

The secretory cells produce a protein-rich mucus that is conveyed along the oviduct to the uterus by the cilia. This ciliary-mucus escalator maintains a healthy epithelium, moves the cumulus-oocyte complex toward the uterus, and may provide directional cues for swimming sperm. The movement of the cumulus-oocyte complex slows at the ampullary-isthmus junction, where fertilization normally takes place. This appears to be due in part to a thick mucus that is produced by the human isthmus and to an increased tone of the muscularis of the isthmus. The composition of oviductal secretions is complex and includes growth factors, enzymes, and oviduct-specific glycoproteins. Note that IVF has shown that the secretions of the oviduct are not absolutely necessary for fertility by in vitro techniques. However, normal oviductal function is absolutely required for both fertilization and implantation from in vivo insemination, and to minimize the risk for ectopic implantation (i.e., implantation outside of the uterus). In fact, the most common site of ectopic implantation is the oviduct.

CLINICAL BOX 10.3

Primary ciliary dyskinesia (also called **immotile cilia syndrome** or **Kartagener syndrome**) is a highly heterogeneous inherited disease caused by the absence or defect of one of the many components of the ciliary-flagellar axoneme. The mutation can cause no beating (ciliary immotility), abnormal beating (ciliary dyskinesia), or loss of cilia (ciliary aplasia). The disease is primarily characterized by infections of the upper respiratory tract, nasal tract, and middle ear. The importance of ciliary transport in the oviduct is indicated by the finding that about 50% of women with primary ciliary dyskinesia are infertile or subfertile.

Hormonal Regulation During the Menstrual Cycle

In general, estrogen secreted during the follicular phase increases endosalpinx epithelial cell size and height. Estrogen increases blood flow to the lamina propria of the oviducts, increases the production of oviduct-specific glycoproteins (whose functions are poorly understood), and increases ciliogenesis throughout the oviduct. Estrogen promotes the secretion of a thick mucus in the isthmus and increases tone of the muscularis of the isthmus, thereby keeping the cumulus-oocyte complex at the ampullary-isthmus junction for fertilization. High progesterone, along with estrogen, during the early to mid-luteal phase decreases epithelial cell size and function. Progesterone promotes deciliation. Progesterone also decreases the secretion of thick mucus and relaxes the tone in the isthmus.

The Uterus

Structure and Function

The uterus is a single organ that sits in the midline of the pelvic cavity between the bladder and the rectum. The mucosa of the uterus is called the **endometrium**, the three-layered, thick muscularis is called the **myometrium**, and the outer connective tissue and serosa are called the **perimetrium**. The parts of the uterus are the **fundus**, which is that portion that rises superiorly from the entrance of the oviducts; the **body**, which makes up most of the uterus; the **isthmus**, a short narrowed part of the body at its inferior end; and the **cervix**, which extends into the vagina (see Figs. 10.1 and 10.15). Because the cervical mucosa is distinct from the rest of the uterus and does not undergo the process of menstruation, it is discussed separately. The established functions of the uterus are related to supporting a **pregnancy** (see Chapter 11). The main functions of the uterus are as follows:

1. Provide a suitable site for attachment and implantation of the blastocyst, including a thick, nutrient-rich stroma
2. Limit the invasiveness of the implanting embryo so that it stays in the endometrium and does not reach the myometrium
3. Provide a maternal side of the mature placental architecture. This includes the basal plate, to which the fetal side attaches, and large, intervillous spaces that become filled with maternal blood after the first trimester
4. Grow and expand with the growing fetus so that the fetus develops within an aqueous, largely nonadhesive environment
5. Provide strong muscular contractions to expel the fetus and placenta at term

An understanding of the function of the uterus and hormonally induced uterine changes during nonfertile menstrual cycles requires a basic knowledge of the fine structure of the endometrium and of the relationship of the uterine blood supply to the endometrium (see Fig. 10.17). The luminal surface of the endometrium is covered by a simple cuboidal-columnar epithelium. The epithelium is continuous with mucosal glands (called **uterine glands**) that extend deep into the endometrium. The mucosa is vascularized by **spiral arteries**, which are branches of the uterine artery that run through the myometrium. The terminal arterioles of the spiral arteries project to a position just beneath the surface epithelium. These arterioles give rise to a subepithelial plexus of capillaries and venules, which have ballooned, thin-walled segments called venous lakes or **lacunae**. The lamina propria (i.e., the connective tissue and stroma of the mucosa supporting the epithelium) itself is densely cellular. The stromal cells of the lamina propria play important roles during both pregnancy and menstruation.

About two thirds of the luminal side of the endometrium is lost during menstruation and is called the **functional zone** (also called the **stratum functionalis**) (see Fig. 10.17). The basal one third of endometrium that remains after menstruation is called the **basal zone** (also called the **stratum basale**). The basal zone is fed by straight arteries that are separate from the spiral arteries and contains all of the cell types of the endometrium (i.e., epithelial cells from the remaining tips of glands, stromal cells, and endothelial cells).

Hormonal Regulation of the Uterine Endometrium During the Menstrual Cycle

Phases of the uterine cycle are controlled by ovarian estrogen and progesterone. Thus phases of the endometrial cycle correspond to phases of the ovarian cycle.

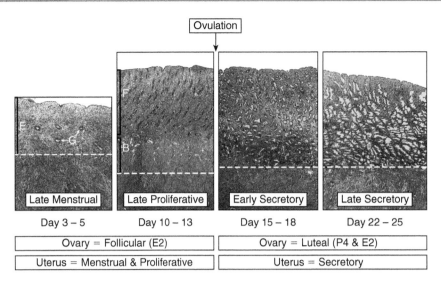

Ovulation

| Late Menstrual | Late Proliferative | Early Secretory | Late Secretory |
| Day 3 – 5 | Day 10 – 13 | Day 15 – 18 | Day 22 – 25 |

| Ovary = Follicular (E2) | Ovary = Luteal (P4 & E2) |
| Uterus = Menstrual & Proliferative | Uterus = Secretory |

Fig. 10.18 Changes in endometrial glands at different phases of the uterine cycle, and the corresponding phases of the ovarian cycle. (Modified partial images from Young B, Lowe J, Stevens A, et al: *Wheater's Functional Histology*, 5th ed., Edinburgh, 2006, Churchill Livingstone.)

The Proliferative Phase. At the end of menses (days 3 to 5), the functional layer of the uterine endometrium has been shed, and the basal layer is undergoing reepithelialization (Fig. 10.18). In the ovary, the follicular phase is underway. By day 5 of the ovarian cycle, FSH has recruited a cohort of 2- to 5-mm antral follicles that begin producing low but increasing levels of estradiol. Once the dominant follicle is selected at midfollicular phase, estradiol production increases dramatically (see Fig. 10.14). The estrogen produced by the follicular phase of the ovary drives the **proliferative phase** of the uterine endometrium. Estrogen induces all cell types in the basal layer to proliferate, thereby rebuilding the functional layer of the endometrium. In fact, the definition of an estrogenic compound has historically been one that is **uterotropic**. It is not clear whether estrogen stimulates the growth and differentiation of pluripotential stem cells or stimulates the growth of cells that are already defined as endothelial, epithelial, and stromal. Estrogen increases cell proliferation directly through **estrogen receptor-α (ERα)** and indirectly through the production of growth factors, such as insulin-like growth factor-I (IGF-I). Estrogen also induces the expression of **progesterone receptors**, thereby **priming** the uterine endometrium so that it can respond to progesterone during the luteal phase of the ovary.

During the proliferative phase, the functional layer of the endometrium increases from about 0.5 to 5 mm in thickness. Mitotic figures are found throughout the tissue. The uterine glands display a straight or coiled shape with narrow lumina (see Fig. 10.18).

The Secretory Phase. By the time of ovulation, the thickness of stratum functionalis has been reestablished under the proliferative actions of estradiol (see Fig. 10.18). After ovulation, the corpus luteum produces high levels of progesterone, along with estradiol. The **luteal phase** of the ovary switches the proliferative phase of the uterine endometrium to the **secretory phase**. In general, progesterone inhibits further endometrial growth and induces the differentiation of epithelial and stromal cells. Progesterone induces the uterine glands to secrete a nutrient-rich product, which will support an implanting blastocyst, thereby increasing embryo viability. As the secretory phase proceeds, the mucosal uterine glands become corkscrewed and sacculated. Progesterone also induces changes in the adhesivity of the surface epithelium, thereby generating the **window of receptivity** for implantation (see Chapter 11). Progesterone also promotes the differentiation of the stromal cells into **predecidual cells,** which must be prepared to form the **decidua** of pregnancy, or to orchestrate menstruation in the absence of pregnancy.

Of importance, progesterone opposes the proliferative actions of estradiol. Progesterone downregulates the estrogen receptor. Progesterone also induces **inactivating isoforms of 17β-HSD**, thereby converting the active **estradiol** into the inactive **estrone**. Progesterone also upregulates the expression of a steroid **sulfotransferase** that sulfates and inactivates estrogen. This opposition of the mitogenic actions of estradiol by progesterone is extremely important in protecting the uterine endometrium from estrogen-induced uterine cancer. By contrast, the administration of unopposed estrogen significantly increases the risk for uterine cancer in women.

The Menstrual Phase. In a nonfertile cycle, death of the corpus luteum leads to a sudden withdrawal of progesterone and estrogen, which leads to changes in the uterine endometrium that result in the loss of the stratum functionalis. Menstruation normally lasts 3 to 5 days (called a period), and the volume of blood loss ranges from 25 to 35 mL. Menstruation coincides with the early follicular phase of the ovary.

The breakdown of the stratum functionalis is due to the upregulation of hydrolytic enzymes, called matrix metalloproteases, which destroy the extracellular matrix and basal lamina of the endometrium. These enzymes are produced by the three resident cell types of the endometrium: the epithelial cell, the stromal cell, and the endothelial cell. Matrix metalloproteases are also produced by leukocytes, which infiltrate into the endometrium just before menstruation. The other major component that leads to menstruation is the production of prostaglandins. The inducible enzyme required for prostaglandin synthesis, cyclooxygenase-2 (COX-2), is increased in endothelial cells on progesterone withdrawal. This increases production of inflammatory prostaglandins, especially PGF2α, which, in turn, promotes contraction of the smooth muscle cells of the myometrium and the vascular smooth muscle cells of the spiral arteries. Intermittent spiral artery contraction and dilation cause hypoxic necrosis, followed by reperfusion injury of weakened tissue. The degree of tissue loss and the onset of tissue repair appear to be dependent on increasing estrogen levels during the early follicular phase.

CLINICAL BOX 10.4

Disorders of menstruation are relatively common and include menorrhagia (loss of > 80 mL of blood) and dysmenorrhea (painful periods). The existence of few, irregular periods, called oligomenorrhea, and the absence of periods, called amenorrhea, often are due to dysfunction or cessation of the hypothalamus-pituitary-ovarian axis, as opposed to local pelvic pathophysiology.

Hormonal Regulation of the Myometrium

The smooth muscle cells of the myometrium are also responsive to changes in steroid hormones. Peristaltic contractions of the myometrium favor movement of luminal contents from the cervix to the fundus at ovulation, and these contractions may play a role in rapid bulk transport of ejaculated sperm from the cervix to the oviducts. During menstruation, contractions propagate from the fundus to the cervix, thereby promoting expulsion of sloughed functional zone. The size and number of smooth muscle cells are determined by estrogen and progesterone. Healthy, cycling women maintain a robust myometrium, whereas the myometrium progressively thins in postmenopausal women.

The Cervix
Structure and Function

The cervix represents the inferior extension of the uterus that projects into the vagina (see Figs. 10.1 and 10.15). It has a mucosa that lines the endocervical canal, which has a highly elastic lamina propria, and a muscularis that is continuous with the myometrium. The cervix acts as a gateway to the upper female tract; at midcycle, the endocervical canal facilitates sperm viability and entry. During the luteal phase, changes in the endocervical canal serve to impede the passage of sperm and microbes, thereby minimizing the chance of superimplantation of a second embryo, as well as inhibiting ascending infections into the placenta, fetal membranes, and fetus. The cervix physically supports the weight of the growing fetus. At term, cervical softening and dilation allow passage of the newborn and placenta from the uterus into the vagina.

Hormonal Regulation of Cervical Mucus During the Menstrual Cycle

The endocervical canal is lined by a simple columnar epithelial gland that secretes cervical mucus in a hormonally responsive manner. Estrogen stimulates production of a copious quantity of thin, watery, "egg white" mucus that aids passage of sperm through the cervix by forming channels in a "ferning" pattern. In addition, the slightly alkaline pH of the mucus makes it an ideal environment for sperm. Progesterone stimulates production of a scant, viscous, slightly acidic mucus that is hostile to sperm and does not "fern." This thick mucus forms a barrier within the endocervical canal during the secretory phase of the endometrium and during pregnancy, when the placenta produces high amounts of progesterone (see Chapter 11).

The Vagina
Structure and Function

The vagina is the main copulatory structure in women (the clitoris being the other) and serves as the birth canal (see Fig. 10.16). Its mucosa is lined by a nonkeratinized, stratified squamous epithelium. The mucosa has a thick lamina propria enriched with elastic fibers and is well vascularized. There are no glands in the vagina, so lubrication during intercourse comes from the following elements:

- Cervical mucus (especially during midcycle)
- A transudate (i.e., ultrafiltrate) from the blood vessels of the lamina propria

- From the **vestibular glands** (see later in the text)

The mucosa is surrounded by a relatively thin (i.e., relative to the uterus and cervix) two-layered muscularis and an outer connective tissue. The vaginal wall is innervated by branches of the pudendal nerve, which contribute to sexual pleasure and orgasm during intercourse.

Hormonal Regulation During the Menstrual Cycle

The superficial cells of the vaginal epithelium are continually desquamating and the nature of these cells is influenced by the hormonal environment. Estrogen stimulates proliferation of the vaginal epithelium and increases its glycogen content. Estradiol also induces minimal keratinization of the apical layers. Progesterone increases the desquamation of the epithelial cells. The glycogen is metabolized to lactic acid by commensal lactobacilli, thereby maintaining an acidic environment. This relative acidity inhibits infections by noncommensal bacteria and fungi.

The External Genitalia

Structure and Function

The female external genitals are surrounded by the **labia majora** (homologs of the scrotum) laterally and the **mons pubis** anteriorly (see Fig. 10.16). The **vulva** collectively refers to an area that includes the labia majora and the mons pubis, plus the labia minora, the clitoris, the vestibule of the vagina, the vestibular bulbs (glands), and the external urethral orifice (Fig. 10.19). The vulva also is referred to as the **pudendum** by clinicians. The structures of the vulva

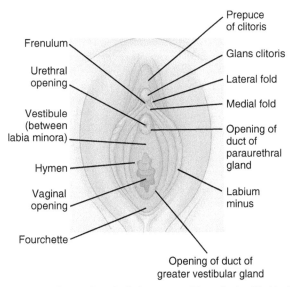

Fig. 10.19 External genitalia in women. (From Drake RL, Vogl W, Mitchell AWM: *Gray's Anatomy for Students*, Philadelphia, 2005, Churchill Livingstone.)

serve the functions of **sexual arousal** and **orgasm**, direct the flow of urine, and provide a partial cover of the opening of the vagina, thereby inhibiting the entry of pathogens.

The **clitoris** is the homolog of the penis. The clitoris is composed of erectile tissue that undergoes the process of erection in essentially the same manner as the penis. Unlike the penis, clitoral tissue is completely separate from the urethra. Thus the only function of the clitoris is involved with sexual arousal and climax at orgasm.

Hormonal Regulation During the Menstrual Cycle

The structures of the vulva do not show marked changes during the menstrual cycle. The health and function of these structures, however, are dependent on hormonal support. The external genitalia and vagina appear to be responsive to androgens (testosterone and dihydrotestosterone), as well as estrogen. Androgens also act on the central nervous system (CNS) to increase libido in women.

BIOLOGY OF ESTRADIOL AND PROGESTERONE

Mechanisms of Estrogen and Progesterone Hormone Action

Estrogen and progesterone are steroid hormones; accordingly, their cognate receptors belong to the nuclear hormone receptor superfamily (see Chapter 1).

Biologic Effects of Estrogen and Progesterone

Although the levels of estradiol and progesterone fluctuate during the menstrual cycle, estrogen and progesterone levels are always higher in women than in men. Estradiol and progesterone have multiple effects that can be categorized according to whether they are directly related to the reproductive system. As discussed previously, both steroid hormones have profound effects on the ovary, oviduct, uterus, cervix, vagina, and external genitalia, and on the hypothalamus and pituitary. Estrogen and progesterone also have important effects on the following nonreproductive tissues:

> **Bone: Estrogen** is required for closure of the epiphyseal plates of long bones in both sexes. **Estradiol** has a bone anabolic effect and a calciotropic effect at several sites. Estrogen stimulates intestinal calcium absorption and renal tubular calcium reabsorption. Estrogen is also one of the most potent regulators of osteoblast and osteoclast function. Estrogen promotes survival of osteoblasts and apoptosis of osteoclasts, thereby favoring bone formation over resorption. Loss of estradiol at menopause is frequently associated with osteoporosis.

Liver: The overall effect of estrogen on the liver is to improve circulating lipoprotein profiles. Estrogen increases expression of the LDL receptor, thereby increasing clearance of cholesterol-rich LDL particles by the liver. Estrogen also increases circulating levels of high-density lipoprotein (HDL) levels. Estrogen regulates hepatic production of several transport proteins, including cortisol-binding protein, thyroid hormone–binding protein, and sex hormone-binding protein.

Cardiovascular organs: Premenopausal women have significantly lower cardiovascular disease than men or postmenopausal women. Estrogen promotes vasodilation through increased production of nitric oxide, which relaxes vascular smooth muscle and inhibits platelet activation. Estrogen promotes angiogenesis in target tissues.

Integument: Overall, estrogen and progesterone maintain a healthy, smooth skin with normal epidermal and dermal thickness. Estrogen stimulates proliferation and inhibits apoptosis of keratinocytes. In the dermis, estrogen increases collagen synthesis and inhibits (along with progesterone) the breakdown of collagen by suppressing matrix metalloproteases. Estrogen increases glycosaminoglycan production and deposition in the dermis. Estrogen also promotes wound healing.

CNS: In general, estrogen is neuroprotective—that is, it inhibits neuronal cell death in response to hypoxia or other insults. The positive effects on angiogenesis may account for some of the beneficial and stimulant-like actions of estrogen on the CNS. Currently, the proposed benefits of estrogen for the onset and severity of Parkinson disease and Alzheimer disease are controversial. Progesterone acts on the hypothalamus to increase the setpoint for thermoregulation, thereby elevating body temperature by approximately 0.5°F. This is the basis for using body temperature measurements to determine whether ovulation has occurred. Progesterone generally acts as a depressant on the CNS. Loss of progesterone on demise of the corpus luteum of menstruation is the basis for premenstrual syndrome (PMS) and the severe variant premenstrual dysphoria disorder (PMDD) experienced by some women.

Adipose tissue: Estrogen decreases adipose tissue by decreasing lipoprotein lipase activity and increasing hormone-sensitive lipase (i.e., it has a lipolytic effect). Loss of estrogen results in an accumulation of adipose tissue, especially in the abdomen.

The actions of estrogen and progesterone on the maternal physiology and breast development and function are discussed in Chapter 11.

Transport and Metabolism of Ovarian Steroids

Steroid hormones are sparingly soluble in blood and are carried primarily in association with plasma proteins. About 60% of the estrogen is transported bound to sex hormone–binding globulin (SHBG), 20% is bound to albumin, and 20% is in the free form. Progesterone binds primarily to cortisol-binding globulin (CBG) (i.e., transcortin) and albumin. Because it has a relatively low binding affinity for these proteins, its circulating half-life ($t_{1/2}$) is about 5 min.

Although the ovary is the primary site of estrogen production, it is important to understand that peripheral aromatization of androgens to estrogens can generate locally high levels of estradiol in specific tissues. For example, the fact that CYP19 (aromatase) is expressed in the adipose tissue of the breast is the basis for the use of aromatase inhibitors in the treatment of estrogen-dependent breast cancer.

Estrogens and progestins are degraded in the liver to inactive metabolites, conjugated with sulfate or glucuronide, and excreted in the urine. Major metabolites of estradiol include estrone, estriol, and catecholestrogens (2-hydroxyestrone and 2-methoxyestrone). The major metabolite of progesterone is pregnanediol, which is conjugated with glucuronide and excreted in the urine.

OVARIAN PATHOPHYSIOLOGY

Turner Syndrome

Turner syndrome, or gonadal dysgenesis, is the most common cause of congenital hypogonadism. In about 50% of cases, it results from the complete absence of the second X chromosome, so the karyotype of the affected person is 45,XO. The germ cells do not develop, and each gonad consists of a connective tissue–filled streak. The major clinical characteristics include short stature, a characteristic webbed neck, low-set ears, a shield-shaped chest, short fourth metacarpals, and sexual infantilism resulting from gonadal dysgenesis (Fig. 10.20). Internal and external genitalia typically are female.

Polycystic Ovarian Syndrome

Chronically anovulatory women with high circulating androgen, estrogen, and LH levels often have the disorder called polycystic ovarian syndrome (PCOS). This syndrome may be caused by any of a broad array of underlying

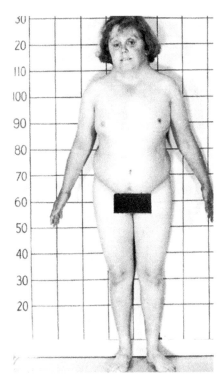

Fig. 10.20 Female with Turner syndrome. Note the characteristically broad, webbed neck. Stature is reduced, and sexual secondary characteristics are poorly developed. (From Goodman RM, Gorlin RJ: *Atlas of the Face in Genetic Disorders*, 2nd ed., St. Louis, 1977, Mosby.)

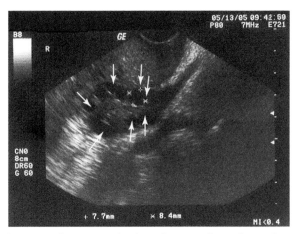

Fig. 10.21 Sonogram of polycystic ovary. Cysts *(arrows)* are due to large antral follicles in the cortex that failed to ovulate. (Courtesy of Dr. Andrea DiLuigi, Department of Obstetrics and Gynecology, University of Connecticut Health Center, Farmington, Conn.)

FSH levels are low, which inhibits granulosa cell function, and the high intrafollicular androgen level inhibits follicular maturation. A significant proportion of the circulating estrogen, present in high levels, is estrone formed from peripheral aromatization of androstenedione. These high androgen levels can produce hirsutism and acne. Hirsutism is the abnormal formation of coarse sexual hair in regions atypical for a woman, such as the face, back, and chest.

The exact cause of PCOS is not well understood, but the primary defect appears to be inappropriate signals between the hypothalamic-pituitary axis and the ovary. A significant subset of patients with PCOS are overweight or obese and have insulin resistance and hyperinsulinemia. Insulin promotes ovarian androgen production, and hyperinsulinism may account for increased androgen production. Reduction of insulin levels (such as by weight loss, exercise, or metformin administration) ameliorates the hyperandrogenism and PCOS in these patients. Alternatively, an inadequate response of the follicle to FSH may be due to impaired IGF-I or insulin signaling.

problems, and PCOS accounts for 75% of **anovulatory infertility**. Currently, the diagnosis of PCOS requires two of the following three conditions: **amenorrhea**, evidence of **excessive androgen secretion** (i.e., acne, hirsutism), and **polycystic ovaries**, as usually detected by sonogram (Fig. 10.21). The ovarian cysts represent large antral follicles that have failed to ovulate and luteinize. The continuous gonadotropin secretion leads to ovarian enlargement, and the ovaries typically show a thickened capsule and numerous follicles, many of which are undergoing atresia.

SUMMARY

1. The female reproductive system includes the ovary, oviducts, uterus, cervix, vagina, and external genitalia, along with the pituitary gonadotropes and hypothalamic GnRH neurons. The mammary glands (breasts) also can be considered a part of the female reproductive system.

2. The ovarian phases of the human menstrual cycle are the follicular phase, the periovulatory period, and the luteal phase.

3. The ovarian follicle contains a primary oocyte arrested in meiotic prophase and variable layers of granulosa and theca cells. Preantral and early antral follicular growth is gonadotropin independent. Intermediate

antral follicular growth is dependent on a basal level of FSH, but not affected by fluctuations in FSH associated with the menstrual cycle. Large antral follicular development is exquisitely dependent on fluctuations of FSH. Follicles can degenerate at any phase during the process of atresia.

4. The dominant follicle is selected based on its size, number of FSH receptors, aromatase activity, and blood supply. The dominant follicle is the endocrine structure of the follicular phase. The theca cells express the LH receptor, and LH stimulates the production of androgens (primarily androstenedione). The granulosa cells express the FSH receptor, and FSH promotes the aromatization of androgens to estrogens (primarily estradiol). FSH also induces the expression of the LH receptor in granulosa cells of the dominant follicle.

5. The dominant follicle signals that it is ready to ovulate by its estrogen production. High sustained levels of estrogen induce the midcycle LH surge through a positive feedback mechanism. This is due, in part, to a marked increase in the sensitivity of the pituitary gonadotropes to GnRH pulses.

6. The periovulatory period involves the meiotic maturation of the primary oocyte to a secondary oocyte (egg) arrested at metaphase II. Ovulation involves the rupture of the follicular wall at the stigma, release of the cumulus-oocyte complex, and differentiation of the remaining follicular cells into a corpus luteum.

7. The luteal phase is characterized by high progesterone production. The corpus luteum is programmed to die in 14 days, unless rescued by hCG.

8. The oviduct functions to capture the cumulus-oocyte complex, transport and nurture both male and female gametes, promote fertilization and early embryonic development, and determine the timing of the movement of the blastocyst into the uterine cavity.

9. The mucosa of the uterus is called the endometrium. The function of the endometrium is to allow implantation and placentation. Estrogen produced during the mid- to late follicular phase of the ovary drives the proliferative phase of the uterus, during which the endometrium grows in thickness. The progesterone produced by the luteal phase of the ovary drives the secretory phase of the uterus. Progesterone opposes the estradiol-dependent proliferation of the endometrial functional zone. Loss of progesterone after the death of the corpus luteum causes the endometrium to break down. This represents the menstrual phase of the uterus. The cyclic changes in ovarian steroids also alter cervical mucus and vaginal epithelium. The external genitalia are responsive to estrogen and androgens.

10. Estrogen and progesterone regulate numerous processes directly associated with reproduction. However, these steroids also regulate nonreproductive aspects of physiology, including bone growth and health, cardiovascular function, hepatic function, and others. Estrogen and progesterone act primarily through interaction with classic estrogen and progesterone receptors, which belong to the family of nuclear hormone receptors. Estrogen and progesterone also have rapid, membrane-initiated actions.

11. Turner syndrome (gonadal dysgenesis) is the most common cause of congenital hypogonadism. It typically results from the absence of the second X chromosome, so the karyotype of the affected person is 45,XO.

12. Polycystic ovarian syndrome produces chronic anovulation. Circulating androgen, estrogen, and LH levels typically are high.

SELF-STUDY PROBLEMS

1. During treatment of in vitro fertilization, the patient receives a daily injection of FSH for 8 to 10 days, followed by one injection of hCG. Cumulus-oocyte complexes are retrieved 35 hours after the hCG injection from ovarian follicles just before they ovulate. Because oocytes are retrieved before ovulation, and patients are treated with progesterone after retrieval, what is the purpose of the hCG injection?

2. When and in what cells is the LH receptor expressed during the menstrual cycle?

3. Describe the major ovarian processes that occur during the periovulatory period.

4. What is meant by the "two-cell model" of ovarian steroidogenesis?

5. Name three effects of estrogen on reproductive tissue and three effects on nonreproductive tissue.

6. What would be the outcome of a truncated luteal phase with early death of the corpus luteum on the uterine endometrium?

7. What is the ovarian reserve?

8. What is the response of the pituitary gonadotropes to the death of a corpus luteum of menstruation?

9. What is the response of the ovary to declining FSH levels during the early follicular phase?

KEYWORDS AND CONCEPTS

Anatomy of female reproductive system
Corpus luteum
Estrogen
Gonadotropin-releasing hormone (GnRH)
Granulosa cells
Menstrual cycle: follicular and luteal phases
Secretion of pituitary and ovarian hormones
LH surge
Luteinization
Menstruation

Ovarian follicles: histology, follicular development
Ovulation
Pituitary gonadotropes (FSH and LH)
Phases of uterine cycle: proliferative, secretory:
Structure of uterine endometrium: functional zone, basal zone, spiral arteries, uterine glands
Steroid hormones (estrogen, progesterone)
Theca cells
Two-cell model of ovarian steroidogenesis during follicular and luteal phases

Fertilization, Pregnancy, and Lactation

OBJECTIVES

1. Describe the synchronization among fertilization, early embryonic events, and the human menstrual cycle.
2. Describe the events involved in fertilization.
3. Explain how implantation and placentation occur.
4. Discuss the endocrine and transport functions of the placenta.
5. Describe the development of the fetal endocrine system.
6. Discuss maternal endocrine changes during pregnancy.
7. Discuss the current models for the initiation and progression of labor (parturition) in humans.
8. Describe the development and regulation of the mammary glands.
9. Discuss the endocrine basis for contraception, the "morning after" pill, and the abortion pill.

Human reproduction involves internal insemination, internal fertilization, and internal gestation, all within the female tract. Internal gestation also involves the development of a transient organ, the placenta. The placenta is remarkable in that it is composed of tissues from two organisms:

- An extraembryonic membrane (called the *chorion*) of the fetus
- Endometrial tissue (called *decidua*) of the mother

From an endocrine point of view, pregnancy represents a state in which three separate endocrine systems—**maternal, fetal, and placental**—interact to promote adequate growth and nutrition of the fetus, the timing of parturition, and preparation of the maternal mammary glands to support extrauterine life of the fetus.

FERTILIZATION, EARLY EMBRYOGENESIS, IMPLANTATION, AND PLACENTATION

Synchronization With Maternal Ovarian and Reproductive Tract Function

Fertilization, early embryogenesis, implantation, and early gestation are all synchronized with the human menstrual cycle (Fig. 11.1). Just before ovulation, the ovary is in the late follicular stage and produces high levels of estrogen. Estrogen promotes growth of the uterine endometrium and induces expression of the progesterone receptor. Estrogen ultimately induces the luteinizing hormone (LH) surge, which in turn induces meiotic maturation of the oocyte and ovulation of the cumulus-oocyte complex.

The events between fertilization and implantation take about 6 days to complete, and implantation occurs at about day 21 of the menstrual cycle. At this time, the ovary is in the midluteal phase, secreting large amounts of progesterone. Progesterone stimulates secretion from uterine glands, which provide nutrients to the embryo. This is referred to as histotrophic nutrition and is an important mode of maternal-to-fetal transfer of nutrients for about the first trimester of pregnancy, after which it is replaced by hemotrophic nutrition. Progesterone inhibits myometrial contraction and prevents the release of paracrine factors that lead to menstruation.

Progesterone induces the window of receptivity in the uterine endometrium, which exists from about day 20 to 24 of the menstrual cycle. This receptive phase is associated with increased adhesivity of the endometrial epithelium and involves the formation of cellular extensions, called pinopodes, on the apical surface of endometrial epithelia, along with increased expression of adhesive proteins (e.g., integrins, cadherins) and decreased expression of antiadhesive proteins (e.g., mucins) in the apical cell membrane.

Thus during the time it takes a fertilized egg to implant in the uterus, the uterine endometrium is at its full thickness,

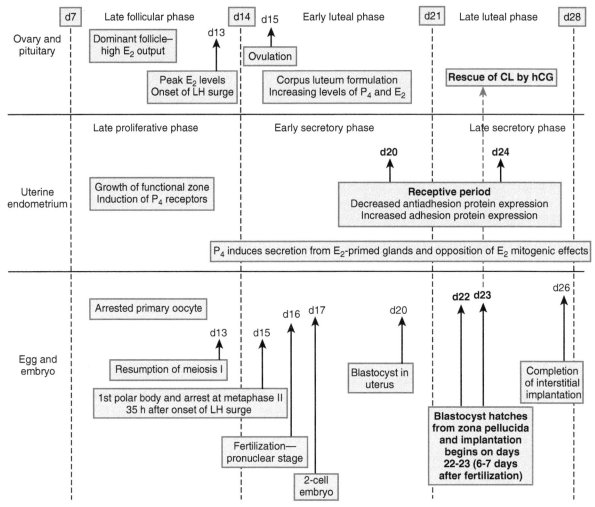

Fig. 11.1 Synchronization of the human menstrual cycle with fertilization and early embryogenesis. *CL,* Corpus luteum; *E,* estrogen; *E2,* estrone; *hCG,* human chorionic gonadotropin; *LH,* luteinizing hormone; *P4,* progesterone.

actively secretory, and capable of tightly adhering to the implanting embryo. It should also be noted that the uterine endometrium is well vascularized at the time of implantation. Spiral arteries extend to the basal lamina of the surface epithelium (see Fig. 10.17 in Chapter 10) and give rise to rich capillary beds and postcapillary venous lakes (also called lacunae). Apart from its nutrient supply to all cells of the endometrium, the extensive blood supply immediately adjacent to the surface epithelium plays a critical role in capturing embryonic human chorionic gonadotropin (hCG) and transporting hCG to the ovary, where it *rescues* the corpus luteum. The rich endometrial blood supply is also important for efficient delivery of progesterone to the endometrium.

Fertilization

Fertilization accomplishes both the recombination of genetic material to form a new, genetically distinct organism and the initiation of events that begin embryonic development. There are several steps that must occur for successful fertilization to be achieved. The sperm must find its way to the egg, and the sperm and the egg must contact, recognize one another, and fuse. After sperm-egg fusion, an intracellular signaling cascade occurs within the egg that has two major consequences. First, it allows the egg to regulate sperm entry such that only one sperm can fuse with the egg. This prevents polyspermy, which is lethal. Second, it "wakes up" the metabolically quiescent egg so that it can resume meiosis and begin embryonic development. This process is called **egg activation**.

Spermatozoa present in the male ejaculate enter the vagina near the cervix and must reach the **ampulla of the oviduct** where fertilization occurs. Sperm transport is largely dependent on the female reproductive tract and, while the sperm are still in the uterus, is essentially independent of swimming. Large numbers of sperm in the ejaculate generally are required for successful fertilization of the egg by a single sperm—of the 300 million sperm typically ejaculated, only about 200 reach the oviduct. Clinically, males with fewer than 20 million sperm per mL of ejaculate are considered to be **infertile**.

The female reproductive tract is an important regulator of sperm transport. Toward the end of the follicular phase of the menstrual cycle, before ovulation, estrogen levels are high. Estrogen causes the cervix to produce a **watery mucus**, often called "egg white cervical mucus" because of its consistency. This mucus forms channels to aid the passage of sperm through the cervix, and only motile sperm can pass through this barrier. Estrogen also causes contractions of the **myometrium** to help propel sperm upward toward the oviduct (i.e., cervical-to-fundal contractions).

Sperm must undergo a process called **capacitation** in the female reproductive tract before they are able to fertilize the egg. Sperm capacitation is an incompletely understood, transient event that occurs largely in the **oviduct** and modifies the spermatozoan in several ways so that it becomes capable of fertilizing the egg. These changes include the following:

1. An altered membrane fluidity due to the removal of cholesterol from the sperm membrane
2. The removal of proteins and carbohydrates from the membrane that may otherwise block sites that bind to the egg
3. A change in membrane potential that may permit Ca^{2+} to enter the sperm and thereby facilitate the **acrosome reaction** (see later in the text)
4. Phosphorylation of numerous proteins

Incapacitated sperm bind actively to the epithelial cells of the **oviductal isthmus** and become unbound when they are capacitated. This binding slows the capacitation process, extends the sperm life span, prevents too many sperm from reaching the egg, and increases the probability that sperm will be in the oviduct when the egg is ovulated. Sperm can therefore survive in the female reproductive tract for several days. **Hyperactivation** is another phenomenon that occurs in the oviduct. Hyperactivation involves a change in flagellar motion from a wavelike to a whiplike motion and is caused by Ca^{2+} entry through sperm-specific Ca^{2+} channels called **CatSper channels**, which are activated by progesterone produced by the cumulus cells. This whiplike flagellar movement is necessary for the sperm to detach from the oviductal epithelium, is well suited to swimming through the thick oviductal fluid, and helps propel the sperm through the outer layers of the egg to reach the egg's plasma membrane.

Capacitated sperm reach the egg, surrounded by its expanded **cumulus cells**, in the ampulla of the oviduct. Fertilization involves the penetration of the egg by the sperm. To do this, the sperm must breach three barriers (Fig. 11.2):

- Expanded cumulus
- Zona pellucida
- Plasma membrane of the egg (called the *oolemma*)

The cumulus cell matrix is composed predominantly of **hyaluronic acid**, and the sperm are able to digest through this layer with a membrane-bound hyaluronidase called **PH-20** (also called **sperm adhesion molecule 1, or SPAM1**) (see Fig.11.2, step 1). The next obstacle the sperm encounters is the **zona pellucida,** an extracellular coat made up of four glycoproteins (**ZP1, ZP2, ZP3, and ZP4**). Sperm transport through the zona is achieved by the **acrosome reaction**, a Ca^{2+}-dependent event in which the sperm plasma membrane fuses with the outer acrosomal membrane to release the contents of the **acrosomal vesicle** (see Fig. 11.2, step 2). The enzymes released from the acrosomal vesicle then digest the zona pellucida. The acrosome reaction appears to begin while the sperm is in contact with the cumulus cells and may be enhanced through the binding to zona pellucida proteins.

The molecular mechanisms involved in the interactions of the sperm and egg plasma membranes are not completely understood. Sperm and eggs recognize and bind to each other through the proteins **IZUMO1** and **JUNO**, respectively. **Sperm-egg fusion** is likely to involve **tetraspanin proteins**, such as CD9, in the egg (see Fig. 11.2; step 3).

The entire sperm enters the egg during fusion. The flagellum and mitochondria disintegrate, so most of the mitochondrial DNA in cells is maternally derived. Once the sperm is inside the egg, protamines associated with the tightly condensed sperm DNA are uncoiled by the highly reducing egg cytoplasm, causing **decondensation** of the sperm DNA. A membrane called the **pronucleus** forms around the sperm DNA while the newly activated egg completes the **second meiotic division**.

The egg is a metabolically quiescent cell that is "woken up" as a result of sperm-egg fusion, in a process called **egg activation**. All of the events associated with egg activation depend on **intracellular release of Ca^{2+} in the egg**. Ca^{2+} release is stimulated by the production of **inositol 1,4,5-trisphosphate (IP3)** in response to the sperm-specific phospholipase C enzyme, **PLCζ** which is introduced into the egg upon sperm-egg fusion (see Fig. 11.2, step 3). PLCζ

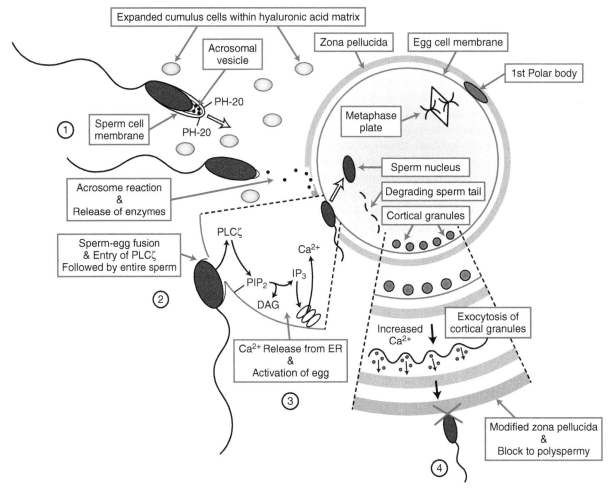

Fig. 11.2 Events of fertilization: (1) penetration of expanded cumulus; (2) acrosome reaction; (3) fusion of sperm membrane with egg membrane and egg activation; (4) exocytosis of cortical granules and block to polyspermy. *PH-20*, hyaluronidase; *DAG*, diacylglycerol; *IP₃*, inositol 1,4,5-trisphosphate; *PIP₂*, phosphatidylinositol 4,5-biphosphate; *PLCζ*, phospholipase Cζ; *ZP2*, zona pellucida glycoprotein 2.

cleaves the egg membrane phospholipid, phosphatidylinositol-4,5-bisphosphate (PIP_2), to form IP_3 and diacylglycerol. IP_3 binds to its receptor on the endoplasmic reticulum and opens Ca^{2+} channels (see Chapter 1). In human eggs, an initial burst of Ca^{2+} occurs soon after sperm-egg fusion that is followed by a series of Ca^{2+} oscillations that last for several hours after fertilization. These Ca^{2+} pulses are absolutely required for all the major events of egg activation.

One of the earliest Ca^{2+}-dependent events that occurs at fertilization of mammalian eggs is the prevention of polyspermy. Enzyme-filled vesicles, called **cortical granules**, reside in the outermost, or cortical, region of the unfertilized egg (see Fig. 11.2, step 4). In response to increases in intracellular Ca^{2+}, these vesicles translocate to the plasma membrane and release hydrolytic enzymes through exocytosis. These enzymes modify ZP2, generating ZP_f, which blocks binding of any more sperm. Thus only one sperm usually enters the egg. Occasionally, more than one sperm does enter the egg. This results in a **triploid cell**, which is lethal. It is thought that up to 10% to 15% of miscarriages are caused by polyspermy.

Ca^{2+} release also stimulates the egg to reenter the cell cycle, **complete meiosis**, and recruit **maternal messenger RNAs (mRNAs)** after fertilization. The unfertilized egg is held in meiotic arrest at **metaphase of meiosis II** by the cell cycle regulatory protein complex, **maturation-promoting**

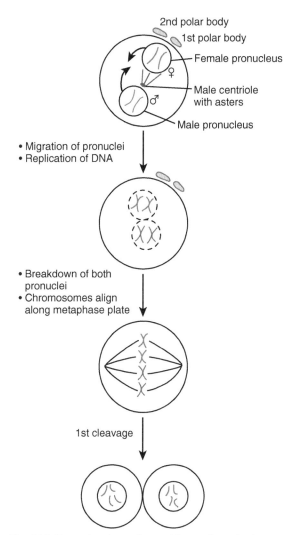

- Migration of pronuclei
- Replication of DNA

- Breakdown of both pronuclei
- Chromosomes align along metaphase plate

1st cleavage

Fig. 11.3 Pronuclear formation and first embryonic cleavage.

factor (MPF), as well as **cytostatic factor (CSF)**, which contains components of the **mitogen-activating protein kinase (MAPK) pathway**. Ca^{2+}-calmodulin–dependent pathways inactivate both MPF and CSF so that the metaphase II chromosomes decondense, the anaphase-promoting complex becomes active, and the egg can form a **pronucleus**. The unfertilized egg is transcriptionally inactive, and Ca^{2+} release at fertilization is also needed for the recruitment of **stored maternal mRNAs** for translation into **maternally derived proteins** needed for early embryonic development.

The activated egg completes the second meiotic division while the sperm DNA decondenses and a pronucleus forms around it (Fig. 11.3). Once the egg has completed meiosis,

a pronucleus forms around the female chromosomes as well. A **centrosome**, contributed by the sperm, becomes a **microtubule-organizing center** from which microtubules extend until they contact the female pronucleus. The male and female DNAs replicate while the two pronuclei are pulled together. Once the pronuclei contact each other, the nuclear membranes break down, the chromosomes align on a common metaphase plate, and the **first embryonic cleavage** occurs.

Early Embryogenesis and Implantation

Fertilization typically occurs on day 15 or 16 of the menstrual cycle, and implantation occurs about 6 days later. Thus the first week of embryogenesis occurs within the lumina of the oviduct and uterus (Fig. 11.4). For most of this time, the embryo remains encapsulated by the zona pellucida. The first two cleavages take about 2 days, and the embryo reaches a 16-cell **morula** by 3 days. The outer cells of the morula become tightly adhesive with each other and begin transporting fluid into the embryonic mass. During days 4 and 5, the transport of fluid generates a cavity, called the *blastocyst cavity* (blastocoele), and the embryo is now called a **blastocyst** (Fig. 11.5). The blastocyst is composed of two subpopulations of cells:

- The eccentric inner cell mass
- An outer, epithelial-like layer of trophoblasts. The region of trophoblast layer immediately adjacent to the inner cell mass is referred to as the embryonic pole, and it is this region that attaches to the uterine endometrium at implantation.

The embryo resides within the oviduct during the first 3 days and then enters the uterus. By 5 to 6 days of development, the trophoblasts of the blastocyst secrete proteases that digest the outer-lying zona pellucida. At this point, corresponding to about day 22 of the menstrual cycle, the **hatched blastocyst** (Fig. 11.6) is able to adhere to and implant into the receptive uterine endometrium.

At the time of attachment and **implantation**, the trophoblasts differentiate into two cell types: an inner layer of **cytotrophoblasts** and an outer layer of multinuclear and multicellular **syncytiotrophoblasts** (Fig. 11.7). The cytotrophoblasts initially provide a feeder layer of continuously dividing cells. Syncytiotrophoblasts perform three general types of functions: **adhesive, invasive,** and **endocrine**. Syncytiotrophoblasts express adhesive surface proteins (i.e., cadherins and integrins) that bind to uterine surface epithelia, and as the embryo implants, these bind to components of the uterine extracellular matrix. In humans, the embryo completely burrows into the superficial layer of the endometrium (see Fig. 11.7). This mode of implantation, called **interstitial implantation**, is the most invasive among placental mammals. Interstitial

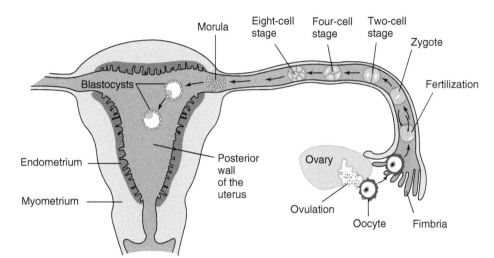

Fig. 11.4 Fertilization and human development during the first week.

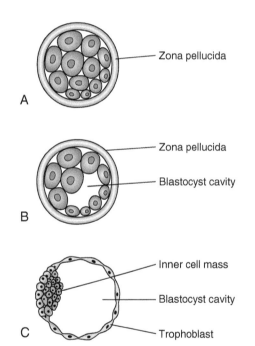

Fig. 11.5 Early cleavage stages in embryos. (A) Morula. (B) Early blastocyst with zona pellucida intact. (C) Late blastocyst shows inner cell mass and blastocyst cavity.

implantation involves adhesion-supported invasion and migration of syncytiotrophoblasts into the endometrium, along with the breakdown of extracellular matrix by the secretion of matrix metalloproteases and other hydrolytic enzymes.

The endocrine function begins with the onset of implantation, when syncytiotrophoblasts begin secreting the LH-like protein **hCG** (see later in the text), which maintains the viability of the corpus luteum (**corpus luteum of pregnancy**) and, thus, maintains **progesterone** secretion. Syncytiotrophoblasts become highly steroidogenic by 10 weeks and make progesterone at sufficient levels to maintain pregnancy independently of the corpus luteum. Syncytiotrophoblasts produce several other hormones, as well as enzymes that modify hormones (see later in the text).

While implantation and placentation progress, syncytiotrophoblasts take on the important functions of **phagocytosis** (during histotrophic nutrition) and **bidirectional placental transfer** of gases, nutrients, and wastes. Exchange across the syncytiotrophoblasts involves diffusion (e.g., gases), facilitated transport (e.g., GLUT1-mediated transfer of glucose), active transport (e.g., amino acids by specific transporters), and pinocytosis-transcytosis (e.g., of iron-transferrin complexes).

There also is a maternal response to implantation, called **decidualization**, which involves the transformation of the **endometrial stroma** into enlarged and glycogen-filled **decidual cells** (the endometrium is now referred to as the **decidua**). The decidua forms an epithelial-like sheet with adhesive junctions that inhibit migration of the implanting embryo. The decidua also secretes factors, such as tissue inhibitors of metalloproteases (TIMPs), which moderate the activity of syncytiotrophoblastic-derived hydrolytic enzymes in the endometrial matrix. Consequently, decidualization allows for regulated invasion during implantation.

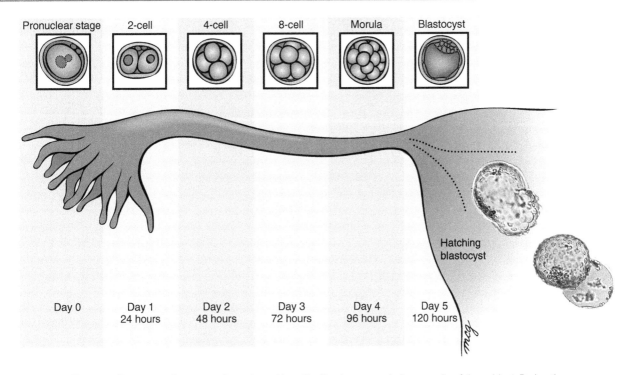

Fig. 11.6 Cleavage and transport down the oviduct. Fertilization occurs in the ampulla of the oviduct. During the first five days, the zygote undergoes cleavage while it travels down the oviduct and enters the uterus. On day five, the blastocyst hatches from the zona pellucida and is then able to implant in the uterine endometrium. (From Schoenwolf GC, Bleyl SB, Brauer PR, et al: *Larsen's Human Embryology*, 6th ed., Philadelphia, 2015, Elsevier.)

CLINICAL BOX 11.1

Normally, the implanting embryo and placenta do not extend to and involve the **myometrium**. Placental **accreta** is the destruction of the endometrium and adherence of the placenta to the myometrium, a condition associated with potentially life-threatening **postpartum hemorrhage**. It is important to note that the decidual response occurs only in the uterus. Thus the highly invasive nature of the human embryo poses considerable risk to the mother in the case of **ectopic implantations**. The most common site of ectopic implantation is the oviduct (giving rise to a **tubal pregnancy**), but implantations also rarely occur in the ovary and cervix and within the abdominal cavity.

Structure of the Mature Placenta

The progression of placental development is complicated, and the reader is referred to embryology texts for a more complete discussion than the one presented here. It is useful to consider placental development with a focus first on the entire gravid uterus and then on the fine structure of the mature placenta.

Initially, the growing syncytiotrophoblasts extend evenly from the embryo into the outer-lying decidua. At about 9 days, spaces appear within the syncytiotrophoblast layer, called lacunae. These spaces become filled with the secretions of endometrial glands, maternal blood from degraded vessels, and the remnants of enzymatically digested matrix, referred to as the **embryotroph**, which provides for histotrophic nutrition (Fig. 11.8).

By the end of the second week of development, the columns of syncytiotrophoblasts with a core of cytotrophoblasts are distinguishable as primary villi (Fig. 11.9). By this time, a new extraembryonic layer, called **extraembryonic mesoderm**, becomes associated with the cytotrophoblast and syncytiotrophoblast layers. The three layers are now referred to as the **chorionic membrane**. After primary villi gain a mesodermal core, they are referred to as secondary villi. The extraembryonic mesoderm provides a connection, called the **connecting stalk**, between the chorion and the embryo. It is within this mesoderm that the

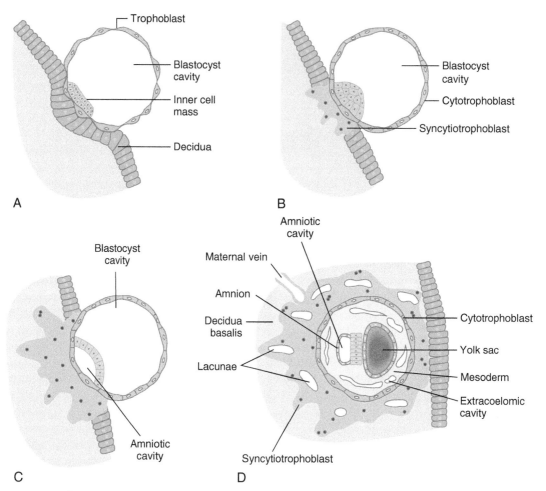

Fig. 11.7 Steps in implantation. (A) Early implantation of blastocyst. (B) Formation of cytotrophoblast and syncytiotrophoblast. (C) Formation of amniotic cavity. (D) Formation of lacunae with maternal venous penetration.

fetal (**umbilical**) **circulation** develops. Once villi contain umbilical blood vessels, they are referred to as **tertiary villi** (see Fig. 11.9). **Chorionic villi** represent the functional unit of the placenta and, through extensive branching, greatly increase the surface area for maternal-fetal exchange.

Although villi develop from the entire spherical chorionic membrane, they quickly degenerate around most of the chorion, forming a smooth chorion, or the **chorion laeve** (Fig. 11.10). In the region of the original embryonic pole, however, the chorion develops into a highly branching villous chorion, called the **chorion frondosum** (see Fig. 11.10). The chorion frondosum represents the fetal side of the mature placenta.

The uterine decidua immediately apposed to the chorion frondosum is called the **decidua basalis** and forms the maternal side of the mature placenta (see Fig. 11.10). The decidua that is subjacent to the chorion laeve is called the **decidua capsularis**. With time, the decidua capsularis fuses with the **decidua parietalis**, which is the part of the uterine endometrium that is not directly associated with the chorionic membrane (see Fig. 11.10). This means that the original uterine lumen is obliterated. The decidua capsularis ultimately degenerates.

Another extraembryonic membrane, called the **amnion**, grows and surrounds the developing fetus. The amnion becomes a fluid-filled sac, allowing for a nonadhesive environment in which the fetus can develop. By the beginning of the third trimester, the amnion fuses with the chorion, forming the **amniochorionic membrane**, which in turn fuses with the decidua parietalis (see Fig. 11.10).

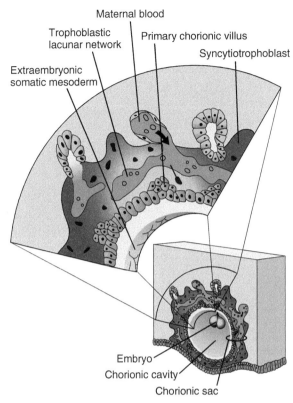

Fig. 11.8 Histotrophic nutrition *(arrows)* while the endometrial glands and spiral arteries are invaded and eroded by advancing syncytiotrophoblasts (at 14 days). (Modified from Moore KL, Persaud TVN: *The Developing Human: Clinically Oriented Embryology,* Philadelphia, 2003, Saunders.)

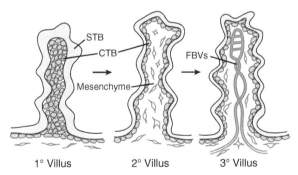

Fig. 11.9 Development of primary (1°), secondary (2°), and tertiary (3°) villi. *CTB,* Cytotrophoblast; *FBVs,* fetal blood vessels; *STB,* syncytiotrophoblast.

With the disappearance of the decidua capsularis, only the fetal amniochorionic membrane stretches across the internal opening of the cervical canal, and it is the amniochorionic membrane that ruptures during childbirth.

The mature placenta (Fig. 11.11) is composed of three major structures:

1. The **chorionic villi**, which are lined externally by the syncytiotrophoblast layer and contain the termini of umbilical blood vessels within their core. While chorionic villi branch, they become increasingly smaller, thinner, and more involved in maternal-fetal exchange. The smallest villi, called **terminal villi**, are the predominant sites of maternal-fetal exchange (Fig. 11.12). Terminal villi have an outer layer of syncytiotrophoblasts, which becomes extremely thin in certain regions. Subjacent to the thinnest regions of syncytiotrophoblasts, the cytotrophoblasts disappear, and an umbilical capillary presses against the syncytiotrophoblast layer. Thus nutrients from the maternal blood that bathes the terminal villi (see intervillous space in next entry) have to cross only a single, flat layer of syncytiotrophoblast, the fused basal lamina of the syncytiotrophoblast and capillary endothelium, and a flattened umbilical endothelial cell. This barrier between maternal blood and the umbilical circulation is called the **placental membrane** (see Fig. 11.12) and is also called a **vasculosyncytial membrane**. It represents the thinnest barrier to maternal-fetal exchange among placental (i.e., eutherian) mammals.

2. The **intervillous space,** into which maternal blood flows from the open ends of **spiral arteries** (see Fig. 11.11). This blood bathes the chorionic villi and returns to maternal circulation through **endometrial veins**. Because the maternal side of the placenta is represented by maternal blood within the intervillous space, and the fetal side is represented by the chorionic vasculosyncytial membrane, human placentation is referred to as **hemochorial placentation**.

3. The **decidua basalis.** Some villi, called **anchoring villi**, extend through the intervillous space and anchor onto the decidua (see Fig. 11.11). Columns of cytotrophoblasts migrate out of the end of the anchoring villi and spread across the decidua basalis. These **extravillous cytotrophoblasts** form an adhesive layer, called the **cytotrophoblastic shell**, that anchors the **chorion frondosum** to the **decidua basalis** (see Fig. 11.11). Spiral arteries extend through the decidua basalis and open into the intervillous space through breaks in the cytotrophoblastic shell. During the first trimester, extravillous cytotrophoblasts migrate into the spiral arteries and plug them up. Thus embryonic and early fetal development is supported primarily by histotrophic nutrition within a **hypoxic environment**. During

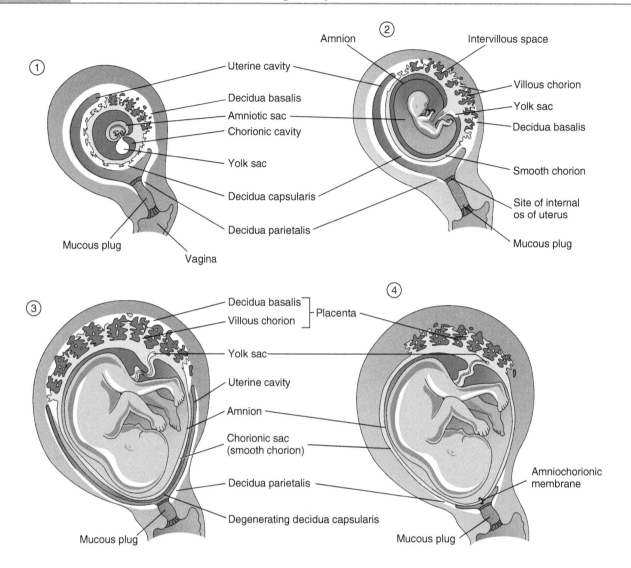

Fig. 11.10 Development and fusion of fetal membranes and decidua. (From Moore KL, Persaud TVN: *The Developing Human: Clinically Oriented Embryology,* Philadelphia, 2003, Saunders.)

this time, the cytotrophoblasts that have invaded the spiral arteries replace the **tunica media** (i.e., the vascular smooth muscle layer) and **tunica intima** (i.e., the endothelia and their lamina propria), thereby converting the arteries into **low-resistance, high-capacitance vessels.** At the beginning of the second trimester, coincident with entry of the fetus into a rapid growth phase, the converted spiral arteries become unplugged, and **hemotrophic nutrition predominates** until parturition.

CLINICAL BOX 11.2

Preeclampsia, which is a form of hypertension and proteinuria of pregnancy, is often accompanied by a shallow invasion of the placenta and an inability of the cytotrophoblasts to convert the spiral arteries. This condition leads to **intrauterine growth restriction (IUGR)** of the fetus, increasing the risk for perinatal mortality.

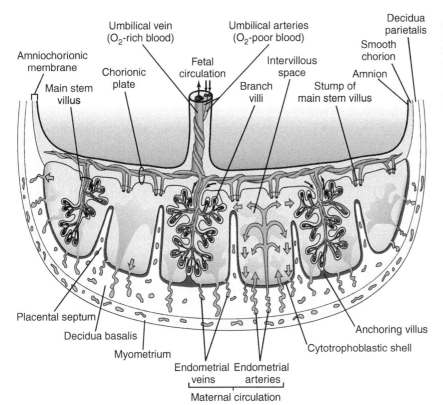

Fig. 11.11 Structure of the mature hemochorial placenta. Villi have been removed in some segments to show flow of maternal blood. (From Moore KL, Persaud TVN: *The Developing Human: Clinically Oriented Embryology*, Philadelphia, 2003, Saunders.)

Labels in figure:
Umbilical vein (O₂-rich blood)
Umbilical arteries (O₂-poor blood)
Decidua parietalis
Amniochorionic membrane
Smooth chorion
Chorionic plate
Fetal circulation
Intervillous space
Amnion
Main stem villus
Branch villi
Stump of main stem villus
Placental septum
Anchoring villus
Decidua basalis
Cytotrophoblastic shell
Myometrium
Endometrial veins
Endometrial arteries
Maternal circulation

Endocrine Function of the Placenta

The syncytiotrophoblasts of the placenta produce several steroid and protein hormones. The general functions of these hormones in pregnancy include the following:

- Maintaining the pregnant state of the uterus
- Stimulating lobuloalveolar growth and function of maternal breasts
- Adapting aspects of maternal metabolism and physiology to support a growing fetus
- Regulating aspects of fetal development
- Regulating the timing and progression of parturition

Human Chorionic Gonadotropin

The first hormone produced by the syncytiotrophoblasts is hCG. This hormone is structurally related to the pituitary glycoprotein hormones (see Chapter 5). As such, hCG is composed of a common α-glycoprotein subunit (α-GSU) and a hormone-specific β-subunit, β-hCG. Antibodies used to detect hCG (as in laboratory assays and over-the-counter pregnancy tests) are designed to specifically detect the β-subunit. hCG is most similar to LH and binds with high affinity to the LH receptor. The β-subunit of hCG is longer than that of LH and contains more sites for glycosylation, which greatly increases the half-life of hCG to up to 30 hours. The stability of hCG allows it to rapidly accumulate in the maternal circulation, so hCG is detectable within maternal serum within 24 hours of implantation. Serum hCG levels double every 2 days for the first 6 weeks until they peak at about 10 weeks. Serum hCG then declines to a constant level at about 50% of the peak value (Fig. 11.13).

The primary action of hCG is to stimulate LH receptors on the corpus luteum. This prevents luteolysis and maintains a high level of luteal-derived progesterone production during the first 10 weeks, after which the syncytiotrophoblasts take over progesterone production. The rapid increase in hCG is responsible for the nausea of morning sickness

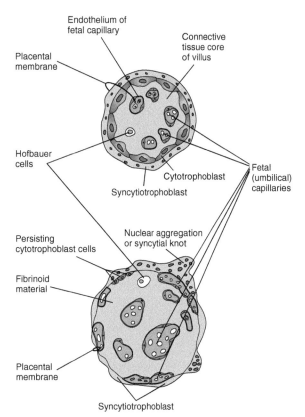

Fig. 11.12 Cross section of early *(upper)* and mature *(lower)* terminal villi. In the mature terminal villus, the cytotrophoblast layer becomes discontinuous, the fetal vessels assume an eccentric position subjacent to the syncytiotrophoblast layer, and the syncytiotrophoblast becomes very thinned out except for nuclear aggregations (also called *syncytial knots*). (From Moore KL, Persaud TVN: *The Developing Human: Clinically Oriented Embryology,* Philadelphia, 2003, Saunders.)

associated with early pregnancy. hCG binds weakly to the thyrotropin (thyroid-stimulating hormone [TSH]) receptor, so early pregnancy can be associated with a **transient gestational hyperthyroidism**. A small amount (i.e., 1% to 10%) of hCG enters into the fetal circulation. The hCG stimulates **fetal Leydig cells** to produce **testosterone** before the fetal gonadotropic axis is fully mature. hCG may also stimulate the fetal adrenal cortex during the first trimester.

CLINICAL BOX 11.3

Human chorionic gonadotropin is produced in high levels by cancers derived from **trophoblastic cells**, such as **molar disease** and **choriocarcinoma**. Thus hCG levels can be used as a measure of the efficacy of chemotherapy.

Progesterone

The syncytiotrophoblasts express high levels of CYP11A1 (side-chain cleavage enzyme) and a placenta-specific 3β-hydroxysteroid dehydrogenase type 1 (3β-HSD1) but do not express CYP17 (Fig. 11.14). Syncytiotrophoblasts also express the receptors (e.g., low-density lipoprotein [LDL] receptor) that import cholesterol from the maternal blood. Consequently, the placenta produces a high amount of **progesterone**, which is absolutely required to maintain a quiescent myometrium and a pregnant uterus. Progesterone production by the placenta is largely unregulated—the placenta produces as much progesterone as the supply of cholesterol and the levels of CYP11A1 and 3β-HSD will allow. Of note, placental steroidogenesis differs from that in the adrenal cortex, ovaries, and testis, in that cholesterol is transported into the placental mitochondria by a mechanism that is independent of the labile **steroidogenic acute regulatory (StAR) protein**. Thus this first step in steroidogenesis is not a regulated, rate-limiting step in the placenta as it is in other steroidogenic glands. This means that a fetus with an inactivating mutation in StAR protein will develop lipoid congenital adrenal hyperplasia (see Chapter 7) and hypogonadism but will have normal progesterone levels produced by their placenta. It also should be noted that progesterone production by the placenta does not require fetal tissue. Consequently, progesterone levels are largely independent of fetal health status and cannot be used as a measure of fetal well-being. Maternal progesterone levels continue to increase throughout pregnancy (see Fig. 11.13).

Progesterone is released primarily into the maternal circulation and is required for implantation and the maintenance of pregnancy. Progesterone also has several effects on maternal physiology and induces breast growth and differentiation (discussed later in the text). The switch from corpus luteum–derived progesterone to placenta-derived progesterone (referred to as the **luteal-placental shift**) is complete at about the eighth week of pregnancy. Progesterone and pregnenolone are used by the definitive zone of the fetal cortex (see later in the text) to make cortisol late in pregnancy.

Estrogen

Estrogens are produced by the syncytiotrophoblasts. Syncytiotrophoblasts lack CYP17 and are dependent on another cell type to provide 19-carbon androgens for aromatization. The ancillary, androgen-producing cell resides in the **fetal adrenal cortex**.

The cells of the fetal adrenal cortex emerge at week 5, and by 8 weeks there exists a distinct cortex and medulla. Initially, the cortex is composed of one zone, the **fetal zone** (Fig. 11.15). The fetal zone becomes surrounded by cells

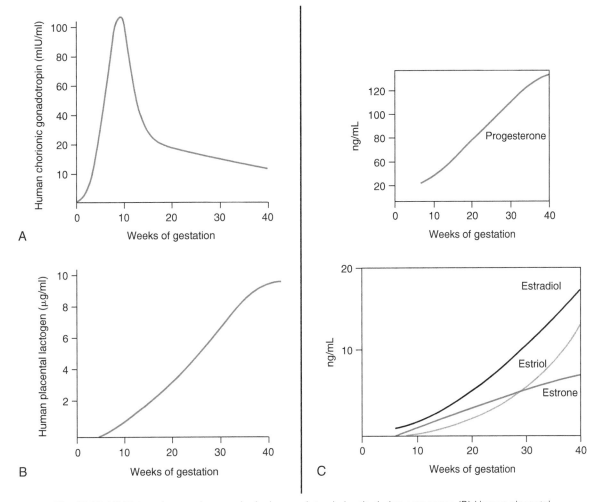

Fig. 11.13 (A) Maternal serum human chorionic gonadotropin levels during pregnancy. (B) Human placental lactogen levels during pregnancy. (C) Progesterone and estrogen. (C, From Koeppen B, Stanton B: *Berne and Levy Physiology,* updated 6th ed., Philadelphia, 2010, Mosby.)

that make up the **definitive cortex**, which will differentiate into the adult zona glomerulosa and zona fasciculata. The fetal zone constitutes as much as 80% of the bulk of the large fetal adrenal gland. The fetal zone recedes after birth (see Fig. 11.15). The zona reticularis develops after 1 to 3 years, but does not secrete hormones until adrenarche at 6 to 8 years of age.

The fetal zone does not express **3β-HSD** and releases the sulfated form of the inactive androgen, **dehydroepiandrosterone sulfate (DHEAS)**, throughout most of gestation (Fig. 11.16). The production of DHEAS from the fetal adrenal is absolutely dependent on **fetal adrenocorticotropic hormone (ACTH)** from the fetal pituitary by the end of the first trimester.

The DHEAS released from the fetal zone has two fates (see Fig. 11.16). First, DHEAS can go directly to the **syncytiotrophoblast**, where it is desulfated by a placental **steroid sulfatase** and used as a 19-carbon substrate for the synthesis of **estradiol-17β** and **estrone**. The second fate of DHEAS is 16-hydroxylation in the **fetal liver** by the enzyme CYP3A7. 16-Hydroxyl-DHEAS is then converted by the syncytiotrophoblasts to the major estrogen of pregnancy, **estriol** (see Fig. 11.16).

Because estrogen production is dependent on a healthy fetus, estriol levels can be used to assess fetal well-being. The **fetoplacental unit** represents the collective term for the tissues that make estrogen. Estrogens increase uteroplacental blood flow, enhance LDL receptor expression in

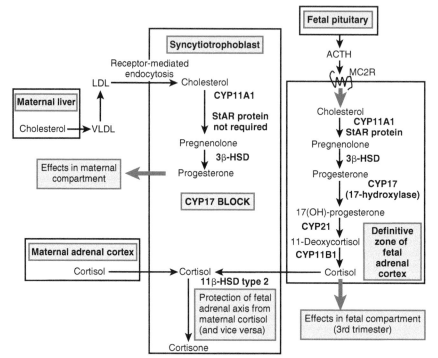

Fig. 11.14 Progesterone biosynthesis by the syncytiotrophoblast. *ACTH*, Adrenocorticotropic hormone; *3β-HSD*, 3β-hydroxysteroid dehydrogenase; *11β-HSD*, 11β-hydroxysteroid dehydrogenase; *LDL*, low-density lipoprotein; *MC2R*, melanocortin-2 receptor (ACTH receptor); *StAR protein*, steroidogenic acute regulatory protein; *VLDL*, very-low-density lipoprotein.

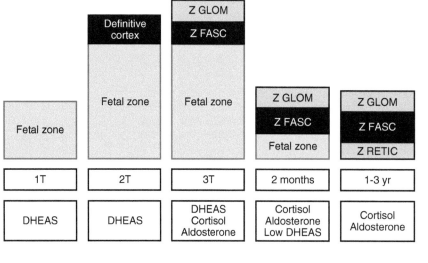

Fig. 11.15 The zones of the fetal adrenal cortex.

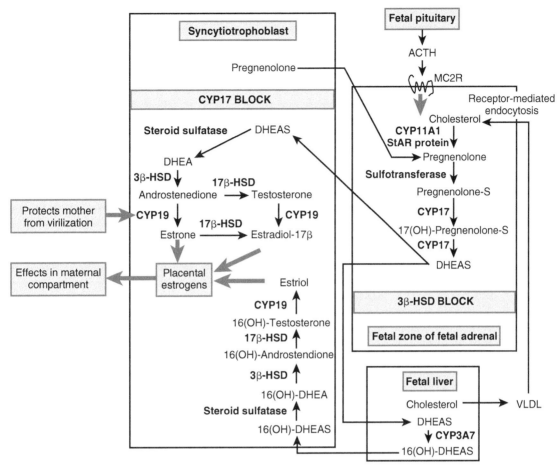

Fig. 11.16 Estrogen biosynthesis by the fetoplacental unit. *ACTH*, adrenocorticotropic hormone; *DHEA*, dehydroepiandrostenedione; *DHEAS*, dehydroepiandrostenedione sulfate; *3β-HSD*, 3β-hydroxysteroid dehydrogenase; *17β-HSD*, 17β-hydroxysteroid dehydrogenase; *MC2R*, melanocortin-2 receptor (ACTH receptor); *16(OH)-*, 16-hydroxy-; *StAR protein*, steroidogenic acute regulatory protein; *VLDL*, very-low-density lipoprotein.

syncytiotrophoblasts, and induce several components (e.g., prostaglandins, oxytocin receptors) involved in parturition. Estrogens increase the growth and development of the **mammary glands** directly, and also indirectly through the stimulation of **maternal pituitary prolactin** production (see later in the text). Estrogens are not necessary for a normal pregnancy but are required for labor and parturition.

Human Placental Lactogen

Human placental lactogen (hPL), also called *human chorionic somatomammotropin* (hCS), is a 191-amino acid protein hormone produced in the syncytiotrophoblast that is structurally similar to growth hormone (GH) and prolactin

(PRL). It can be detected within the syncytiotrophoblast by 10 days after conception and in maternal serum by 3 weeks of gestation (see Fig. 11.13). Maternal serum levels rise progressively throughout the remainder of the pregnancy. As much as 1 g/day of hPL can be secreted late in gestation! Like GH, hPL is protein-anabolic and lipolytic. Its antagonistic action to insulin contributes to the **diabetogenicity of pregnancy**. Glucose is a major energy substrate for the fetus, and hPL increases glucose availability by inhibiting maternal glucose uptake (Fig. 11.17). The lipolytic actions help the mother to shift to the use of free fatty acids for energy. Despite its very high levels in the maternal blood, hPL is probably not essential for normal pregnancy.

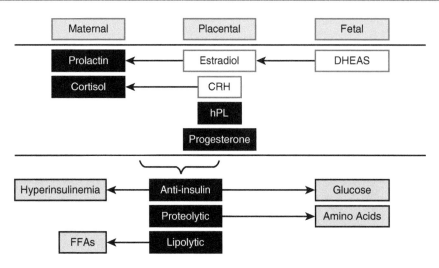

Fig. 11.17 Role of human placental lactogen *(hPL)*, prolactin (PRL), and cortisol in altering maternal metabolism to provide amino acids and glucose to fetus during the second half of pregnancy.

Other Placental Hormones

The placenta is a source of many other hormones. The placenta produces parathyroid hormone–related protein (PTHrP), which increases placental calcium transport (see later in the text). The role of placental corticotropin–releasing hormone (CRH) in the induction of labor is discussed later.

PLACENTAL TRANSPORT

As discussed earlier, the thickness of placental membrane is minimized and the surface area maximized. Depending on the substance involved, transport can occur by simple diffusion, facilitated diffusion, active transport, or endocytosis.

Gases, water, and many electrolytes cross the placenta by simple diffusion. Because the placental membrane is considerably thicker than the diffusional surface of the lungs, placental gas transport efficiency is only about 1/50th that of the lung on a per-unit weight basis. A sizable gradient exists for oxygen between maternal and fetal blood. Fetal compensation for the low Po_2 is aided by a high fetal blood flow rate and the high oxygen affinity of fetal hemoglobin.

Carbon dioxide, on the other hand, is more soluble in body tissues, and the diffusion capacity is greater.

Amino acids are transported by selective active transporters. Glucose is transported by facilitated diffusion, primarily by GLUT1. Neutral fats do not cross the placenta, and LDLs are transported into the placenta by LDL receptor–mediated endocytosis.

The fat-soluble steroid hormones cross relatively readily, but protein hormone transport is minimal.

THE FETAL ENDOCRINE SYSTEM

The timing and some key aspects of the fetal endocrine system are listed in Table 11.1. The details of the development of the reproductive systems are presented in Chapter 8.

MATERNAL ENDOCRINE CHANGES DURING PREGNANCY

Pituitary Gland

PRL levels rise during pregnancy because estrogen stimulates PRL synthesis and secretion (see later in the text). The pituitary gland increases significantly (i.e., more than twofold) in size during pregnancy. This pituitary enlargement is due to lactotroph hypertrophy and hyperplasia. Pituitary enlargement during pregnancy can cause dizziness and visual problems if the pituitary presses against the optic chiasm, and makes the pituitary susceptible to vascular insult and necrosis at parturition (Sheehan syndrome).

Pituitary production of LH and follicle-stimulating hormone (FSH) decreases during pregnancy because of negative feedback inhibition by the high levels of placentally produced estrogens plus progesterone.

Thyroid Gland

Thyroid size increases during pregnancy, and serum total T_4 and total T_3 levels can double. The primary basis for the increase in total thyroid hormone levels is an estrogen-induced increase in liver thyroxine-binding globulin (TBG) production, which leads to an increase in hormone binding. Serum free T_4 and T_3 levels do not increase

TABLE 11.1   Development of the Fetal Endocrine System

Endocrine Gland	Timing of Development	Comments
Hypothalamus and pituitary gland	All **pituitary hormones** produced by 12 wk All **hypothalamic-releasing hormones** being produced by 12 wk	**Hypothalamohypophyseal portal system** is functional at 18 wk
Thyroid gland	T_4 produced by 10 to 12 wk	Early neural development is dependent on some **maternal T_3**; even mild maternal hypothyroidism can cause neurologic deficits in fetus (e.g., lower IQ) Fetal blood T_3 increases significantly after 30 wk due to **type 1 deiodinase** expression Fetus is protected from maternal hyperthyroidism by **placental type 3 (inner ring) deiodinase**
Parathyroid glands	Parathyroids form by 8 to 10 wk, secretion of **PTH** is inhibited by relative hypercalcemic state	**Decidual 1,25-dihydroxyvitamin D3** promotes calcium absorption by maternal intestine and **placental PTHrP** promotes placental transfer of calcium into fetal compartment
Pancreatic islets	Secrete **insulin** and **glucagon** by 15 wk	**Fetal glucose** mostly determined by placental transport rather than fetal pancreatic hormones In latter half of pregnancy, maternal diabetes with poor glycemic control can induce hyperplasia of fetal islet cells and fetal hyperinsulinemia
Adrenal glands	Fetal cortex produces **DHEAS** by 7 wk, **cortisol** during second half or pregnancy and **aldosterone** near term Neural crest cells migrate into center of adrenal and differentiate into **chromaffin cells** before adrenal capsule forms by end of first trimester	As discussed earlier, fetal adrenal cortex is composed of large **fetal zone** and small **definitive cortex**; refer to Fig. 11.15 One major role of fetal cortisol is to induce production of **surfactant** in lung; untreated preterm deliveries are associated with **respiratory distress syndrome** Complete or partial loss of **21-hydroxylase** activity encoded by the **CYP21A2** gene is the most common cause of **congenital adrenal hyperplasia (CAH)**. Loss of fetal **cortisol** during second half of pregnancy induces high fetal **ACTH** levels, hypertrophy of definitive cortex, and an increase in **adrenal androgen** production. In a female fetus, CAH causes **virilization** of external genitalia. Severe deficiency of 21-hydroxylase causes dangerous salt wasting and **hyponatremia** in neonate because of **aldosterone** deficiency.

markedly during gestation. The effects of hCG on the maternal thyroid gland were discussed earlier.

Adrenal Gland

Estrogens not only stimulate liver TBG production but also nonspecifically stimulate liver production of many other serum proteins, such as cortisol-binding globulin (CBG) (also called transcortin). Consequently, total serum cortisol levels rise. Although maternal serum ACTH levels increase slightly during pregnancy, they typically remain within the normal nonpregnant range. Late in pregnancy,

however, serum free cortisol levels rise steadily to a peak at parturition that is about twice nonpregnancy levels. The fetus is protected from maternal cortisol levels (and vice versa) by the presence of placental 11β-dehydrogenase type 2, which converts cortisol to the inactive cortisone (see Fig. 11.14).

Estrogen stimulates liver angiotensinogen production and renal renin production. Consequently, synthesis of angiotensin II and aldosterone increases. Estrogens potentiate the adrenal action of angiotensin II but antagonize the vasopressive actions. Aldosterone supports the volume expansion in the mother by increasing NaCl retention (by as much as 1000 mEq). However, because of elevated antidiuretic hormone (ADH) and decreased threshold for thirst, the osmolality of the blood falls slightly.

MATERNAL PHYSIOLOGIC CHANGES DURING PREGNANCY

Physiologic changes occur in the pregnant woman both as a consequence of the size of the developing fetus and as a result of the endocrine and cardiovascular changes associated with the pregnancy (Box 11.1).

Cardiovascular Changes

Pregnancy is associated with an increase in cardiac output coupled to a reduction in peripheral resistance and an expansion of total body and plasma volume.

The **cardiac output** during pregnancy increases to about 40% more than preconception levels, with most of this increase occurring by 8 weeks of gestation. Cardiac output is due to both positive chronotropic and inotropic effects of pregnancy. These may be due to increased sympathetic tone and an increased sensitivity to catecholamines.

Peripheral resistance declines in response to several factors. As discussed previously, the spiral arteries are converted to low-resistance, highly compliant vessels, allowing the uteroplacental blood flow to increase by

---

BOX 11.1   Physiologic Changes in Pregnancy

Cardiovascular Changes
- Vascular volume
- Peripheral resistance
- Stroke volume
- Heart rate
- Contractility
- Cardiac output

Respiratory Changes
- Minute volume
- Tidal volume
- Pco_2
- Functional residual capacity
- Inspiratory reserve volume

Renal Changes
- Antidiuretic hormone, renin, angiotensin II, aldosterone secretion
- Respiratory alkalosis

---

an order of magnitude from the end of the first trimester to term (about 60 to 600 mL per minute). Overall, vascular resistance decreases throughout the maternal circulatory system, and diastolic pressure tends to drop. Blood pressure typically does not rise until late in pregnancy.

Total body volume increases by the retention of up to 8 L of water, which is partitioned among the maternal and growing fetal circulatory systems, uteroplacental circulation, and an enlarging amniotic sac. **Blood volume** increases by up to 50% during pregnancy to accommodate an increasing uteroplacental circulation. Bloating or mild edema is common in pregnancy.

CLINICAL BOX 11.4

Because the growing uterus exerts pressure on the veins of the legs where these veins enter the abdomen, venous pressure in the lower extremities rises on standing, and edema and venous damage can occur. Lying in the supine position can result in compression of the inferior vena cava by the uterus, followed by maternal hypotension.

Respiratory Changes

While pregnancy proceeds, the **functional residual capacity** (volume of air in the lungs at the end of a quiet expiration) and the **residual volume** (volume remaining at the end of a maximal expiration) decrease, and respiratory rate remains unchanged. **Minute volume increases** and **tidal volume increases**, so Pco_2 decreases.

There are three major causes of the respiratory changes associated with pregnancy. The bulk of the growing fetus and uterus increases intraabdominal pressure and forces the diaphragm upward. The high metabolic rate of the growing fetus increases maternal oxygen consumption and carbon dioxide production. In addition, **progesterone** acts on the central nervous system to lower the setpoint for regulation of respiration by carbon dioxide, thereby increasing ventilation.

Renal Changes

The glomerular filtration rate increases about 60% over nonpregnant levels, causing the filtered load to increase, which can lead to **glucosuria** and **aminoaciduria** in pregnancy.

Maternal serum levels of the mineralocorticoid deoxycorticosterone (DOC) increase during pregnancy. This increase in circulating DOC levels results not from increased adrenal secretion but from renal conversion of placental progesterone to DOC. Increased levels of DOC and aldosterone (see earlier in the text) stimulate renal salt and water retention.

Gastrointestinal Changes

Heartburn, or reflux of acidic gastric secretions into the esophagus, occurs for multiple reasons. The increased intraabdominal pressure increases intragastric pressure, which increases the likelihood of reflux into the esophagus. Progesterone also decreases lower esophageal sphincter tone, thereby increasing reflux tendency.

Diabetogenicity of Pregnancy

Pregnancy represents an insulin-resistant, hyperinsulinemic state (see Fig. 11.17). During the last half of pregnancy, maternal energy metabolism shifts from an anabolic state in which nutrients are stored to a catabolic state, sometimes described as accelerated starvation, in which maternal energy metabolism shifts toward fat utilization with glucose sparing. The peripheral responsiveness to insulin decreases and pancreatic insulin secretion increases. β-Cell hyperplasia occurs in pregnancy. Although this usually does not lead to any clinical condition, pregnancy aggravates existing diabetes mellitus, and diabetes mellitus can develop for the first time in pregnancy. If the diabetes resolves spontaneously with delivery, the condition is referred to as gestational diabetes. Hormones contributing to the diabetogenicity of pregnancy are hPL, prolactin, cortisol, and progesterone (see Fig. 11.17).

PARTURITION

Human pregnancy lasts an average of 40 weeks from the beginning of the last menstrual period (gestational age). This corresponds to an average fetal age of 38 weeks. Parturition is the process whereby uterine contractions (labor) lead to childbirth. Labor consists of three stages:

1. Strong uterine contractions that force the fetus against the cervix, with dilation and thinning of the cervix (several hours)
2. Delivery of the fetus (< 1 hour)
3. Delivery of the placenta, along with contractions of the myometrium, which serve to halt bleeding (< 10 minutes).

Parturition control in humans is complex, and the exact mechanisms underlying parturition control are not well understood. In many species, such as sheep, the timing of parturition is controlled by fetus-derived signals, and fetal regulation is at least a factor in humans.

Placental Corticotropin–Releasing Hormone and the Fetal Adrenal Axis

The placenta produces CRH, which is identical to the 41-amino acid peptide produced by the hypothalamus. Placental CRH production and maternal serum CRH levels increase rapidly during late pregnancy and labor. Moreover, circulating CRH is either in the form of free CRH, which is bioactive, or complexed to a CRH-binding protein. Maternal levels of CRH-binding protein plummet during late pregnancy and labor, and free CRH levels increase. Placental CRH also accumulates in the fetal circulation and stimulates fetal ACTH secretion. ACTH stimulates both fetal adrenal cortisol production and fetoplacental estrogen production. In contrast to the inhibitory effect of cortisol on hypothalamic CRH production, cortisol stimulates placental CRH production. This establishes a self-amplifying positive feedback loop. CRH itself promotes myometrial contractions through sensitizing the uterus to prostaglandins and oxytocin. Estrogens also directly and indirectly stimulate myometrial contractility. This model correlates with the onset of parturition with cortisol-induced maturation of fetal systems, including the lungs and gastrointestinal system.

Estrogen

Estrogen is required for labor. It increases receptors and sensitivity of the myometrium to oxytocin and increases prostaglandin production.

CLINICAL BOX 11.5

In male fetuses with X-linked steroid sulfatase deficiency, the fetoplacental unit cannot make estrogens. This results in maternal estrogen levels that are an order of magnitude less than those in normal pregnancies. These babies typically are delivered by cesarean section because the absence of estrogen results in a quiescent myometrium and a pregnancy that goes several weeks beyond the due date. Nevertheless, the pregnancy proceeds normally, and the newborn is normal except for the phenotype associated with sulfatase deficiency (ichthyosis, or scaly skin).

Oxytocin

Oxytocin is released in response to stretch of the cervix, and it stimulates uterine contractions, thereby facilitating delivery (Fig. 11.18). Cervical stretch in response to oxytocin release stimulates the production of more oxytocin, thereby setting up a positive feedback loop that terminates upon childbirth. Oxytocin is sometimes used to induce parturition, and uterine sensitivity to oxytocin increases before parturition.

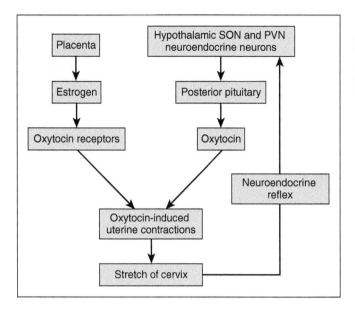

Fig. 11.18 Positive feedback loop between oxytocin-induced uterine contraction and the neuroendocrine loop from the stretched cervix to the hypothalamic supraoptic nucleus (SON) and paraventricular nucleus (PVN), which induces release of oxytocin from the posterior pituitary.

Prostaglandins

Prostaglandins and other cytokines increase uterine motility, and levels of these compounds increase during parturition, thereby facilitating delivery. The prostaglandins PGF2α and PGE$_2$ increase uterine motility. Large doses of these compounds have been used to induce labor.

Uterine Size

Uterine size is thought to be a factor regulating parturition because stretch of smooth muscle, including the uterus, increases muscle contraction. In addition, uterine stretch stimulates uterine prostaglandin production. Multiple births generally occur prematurely.

MAMMOGENESIS AND LACTATION

Structure of the Mammary Gland

The mammary gland is composed of about 20 lobes, each with an excretory lactiferous duct that opens at the nipple (Fig. 11.19). Lobes, in turn, are composed of several lobules, which contain secretory structures called alveoli, and the terminal portions of the ducts. The epithelia of the alveoli and ducts is composed of apical luminal ductal or alveolar cells and a myoepithelial cell layer on the basal side of the epithelium. Myoepithelial cells are stellate,

smooth muscle–like cells, and contraction of these cells in response to oxytocin expels milk from the lumina of the alveoli and ducts. Myoepithelial cells produce the basal lamina of the epithelial layer and oppose the invasion of breast cancer cells from the lumen into the outer-lying stroma.

Lobes and lobules are supported within a connective tissue matrix. The density of this matrix can affect the resolution of mammograms. The other major stromal component of the breast is adipose tissue. The lactiferous ducts empty at the nipple, which is a highly innervated, hairless protrusion of the breast designed for suckling by an infant. The nipple is surrounded by a pigmented, hairless areola, which is lubricated by sebaceous glands. Protrusion of the nipple, called erection, is mediated by sympathetic stimulation of smooth muscle fibers in response to suckling and other mechanical stimulation, erotic stimulation, and cold.

Hormonal Regulation of Mammary Gland Development

The mammary glands develop in utero as rudimentary mammary buds. At puberty, estrogen increases ductal growth and branching. With the onset of luteal phases of the ovary, progesterone and estrogen induce further ductal growth and the formation of rudimentary alveoli. During nonpregnant cycles, the breasts develop somewhat and then regress. Estrogen also increases the deposition

Anatomic structures

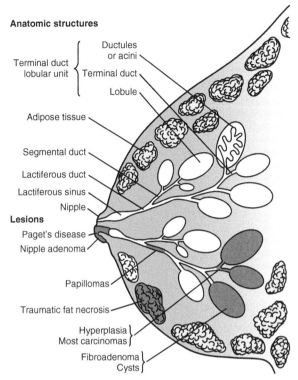

Fig. 11.19 Anatomy of the breast and major lesions at each site within the breast. (From Cotran RS, Kumar V, Robbins SL: *Pathologic Basis of Disease*, 5th ed., Philadelphia, 1994, Saunders.)

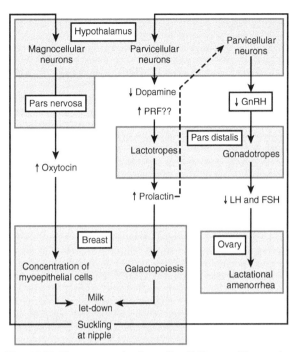

Fig. 11.20 The neuroendocrine reflex linking suckling at the nipple to oxytocin and prolactin release. *FSH*, follicle-stimulating hormone; *GnRH*, gonadotropin-releasing hormone; *LH*, luteinizing hormone; *PRL*, prolactin.

of adipose tissue. Adipose tissue expresses CYP19 (aromatase), and accumulation of this tissue in the breast increases the local production of estrogens from circulating androgens.

The greatest degree of breast development occurs during pregnancy, during which extensive ductal growth and branching and lobuloalveolar development occur. High levels of placental-derived estrogen and progesterone stimulate the extensive development of the breast. Estrogen acts on the breast directly and also indirectly through increasing maternal pituitary PRL production by lactotrophs. Although the luminal alveolar epithelial cells begin to express genes encoding milk proteins and enzymes involved in milk production, progesterone inhibits the onset of milk production and secretion (called *lactogenesis*).

Immediately after parturition, the human breast excretes colostrum, which is enriched with antimicrobial and antiinflammatory proteins. In the absence of placental progesterone, normal breast milk production occurs within a few days. The lobuloalveolar structures produce milk, which is subsequently modified by the ductal epithelium. Lactogenesis and the maintenance of milk production (galactopoiesis) require stimulation by pituitary prolactin, in the presence of normal levels of other hormones, including insulin, cortisol, and thyroid hormone. Whereas placental estrogen stimulates prolactin secretion during pregnancy, the stimulus for prolactin secretion during the nursing period is suckling by the infant (Fig. 11.20). The levels of prolactin are directly correlated with the frequency and duration of sucking at the nipple. The link between suckling at the nipple and prolactin secretion involves a neuroendocrine reflex, in which dopamine (the prolactin-release inhibitory factor; see Chapter 5) secretion at the median eminence is inhibited. It is also possible that suckling increases the secretion of unidentified prolactin-releasing hormones.

Prolactin also inhibits GnRH release; consequently, nursing can be associated with lactational amenorrhea (see Fig. 11.20). This effect of prolactin has been called *nature's contraceptive* and may play a role in spacing out pregnancies. Only very regular nursing over a 24-hour period, however, is sufficient to allow for a prolactin-induced anovulatory state in the mother. Thus lactational amenorrhea is not an effective or reliable form of birth control for most women.

CLINICAL BOX 11.6

The inhibition of GnRH by high levels of prolactin is important clinically. The prolactinoma is the most common form of hormone-secreting pituitary tumor, and hyperprolactinemia is a significant cause of infertility in both sexes. Hyperprolactinemia can also be associated with galactorrhea, or the inappropriate flow of breast milk, in men and women.

Suckling at the nipple also stimulates the release of oxytocin from the posterior pituitary (see Chapter 5) through a neuroendocrine reflex (see Fig. 11.20). Oxytocin receptors on the myoepithelial cells cause contractions that ultimately induce milk letdown, or the expulsion of milk from alveolar and ductal lumina. Oxytocin release and milk letdown can be induced by psychogenic stimuli, such as the sound of a baby crying on a television program or thinking about the baby. Such psychogenic stimuli do not affect prolactin release.

CLINICAL BOX 11.7

The breast epithelium represents a hormonally responsive, highly mitogenic population of cells. Invasive breast cancer (IBC) arises from breast epithelium (primarily from the epithelial cells lining small ducts). IBC represents a very common cancer in women in the United States and is a major cause of death among women older than 45 years. The most commonly diagnosed form of IBC is called luminal A, in which most cells express the α isoform of the estrogen receptor ERα. These tumors are highly dependent on estrogen and regress or fail to recur in response to antiestrogen treatment. This treatment involves the use of a selective estrogen receptor modulator (SERM) such as tamoxifen or aromatase (CYP19) inhibitor. Treatment of an early (not metastasized) form of luminal A IBC usually involves surgical resection of the cancer (lumpectomy, mastectomy), followed by several weeks of radiation therapy, followed by antiestrogen therapy for several years. The overall survival rate for early, lymph node–negative, ERα-positive luminal A IBC is well over 90% in North America.

CONTRACEPTION

Behavioral and Mechanical Approaches

There are multiple methods of contraception. These methods include the age-old rhythm method, which relies on abstinence from sexual intercourse during fertile periods around the time of ovulation. (The fertile period is considered to be the period extending from 3 to 4 days before the time of ovulation until 3 to 4 days afterward.) A second method is withdrawal before ejaculation, coitus interruptus. Both of these methods have higher failure rates (20% to 30%) than the barrier methods (2% to 12%), intrauterine devices (IUDs) (< 2%), and oral contraceptives (< 1%).

Barriers such as condoms or diaphragms are more effective as contraceptives when used with spermicidal jellies.

Among the various methods of contraception, IUDs are the most effective, except for oral contraceptives. These devices are thought to prevent implantation by producing a local inflammatory response in the endometrium. Some forms of IUDs contain copper, zinc, or progestins, which inhibit sperm transport or viability in the female reproductive tract.

Female (tubule ligation) and male (vasectomy) sterilization are also effective options, especially for couples who have children and do not wish for further procreation in the face of continued sexual activity.

Oral Contraceptives

Oral contraceptives have been marketed in the United States since the early 1960s. The doses of steroids used today are many-fold lower than those used in the initial preparations. Properly used, oral contraceptives have a low failure rate.

Many forms of oral contraceptives are marketed today. The trend over the years has been to decrease the dosage of steroids used because the side effects are dose dependent. All oral steroidal contraceptives contain a progestin analog, and some also contain an estrogen analog. The numerous formulations, applications (e.g., pills, patches), and configurations of the timing and duration available are beyond the scope of this chapter.

Oral-contraceptives work through multiple mechanisms. Most block the LH surge that triggers ovulation. However, some pills, such as the progestin-only minipill, block fertility by changing the nature of cervical mucus, by altering endometrial development, and by regulating fallopian tube motility. Because these contraceptives suppress FSH, they impair early follicular development.

Side effects include bloating, breast tenderness, and unscheduled bleeding (breakthrough bleeding). Estrogen-progesterone combination pills appear to increase the risk for venous thrombosis. The effect of combination pills on breast cancer is minimal, and they decrease the incidence of ovarian and uterine cancer. However, cervical cancer is linked to the use of oral contraceptives.

Hormonal Treatment for Emergency Contraception and Abortion

Emergency contraception involves hormonal treatment designed to inhibit or delay ovulation, inhibit corpus luteum function, and disrupt the function of the oviducts and uterus. Candidates for emergency contraception include women who have been sexually assaulted or who experienced a failure of a barrier method (e.g., ruptured condom). The currently preferred medication is levo-norgestrel (Plan B), which is a synthetic progestin-only pill. The efficacy of the pill is inversely correlated with the time it is taken after intercourse. The exact mechanism of action is not known. Treatment has no effect if implantation has occurred.

Medical (hormonal) termination of pregnancy (abortion) can be achieved until up to 49 days of gestation by administration of mifepristone (RU-486). Mifepristone is a progesterone receptor antagonist (i.e., an antiprogestin), which induces collapse of the pregnant endometrium. Mifepristone is followed 48 hours later by ingestion or vaginal insertion of a synthetic prostaglandin E (e.g., misoprostol), which induces myometrial contractions.

IN VITRO FERTILIZATION

The development of in vitro fertilization (IVF) and other assisted pregnancy procedures was made possible through our increased understanding of the basic science of reproduction.

SUMMARY

1. The events of fertilization, early embryogenesis, and implantation are synchronized with the hormonal changes of the human menstrual cycle, ultimately ensuring a receptive uterus at the time of implantation.

2. Spermatozoa bind to the epithelium of the oviductal isthmus, which secretes factors that capacitate the sperm. Hyperactivation allows the sperm to detach and swim to the cumulus-oocyte complex in the ampulla. Fertilization involves the penetration by a spermatozoon of the expanded cumulus as mediated by a membrane hyaluronidase, penetration of the zona pellucida as mediated by the acrosome reaction, and fusion with the oocyte membrane as mediated by specific membrane fusion proteins. The egg is activated, completes the second meiotic division, and releases cortical granule enzymes that prevent polyspermy. The female and male pronuclei are drawn together, line up on a metaphase plate, and undergo the first cleavage.

3. The embryo undergoes cleavage and formation of a morula within the oviduct. The embryo enters the uterus on day 3, forms a blastocyst, degrades the zona pellucida (hatches), and implants on day 6 or 7.

4. The trophoblast layer differentiates into the cytophoblastic layer and an outer syncytiotrophoblastic layer. The syncytiotrophoblasts secrete invasive enzymes, express adhesion molecules, produce protein and steroid hormones, and ultimately become the primary cell involved in maternal-fetal exchange. With the addition of an extraembryonic mesoderm, the trophoblast layers become the chorion. The fetal (umbilical) blood vessels develop within the mesenchyme of the extraembryonic mesoderm. The chorion ultimately gives rise to protrusions, the chorionic villi, which constitute the functional unit of the placenta.

5. The uterine endometrium decidualizes in response to implantation. The decidua impose restraint on the invading embryo.

6. The intervillous spaces become filled with maternal blood from eroded spiral arteries. This gives rise to a hemochorial placenta. Spiral arteries are plugged up by extravillous cytotrophoblasts for the first trimester so that the embryo/early fetus develops in a relatively hypoxic environment and receives histotrophic nutrition. The cytotrophoblasts convert the spiral arteries to low-resistance, high-capacitance vessels that supply blood to the placenta during the second and third trimesters.

7. The first hormone produced by the placenta is hCG. This hormone is structurally similar to LH but has a longer half-life. Its function is to rescue the corpus luteum, which is needed to produce progesterone for the first 10 weeks. hCG also stimulates male fetal gonadal production of testosterone and the early fetal adrenal.

8. Progesterone production is taken over by the placenta. Syncytiotrophoblasts use maternal cholesterol to make progesterone. Because no fetal tissues are involved in progesterone synthesis, progesterone levels are not a measure of fetal health. Progesterone is required for pregnancy. Progesterone maintains a quiescent uterus and affects several aspects of maternal physiology. Progesterone is used by the fetal adrenal cortex for cortisol synthesis.

9. The fetal adrenal cortex is different from the adult. The large inner zone is called the fetal zone. The fetal zone produces DHEAS, which is then converted by the syncytiotrophoblasts to estradiol and estrone. DHEAS

also is converted to 16-hydroxy-DHEAS by the fetal liver, and this steroid is further converted to estriol by the syncytiotrophoblasts. This multiorgan pathway for estrogen synthesis is referred to as the fetoplacental unit. Maternal serum estriol levels can be used as an indicator of fetal health. Estrogen is not required for pregnancy. The primary function of estrogen is to prepare the uterus for parturition. Both estrogen and progesterone play important roles in mammary gland development during pregnancy.

10. The outer definitive zone of the fetal adrenal cortex begins to make cortisol at midgestation and to make aldosterone close to term. Cortisol production increases toward late pregnancy, playing a role in fetal lung surfactant synthesis, fetal gastrointestinal tract maturation, and other aspects of late fetal development.

11. Human placental lactogen (hPL) is structurally and functionally similar to both GH and PRL. It is an insulin antagonist and is lipolytic.

12. Glucose crosses the placenta by GLUT1 carrier-mediated facilitated diffusion. Amino acid transport is by carrier-mediated secondary active transport, and LDL transport is by receptor-mediated endocytosis. Gas transport is by simple diffusion.

13. Cardiovascular changes in pregnancy include increased vascular volume; decreased peripheral resistance; and increased heart rate, cardiac contractility, and cardiac output.

14. Respiratory changes in pregnancy include increased minute volume and increased tidal volume.

15. During pregnancy, ADH, renin, angiotensin II, and aldosterone secretion all increase. These changes produce sodium and water retention.

16. The exact mechanism underlying initiation of parturition in humans has not been defined. Possible stimuli include increases in placental CRH production, fetal ACTH and cortisol production, uterine size, oxytocin receptor concentration, and uterine prostaglandin production. Parturition requires estrogen, which stimulates prostaglandin synthesis and oxytocin receptor expression.

17. Mammary glands are lobuloalveolar structures. Estrogen and progesterone promote ductal and alveolar growth, whereas progesterone and prolactin stimulate alveolar development. The extensive mammary development in pregnancy is driven by PRL, estradiol, and progesterone. Milk production in pregnancy is blocked by progesterone.

18. After parturition, sucking at the nipple is required for prolactin and oxytocin secretion. Prolactin maintains milk production (galactopoiesis), and oxytocin causes the myoepithelial cells to contract. Prolactin inhibits GnRH secretion—the basis for lactational amenorrhea and for both male and female infertility due to a prolactinoma with associated hyperprolactinemia.

19. Breast cancer is often a hormonally responsive cancer in the earlier stages, so antiestrogens and aromatase inhibitors are effective as adjuvant therapy.

20. Elucidation of the basic science of reproductive endocrinology has led to the development of oral contraceptives, emergency contraceptives, medical abortion pills, and in vitro fertilization procedures.

SELF-STUDY PROBLEMS

1. What is meant by *egg activation*?
2. Describe the initial events of implantation.
3. How does placental progesterone synthesis differ from placental estriol synthesis?
4. What is the role of estrogen in pregnancy and parturition?
5. What is the basis for hyperthyroidism during the first trimester of some pregnancies? Why is it transient?
6. How does progesterone affect maternal respiration?
7. What is the relationship between infertility and PRL in a physiologic situation? In a pathologic condition?

KEYWORDS AND CONCEPTS

Amnion
β-hCG
Chorion
Corpus luteum of pregnancy
Early embryogenesis
Estrogens: estradiol-17β
Estriol
Estrone
Events of fertilization: sperm capacitation, acrosome reaction, sperm-egg fusion, egg activation, cortical granule exocytosis

Implantation: blastocyst, cytotrophoblast, syncytiotrophoblast, decidualization
Lactation: Prolactin, oxytocin, neuroendocrine reflex, lactogenesis, galactopoiesis
Lobuloalveolar development
Menstrual cycle: relationship with fertilization and early embryogenesis
Placental steroidogenesis: progesterone, estrogen, fetoplacental unit
StAR protein, Cyp17, 3β-HSD, ACTH, fetal zone, fetal liver, sulfotransferase

Answers to Self-Study Problems

CHAPTER 1

1. Protein hormones are stored within secretory vesicles and are secreted in response to a stimulus. Steroid hormones freely diffuse out of cells. Their synthesis, as opposed to secretion, is regulated by stimuli.

2. Hormone-binding proteins in the serum generally increase the circulating half-life of a hormone. It is the free fraction (i.e., unbound) that is considered to be active.

3. Increasing the GTPase activity of Gs would result in a more rapid inactivation of Gs, thereby decreasing adenylate cyclase activity and cAMP levels. Thus the cell would demonstrate resistance to hormones that act through Gs-coupled GPCRs.

4. The IRS protein is recruited to and phosphorylated by the insulin receptor. The phosphotyrosines within the IRS protein recruit and activate the Ras-Raf-MAPK pathway, which transduces insulin receptor binding into a growth response. Other phosphotyrosines on the IRS protein activate the PI3 kinase–PKB pathway, which is linked primarily to metabolic actions of insulin (including GLUT4 translocation to the membrane).

5. Cytokines and TGF-β–related hormones (e.g., inhibin) signal by phosphorylating a transcription factor (cytokines use STATs, and TGF-β–related hormones use SMADs). The transcription factors then translocate to the nucleus (as dimers) and activate the expression of specific genes.

6. Hormone binding to a GPCR induces a conformational change in the receptor, which makes the receptor a substrate for serine/threonine GPCR kinases (GRKs). β-Arrestins then bind to the phosphorylated residue and link the receptor to clathrin-coated pits and clathrin-mediated endocytosis. Receptors within endosomes may recycle back to the membrane, or may be destroyed by lysosomal enzymes if the endosome fuses with a lysosome.

7. Guanosine nucleotide exchange factors (GEFs) allow a small G protein to exchange a bound GDP (inactive state) for GTP (active state). GPCRs are essentially ligand-activated GEFs for the trimeric G-protein complexes. Without this activity, GPCRs could not activate the α subunits of the trimeric G protein complex.

8. Phospholipase C (PLC) cleaves the membrane phospholipid, phosphatidylinositol, into diacylglycerol (DAG) and inositol-3-phosphate (IP_3). DAG activates certain isoforms of protein kinase C, whereas IP_3 binds to its receptor in the endoplasmic reticulum to induce release of Ca^{2+} into the cytoplasm.

CHAPTER 2

1. Cephalic, gastric, and intestinal. The greatest release of gastrin occurs during the gastric phase. This occurs because (1) the presence of amino acids in the stomach directly stimulates gastrin release from G cells; (2) the presence of food promotes gastrin release through pressor receptors in the stomach wall; (3) the presence of food buffers acidity, thereby decreasing inhibitory somatostatin release; and (4) there is minimal inhibitory signaling from the small intestine and colon.

2. (a) Stimulation. (b) Stimulation. (c) Inhibition. (d) Stimulation. (e) Stimulation.

3. S cells secrete secretin, I cells secrete CCK. CCK inhibits gastric motility. Secretin may act as an enterogastrone to inhibit gastrin secretion but has a minimal effect on gastric emptying.

4. (a) Some stimulation. (b) Strong stimulation. (c) No effect. (d) Increase. (e) Decrease.

5. Both glucagon-like peptide-1 (GLP-1) and glucagon are encoded within the same gene that encodes the preproglucagon prohormone. Glucagon is secreted by α cells of the endocrine pancreas and binds to the glucagon receptor. GLP-1 is released by intestinal L cells and acts through the GLP-1 receptor.

6. An incretin is a hormone (peptide) that is released in response to food (especially glucose) in the intestine and enhances the ability of glucose to promote insulin release from the pancreatic β cells. Two incretins are GIP and GLP-1.

7. Hypertrophy and hyperplasia of the gastric mucosa and rugae (submucosal folds). Enterochromaffin-like (ECL) cells show the greatest degree of proliferation.

8. Erythromycin binds to and activates the motilin receptor.

CHAPTER 3

1. In the fed state, glycolysis in the liver leads to de novo fatty acid and triglyceride synthesis. In the adipose tissue, glycolysis generates glycerol-3-phosphate, which is used to reesterify fatty acids (from the digestion of chylomicrons by LPL) into triglycerides. Glycolysis is also used to generate ATP.

2. Glycogen is a storage form of glucose. In the liver, glycogenolysis contributes directly to blood glucose because the liver can dephosphorylate glucose-6-phosphate to glucose. In the muscle, glycogen is used during exercise to provide ATP by glycolysis. Skeletal muscle cannot dephosphorylate glucose-6-phosphate and thus cannot directly contribute to blood glucose levels.

3. Ketone bodies. The liver produces ketone bodies from free fatty acids and ketogenic amino acids.

4. Accumulation of mitochondrial citrate (in times of plentiful ATP) can be transferred to the cytoplasm, where it can generate cytoplasmic acetyl CoA used for lipogenesis.

5. Lipoprotein lipase (insulin-dependent activation) and hormone-sensitive lipase (insulin-dependent inhibition).

6. LDL particles lose apoprotein E and bind to LDL receptors through apoprotein B100. LDL receptors remove these high cholesterol particles from the blood by receptor-mediated endocytosis. The liver plays the major role in LDL receptor–mediated removal of LDL particles, although steroidogenic cells and proliferating cells (i.e., cells that need cholesterol) also take up LDL particles by the LDL receptor. Loss of LDL receptor results in a high LDL concentration in the blood and, therefore, high cholesterol content in the blood.

7. Malonyl CoA inhibits the carnitine-palmitoyl transferase-I transporter. This prevents the futile cycle of synthesizing fatty acids only to have them transported into the mitochondria for β-oxidation.

8. Decreased glucokinase activity would inhibit glycolysis and therefore ATP production in β cells. Lower ATP would result in less insulin secreted. Heterozygous null mutations of glucokinase cause one form of MODY.

9. a. Glucokinase—insulin increases gene expression through SREBP-1C;

   b. Fructose-1,6-bisphosphatase—insulin represses gene expression through inactivation of FOXO1 and inhibits enzyme activity by increasing the level of fructose-2,6-bisphosphate, which is an allosteric inhibitor of fructose-1, 6-bisphosphatase.

   c. Pyruvate kinase—insulin both increases *PK* gene expression through SREBBP-1C and increases PK activity through protein phosphatase-mediated dephosphorylation.

   d. Acetyl CoA carboxylase—insulin increases *ACC1* and *ACC2* gene expression through SREBP-1C, and increases activity by phosphatase-mediated dephosphorylation.

   e. PEPCK—insulin inhibits *PEPCK* gene expression, at least in part by inactivation of FOXO1.

10. In the presence of a low I/G ratio, more fatty acids are released from adipose tissue. These fatty acids are transported to the liver where they are metabolized. β-Oxidation increases. The low I/G ratio inhibits glycolysis and lipogenesis. Thus malonyl CoA levels remain low. Malonyl CoA is an inhibitor of carnitine-palmitoyl transferase-I: while malonyl CoA levels drop, carnitine-palmitoyl transferase-I activity increases. Hepatocyte mitochondria contain the enzymes for β-oxidation and ketogenesis. The elevated acetyl CoA production from β-oxidation, along with the decreased TCA cycle activity caused by NAD depletion, results in increased ketone body production. T1DM also results in an increased hepatic glucose production; enhanced gluconeogenic flux involves an enhanced efflux of oxaloacetate (as malate) from the mitochondria, further making acetyl CoA available for ketogenesis (as opposed to citrate production).

11. Obesity is associated with the accumulation of ectopic TGs in skeletal muscle and liver. Byproducts of TG synthesis and turnover (especially diacylglycerol and ceramide) activate signaling pathways (serine/threonine kinases) that phosphorylate and desensitize the insulin receptor and insulin-receptor substrate.

CHAPTER 4

1. 1,25-Dihydroxyvitamin D directly represses *PTH* gene expression. 1,25-Dihydroxyvitamin D also increases gene expression of the CaSR, which represses PTH in response to elevated serum calcium. Therefore loss of 1,25-dihydroxyvitamin D would lead to an increase in PTH secretion. PTH would also increase in response to decreases in serum Ca^{2+} resulting from less efficient absorption by the GI tract in the D-deficient state.

2. Vitamin D deficiency would cause increased PTH secretion by the mechanisms outlined earlier in the text.

The increase in PTH secretion would maintain serum Ca^{2+} levels (except in the case of rickets, where skeletal calcium stores may be limited), but would inhibit phosphate reabsorption by the proximal tubule. The resulting hypophosphatemia and decrease in the $Ca^{2+} \times Pi$ product could inhibit bone mineralization resulting in osteomalacia. In rickets, the inability to mobilize Ca^{2+} from bone could result in hypocalcemia as well.

3. Osteoclasts perform the bone resorption phase of bone remodeling. Osteoblasts promote the differentiation of monocyte-macrophage lineage cells into osteoclast precursors (through secretion of M-CSF) and the maturation of osteoclast precursors into actively resorbing osteoclasts (through membrane expression and secretion of RANKL). Note that the PTH1R is expressed by osteoblasts, not osteoclasts.

4. PTH-related peptide (PTHrP) binds to and activates the same receptor as PTH, i.e. PTH1R. PTHrP normally acts as a paracrine factor. However, high levels of PTHrP can be produced by neoplasms, thereby causing hypercalcemia (as in hyperparathyroidism).

5. RANKL binds to RANK on osteoclast progenitors to promote osteoclast differentiation and also prolongs mature osteoclast lifespan and activity. OPG acts as a decoy receptor for RANKL, thereby inhibiting osteoclast-mediated bone resorption. An increase in the RANKL/OPG ratio would therefore cause excess bone resorption and reduced bone density.

6. FGF23, which is produced by osteocytes, acts on the proximal tubule of the kidney to inhibit Pi reabsorption, thereby lowering serum Pi levels.

7. Primary hyperparathyroidism will be characterized by elevated levels of serum PTH in the face of hypercalcemia. Typically, urinary Ca^{2+} will be in the high to high-normal range. In FHH, serum Ca^{2+} levels will be maintained at a higher setpoint due to reduced expression of the CaSR. PTH levels, however, should be in the normal to perhaps high-normal range. Importantly, because expression of the CaSR is also reduced in the thick ascending limb of the kidney, Ca^{2+} will continue to be reabsorbed there despite the hypercalcemia, resulting in hypocalciuria.

8. a. Vitamin D deficiency > Decreased Ca^{2+} absorption > Increased PTH > Ca^{2+} mobilization from bone; Increased Ca^{2+} reabsorption by distal tubule; Increased Pi excretion by kidney > Hypophosphatemia > Deficient bone mineralization

   b. Hyperparathyroidism > Increased PTH > Increased 1,25-dihydroxyvitamin D; Increased serum Ca^{2+} due to PTH actions on bone and kidney, 1,25-dihydroxyvitamin D actions on intestines; Decreased serum Pi due to PTH action on kidney

   c. Hypocalcemia > Increased PTH > Increased 1,25-dihydroxyvitamin D; Increased serum Ca^{2+} due to PTH actions on bone and kidney, 1,25-dihydroxyvitamin D actions on intestines; PTH inhibition of Pi reabsorption maintains normal serum Pi

   d. Hypophosphatemia > Decreased FGF-23 > increased 1,25-dihydroxyvitamin D > Increased Pi and Ca^{2+} uptake by intestines > Decreased PTH secretion to maintain normocalcemia

CHAPTER 5

1. The neurohypophysis (posterior pituitary [pars nervosa], infundibular stalk, and median eminence) is derived from the infundibular downgrowth of the diencephalon. The adenohypophysis (anterior pituitary [pars distalis plus pars tuberalis]) is derived from the Rathke pouch, a cranial outgrowth of the oral ectoderm.

2. The median eminence is where releasing hormones are released and enter the hypothalamohypophyseal portal vessels, which run down the infundibular stalk.

3. Although ADH release can be stimulated by a decrease in blood volume, osmolality is the more sensitive regulator. It is sensed by osmoreceptor neurons in the hypothalamus that stimulate magnocellular neurons of the PVN and SON, causing the secretion of ADH.

4. ADH is synthesized in the hypothalamus, specifically in the cell bodies or magnocellular neurons of the SON and PVN. ADH is synthesized as preprovasophysin, which is proteolytically processed during intraaxonal transport down the stalk. ADH is released from the axonal termini at the pars nervosa.

5. ADH secretion is no longer regulated according to normal servomechanisms. The unregulated, inappropriately high ADH levels lead to excess volume and decrease osmolality. The increased volume stimulates ANP, promoting sodium loss. The decreased osmolality further contributes to hyponatremia.

6. Aquaporin-2 and the vasopressin-2 receptor.

7. Secondary, because the cause of cortisol overproduction occurs at the pituitary.

8. The GHRH receptor is coupled to a Gs-cAMP-PKA pathway and increases *GH* gene expression and somatotrope proliferation.

9. GH is a weak counterregulatory hormone and opposes insulin-dependent glucose uptake.

10. Cortisol and GH are both "stress hormones" that maintain blood glucose during stress. As expected, stress increases CRH and GHRH. TRH is inhibited by cortisol and thus is decreased by stress—this would decrease metabolic demands during stress. Similarly,

the reproductive system imposes significant metabolic demands, and its activity is decreased during stress. Thus GnRH is decreased by stress.

11. After consumption of a balanced meal, the secretion of GH will be stimulated by amino acids. The simultaneous secretion of insulin will help ensure liver responsiveness to GH, resulting in the secretion of IGF-I. Together, GH and IGF-I will stimulate anabolic processes, including bone growth. During fasting, hypoglycemia is the stimulus for GH secretion. GH is a glucose-sparing hormone that helps to mobilize fat as an alternative energy source.

12. ACTH binds to the MC1R on melanocytes with low affinity. However, primary hypercortisolism leads to high ACTH levels, sufficient to activate the MC1R.

13. Acute hypoglycemia increases GHRH and GH secretion. Under fasting conditions, however, when conditions for growth do not exist, IGF-I production by the liver in will be greatly reduced or absent.

14. a. GH stimulates the secretion of IGF-I from the liver.
    b. IGF-I is the primary negative feedback signal on the somatotrope in a classic long-feedback loop.
    c. GH and IGF-I are key positive regulators of bone growth. GH has direct effects on the growth plate to promote chondrocyte differentiation. In addition, GH stimulates both systemic production of IGF-I from the liver and local production of IGF-I in bone. IGF-I is a powerful stimulator of cartilage, bone and organ growth. At the onset of puberty, the GH and IGF-I production are stimulated by sex steroids, contributing to acceleration of growth during puberty.

CHAPTER 6

1. Hypertrophy and hyperplasia of the thyroid leading to goiter is a physical finding that does not predict thyroid status. Patients who are hypothyroid (e.g., iodine deficiency) may have a goiter secondary to high levels of TSH. Iodine deficiency with impaired thyroid hormone synthesis is the most common cause of goiter in parts of the world that do not have access to iodized salt, seafood, kelp, dairy products, or other sources of iodine. Patients with a diffuse goiter may also be euthyroid due to the ability of the gland to compensate for a time. Patients with a nodular goiter may also have TSH and thyroid hormone levels in the normal range. On the other hand, TSH receptor-stimulating antibodies in Graves disease cause hyperthyroidism in the context of thyroid hyperplasia and hypertrophy, possibly leading to goiter.

2. The thyroid hormone receptor (TR) is in fact a gene family encoding TRα1, TRβ1, and TRβ2. TRα1 is expressed primarily in cardiac and skeletal muscle. An inactivating mutation in TRα1 would result in decreased cardiac output and cardiac hypofunction. However, the TRβ2 isoform is expressed in the pituitary thyrotropes and hypothalamic TRH neurons. If this isoform is not mutated, the feedback remains intact.

3. a. TSH-R: Loss of TSH-R function would diminish all aspects of thyroid function, causing greatly diminished RAIU consistent with hypothyroidism
   b. Thyroid peroxidase: Loss of thyroid peroxidase would cause an organification defect. Iodide would be taken up into the thyroid, but would not be incorporated into thyroglobulin. Administration of perchlorate to inhibit further iodide uptake would cause a rapid discharge of unincorporated radioactive iodine from the gland.
   c. NIS: Loss of the sodium-iodide symporter would preclude active iodide uptake into the thyroid gland.

4. The increased estrogen production resulting from the pregnancy increases liver TBG production. As TBG levels increase, serum hormone binding increases. To maintain normal serum free T_4 levels, TSH increases T_4 production until a new equilibrium is established in which free hormone levels are close to normal and total levels (bound plus free) are high. Normal pregnant women have significant thyroidal changes during pregnancy, but they are not considered to be hyperthyroid.

5. The thyroid gland produces primarily T_4 along with some T_3. Thyroid hormones are transported bound to proteins in the blood, primarily thyroid-binding globulin. Peripherally, T_4 can be converted to T_3 by peripheral deiodinases. The most important of these is the type 2 outer ring deiodinase that converts T_4 to T_3, thereby producing active hormone in cells that express this enzyme. This enzyme plays a key role in feedback regulation of TSH secretion in pituitary thyrotropes. There is also a Type 3 inner ring deiodinase that inactivates T_4 and T_3.

6. During severe illness, the thyroid axis is suppressed by central input, causing TRH and TSH levels to fall. Peripherally, type 2 deiodinase activity is reduced, whereas type 3 is increased, resulting in decreased T_4 and T_3 levels. This is not a hypothyroid state, but an energy-sparing adaptation known as nonthyroidal illness syndrome (sick euthyroid syndrome).

7. T_3 increases cardiac output, resting heart rate, and stroke volume. The speed and force of myocardial contractions are enhanced (positive chronotropic and inotropic effects, respectively), and the diastolic relaxation

time is shortened (positive lusitropic effect). T_3 induces a widened pulse pressure due to the combined effects of the increased stroke volume and the reduction in total peripheral vascular resistance that results from blood vessel dilation in skin, muscle, and heart. These effects in turn are partly secondary to the increase in tissue production of heat and metabolites that T_3 induces. T_3 also decreases systemic vascular resistance by dilating resistance arterioles in the peripheral circulation.

8. Neonates who suffer from congenital hypothyroidism due to thyroid dysgenesis or mutation develop normally in utero due to maternal thyroid hormones. However, they must be identified early and receive thyroid hormone replacement to ensure normal postnatal development.

CHAPTER 7

1. Epinephrine acts as a counterregulatory hormone at the liver—it stimulates glycogenolysis, gluconeogenesis, and ketogenesis. At the adipocyte, epinephrine has a strong lipolytic action, through the activation of hormone-sensitive lipase (HSL).

2. Catecholamines act through binding to adrenergic receptors. The β_2-adrenergic receptor is coupled to the Gs-cAMP-PKA pathway, which promotes vascular smooth muscle relaxation (through phosphorylation of myosin light-chain kinase) and, thus, vasodilation. Other vessels have a high density of α_1-adrenergic receptors, which are coupled to a Gq-PLC-IP$_3$-Ca^{2+} signaling pathway that promotes vasoconstriction.

3. Synthetic glucocorticoids inhibit CRH and ACTH production. Low ACTH levels lead to reduced production of endogenous glucocorticoids and adrenal androgens, but also to atrophy of the zona fasciculata and zona reticularis.

4. Excessive ACTH will drive adrenal androgen synthesis in the zona reticularis. The high levels of weak androgens lead to higher levels of testosterone and DHT being produced peripherally in such cells as hair follicle cells, causing hirsutism.

5. Aldosterone increases the synthesis of ENaC (α-subunit). Aldosterone also increases *SGK1* gene expression. SGK1 prevents the ability of a protein, called Nedd 4 to 2, from targeting ENaC for degradation. Thus aldosterone promotes Na$^+$ reabsorption by increasing the synthesis and stability of ENaC in the apical membrane of the distal tubule.

6. A pheochromocytoma produces chronic high levels of catecholamines, which down-regulate all adrenergic receptors. In Addison disease, very low levels of aldosterone deplete the intravascular volume, reducing blood pressure. Low cortisol will decrease angiotensinogen production by the liver, and decreases adrenergic receptor expression (especially α_1) and signaling in blood vessels.

CHAPTER 8

1. (1) Pairing of chromosomes from genetically unrelated individuals. (2) Independent assortment of chromosomes during production of haploid gametes. (3) Crossing-over during prophase of meiosis I.

2. SRY will drive the testicular differentiation of the bipotential gonad. The testis will secrete testosterone and AMH, thereby causing the regression of the Müllerian ducts and development of the Wolffian ducts. Differentiation of the urogenital sinus and external genitalia will also be male. Thus the individual will develop as if they were 46,XY. Psychosexual differentiation is most likely to be male.

3. This individual will have normal male development of the testis, internal tract, and external genitalia. However, the inability to respond to AMH will cause "persistent Müllerian duct syndrome," in which the Müllerian-derived structures will fail to regress. These structures can physically disrupt testicular descent of one or both testes. Treatment involves surgical removal of Müllerian derivatives and correction of an undescended testis.

4. In the testis, meiosis is inhibited in early development by breakdown of retinoic acid. After puberty, meiosis is a continuous process from self-renewing stem cells (spermatogonia) that progress through all steps within about 70 days. In the ovary, all oogonia commit to meiosis, thereby generating a finite number of primary oocytes. Primary oocytes arrest at prophase of meiosis I. Meiosis is continued in response to the LH surge just before ovulation. The secondary oocyte (egg) arrests at metaphase of meiosis II. Meiosis is only completed on fertilization.

5. Kallmann syndrome type 1 is a form of tertiary hypogonadism resulting in low GnRGH, LH, FSH, and testosterone (in males). Early production of testosterone is needed for initial development of Wolffian structures. Placental hCG, as opposed to fetal pituitary LH, stimulates early testicular production of testosterone.

6. Gain of function mutations in the Kiss1R induce gonadotropin-dependent precocious puberty.

7. During the development of the ovary, retinoic acid induces all oogonia to commit to meiosis, and these primary oocytes become surrounded by prefollicle cells. As a result of follicular atresia, and to a lesser extent ovulation, follicles are reduced in number during gestation and throughout infancy, childhood, adolescence,

and adulthood. There is no self-renewal. At menopause, there are too few functional follicles to enter the menstrual cycle. In men, the spermatogonia remain meiotically quiescent owing to the presence of CYP26B1, which degrades retinoic acid. By the time spermatogonia enter meiosis at puberty, their microenvironment regulates their divisions, and they self-renew as well as differentiate into primary spermatogonia by the process of asymmetric division.

8. Menopause is associated with the loss of estradiol and progesterone production by the ovary. This leads to vasomotor instability (hot flashes), decreased bone density (which may progress to osteoporosis), and genital atrophy and vaginal dryness. Postmenopausal women also lose the beneficial effects of estrogen on lipoprotein profile (i.e., high HDL, low LDL) and are at greater risk for cardiovascular disease.

CHAPTER 9

1. The Sertoli cells form occluding junctions just apical to the spermatogonia—these junctions between adjacent Sertoli cells create the basal and adluminal compartments of the seminiferous epithelium.
2. Sertoli cells produce AMH, which cause the regression of the Müllerian ducts and inhibin, which feeds back negatively on FSH production by the pituitary gland.
3. Spermatozoa consist of a head with a condensed and streamlined nucleus, an acrosomal vesicle, and a neck with two centrioles (proximal and distal). The proximal centriole attaches to the nucleus and the distal centriole will generate a "9 + 2" configuration of microtubules that is called the *axoneme*. The tail (also called the *flagellum*), is composed of a middle piece containing a collar of mitochondria, the principal piece and the end piece. Spermiogenesis.
4. 17β-HSD3 is a testis-specific enzyme that catalyzes the conversion of androstenedione to testosterone. Without testosterone production, spermatogenesis would not occur, and the external genitalia would differentiate into female structures. Loss of testicular testosterone production would result in high levels of LH and high levels of circulating androstenedione. Androstenedione will be peripherally converted to estrone and estradiol, as well as to testosterone and DHT. Usually, conversion to estradiol (directly or through estrone) is greater than conversion to testosterone and DHT, resulting in significant breast development.
5. Normal spermatogenesis is absolutely dependent on LH-driven intratesticular production of testosterone, which leads to extremely high levels of testosterone within the seminiferous tubules. Exogenous androgens will increase blood testosterone levels enough to inhibit LH, which will actually result in decreased intratesticular levels of testosterone.

6. (1) Mitosis of spermatogonia. (2) Loss of most cytoplasm. (3) Incapacitation. (4) Mixing of sperm with secretions from seminal vesicles and prostate.
7. The seminal vesicles and the prostate gland produce most of the volume of semen. This contains buffer (citrate), antimicrobial agent (high Zn^+), fructose, etc. Also, semen contains semenogelins that in lower vertebrates create a fibrin-like plug in the vagina. PSA is a prostate-specific serine-protease that eventually breaks down the plug. In humans, these proteins represent evolutionary remnants. However, PSA can enter the blood when the prostate is infected or damaged by a growing prostatic tumor. PSA levels, especially rapid changes in these levels, are used to assess prostate gland health.
8. cGMP increases Ca^{2+} efflux from the vascular smooth muscle cells of the helicine arteries that empty into the cavernous spaces of the penis or clitoris. Decreased intracellular Ca^{2+} promotes vasodilation, allowing blood to enter the cavernous spaces.

CHAPTER 10

1. To induce meiotic maturation of the primary oocyte to an egg (secondary oocyte at metaphase II). Only this cell can be fertilized.
2. The LH receptor is always expressed on theca cells. It is expressed in mural granulosa cells of large preovulatory follicles. The LH receptor is expressed on luteinized theca and granulosa cells. LH expression is induced by FSH during the late follicular phase of the ovary.
3. The LH surge induces the following during the periovulatory period: (1) meiotic maturation of the oocyte; (2) cumulus expansion and breakdown of contact between cumulus and mural granulosa cells; (3) secretion of hydrolytic enzymes that erode the follicular and ovarian wall, and the basal lamina of the mural granulosa, allowing for direct vascularization; and (4) luteinization of the follicle cells, leading to the onset of progesterone secretion.
4. The theca cells convert cholesterol to androstenedione. However, theca cells express little 17β-HSD and essentially no CYP19 aromatase and, thus, cannot produce estradiol. The androstenedione must enter the granulosa cells, which convert it to estradiol.
5. For example, estrogen has a negative and positive feedback on pituitary gonadotropes, stimulates growth of the uterine endometrium, stimulates ductal growth in the breasts, stimulates ciliogenesis in the oviduct, and stimulates secretion of a

thin, watery mucus by the cervix. Nonreproductive actions of estrogen include bone mineralization, growth and epiphyseal plate closure, increased HDL and decreased VLDL and LDL production, increased vasodilation in general, maintenance of healthy skin, and increased lipolysis.

6. The endometrium would not fully develop secretory activity, would not fully express surface proteins involved in implantation, and would undergo early menses.

7. The ovarian reserve indicates the number of primordial follicles in the ovary at any given time.

8. There is a selective rebound in FSH secretion.

9. Selection of recruited follicles.

CHAPTER 11

1. The process by which the sperm induces Ca^{2+} waves in the egg. This induces the cortical reaction, completion of meiosis, and synthesis of proteins involved in early embryogenesis.

2. The trophoblast differentiates into cytotrophoblasts and syncytiotrophoblasts. Syncytiotrophoblasts express adhesion molecules and hydrolytic enzymes that allow for invasion, and secrete hCG.

3. Placental progesterone is completed solely by the syncytiotrophoblast and is independent of fetal viability. Estriol requires the fetal hypothalamus, pituitary, adrenal, and liver, as well as the syncytiotrophoblast of the placenta. Thus fetal and placental health affects estriol synthesis.

4. Estrogen is not needed for a normal pregnancy, except for the development of the breasts for nursing and for a sufficiently responsive myometrium for labor to occur. This latter action involves upregulation of oxytocin receptors and increased prostaglandin synthesis.

5. hCG increases rapidly during the first trimester and cross-reacts with the TSH receptor on the maternal thyroid. hCG production declines to a lower steady level after the first trimester, thereby terminating the hyperthyroidism.

6. Respiratory changes in response to progesterone include increased minute volume and increased tidal volume.

7. Prolactin inhibits GnRH and thus promotes infertility. During very regular nursing, high prolactin levels cause lactational amenorrhea, which inhibits pregnancy while a newborn is being nursed. The most common type of pituitary tumor is the prolactinoma. This is associated with pathologically elevated prolactin, amenorrhea, and infertility.

Comprehensive Multiple-Choice Examination

1. Which receptor resides in the cytoplasm in the absence of hormone?
   a. Insulin receptor
   b. Thyroid hormone receptor
   c. Prolactin receptor
   d. Glucocorticoid receptor

2. One general mode of an intracellular signaling pathway involves:
   a. Exocytosis of matrix molecules
   b. Protein synthesis of a hormone receptor
   c. Covalent phosphorylation of proteins or lipids
   d. Replication of DNA

3. G-protein-coupled receptors (GPCRs) function as ligand-activated:
   a. Protein tyrosine kinases
   b. G-protein exchange factors
   c. Protein phosphatases
   d. Membrane phospholipases

4. GPCRs can be downregulated by:
   a. Ligand-induced endocytosis
   b. Transphosphorylation on tyrosine residues
   c. Dimerization within the cell membrane
   d. Activation of the Gs subunit

5. The transcription factors called STATs are activated by which class of receptor?
   a. Receptor tyrosine kinase
   b. Steroid hormone receptor
   c. GPCR
   d. Cytokine receptor

6. Which of the following is true concerning coactivator proteins?
   a. They modify chromatin coiling
   b. They reside in the cytoplasm
   c. They increase protein translation
   d. They directly bind to steroid hormones

7. During the gastric phase, gastrin secretion is stimulated primarily by:
   a. Histamine
   b. Long-chain fatty acids
   c. Somatostatin
   d. Peptides

8. Erythromycin can be used to treat delayed gastric emptying through acting as an agonist for:
   a. Somatostatin
   b. Motilin
   c. CCK
   d. GLP-1

9. Zollinger-Ellison syndrome (gastrin-secreting tumor) directly causes the overgrowth of which cell type?
   a. S (secretin) cell
   b. Goblet cell
   c. Pancreatic acinar cell
   d. ECL cell

10. The term *incretin* is used to describe a hormone that sensitizes:
    a. G cells to stomach distention
    b. Intestinal K cells to long-chain fatty acids
    c. Pancreatic β cells to glucose
    d. Intestinal L cells to glucose

11. A 25-year-old patient was found to have abnormal overnight fasting blood values during a yearly physical examination. Genetic testing revealed the presence of a partial loss-of-function mutation in *GLUT2* gene. The finding from the initial blood work that ultimately pointed to GLUT2 was:
    a. High liver enzymes
    b. Low cortisol
    c. Elevated LDL
    d. Elevated glucose

12. During acute hypoglycemia, insulin secretion is inhibited by low glucose and:
    a. Cholinergic signaling through the muscarinic receptor
    b. Catecholamine signaling through the α_2-adrenergic receptor
    c. Glucagon signaling through the glucagon receptor
    d. GLP-1 signaling through the GLP-1 receptor

13. The insulin receptor regulates metabolism primarily through a signaling pathway involving:
    a. Akt
    b. cAMP
    c. Ca^{2+}
    d. Ras

14. A primary and direct stimulus for glucagon secretion during the FAST state is:
    a. Low blood sugar
    b. Cholinergic innervation
    c. Low insulin
    d. Low blood free fatty acids

15. Insulin suppresses glucose-6-phosphatase through:
    a. Activation of SREBP-1
    b. Activation of protein phosphatase-1
    c. Inhibition of FOXO1
    d. Activation of cAMP-PKA

16. During the fed state, insulin activates which enzyme/transporter?
    a. Adipose tissue lipoprotein lipase
    b. Hepatic pyruvate carboxylase
    c. Muscle glycogen phosphorylase
    d. Hepatic GLUT2 transporter

17. Quantitatively, insulin maintains glucose tolerance through:
    a. Suppression of hepatic glycolysis
    b. Increased GLUT4-mediated glucose uptake in muscle
    c. Suppression of adipocyte hormone-sensitive lipase
    d. Increased hepatic gluconeogenesis

18. A heterozygous inactivating mutation in the CaSR results in:
    a. Hypercalcemia
    b. Low levels of 1,25-dihydroxyvitamin D_3
    c. Elevated PTH levels
    d. Hypophosphatemia

19. One mechanism by which intermittent treatment with PTH improves bone density is through:
    a. Stimulation of RANKL by osteoblasts
    b. Induction of cell death of osteoclasts
    c. Inhibiting secretion of SOST by osteocytes
    d. Decreasing osteoprotegerin production by osteoblasts

20. The sodium-phosphate cotransporter (NPT) isoform 2a is expressed in the proximal renal tubules. NPT2a is regulated in the following manner:
    a. Increased by PTH
    b. Increased by calciuria
    c. Decreased by PTH
    d. Decreased by 1,25-dihydroxyvitamin D

21. The primary action of 1,25-dihydroxyvitamin D to increase serum Ca^{2+} is to:
    a. Stimulate of osteoblast RANKL production
    b. Increase intestinal Ca^{2+} absorption
    c. Increase renal phosphate excretion
    d. Stimulate PTH production

22. The expression of renal 1α-hydroxylase is directly stimulated by:
    a. FGF23
    b. CaSR

    c. PTH
    d. High serum Ca^{2+}

23. Damage to the pituitary stalk may result in an increase in:
    a. FSH
    b. GH
    c. ACTH
    d. PRL

24. The pituitary cell that produces two hormones is the:
    a. Thyrotrope
    b. Gonadotrope
    c. Corticotrope
    d. Somatotrope

25. Provasophysin in synthesized in magnocellular cells within the:
    a. Anterior pituitary
    b. Posterior pituitary
    c. Hypothalamus
    d. Infundibular stalk

26. During a fast, GH secretion is stimulated by:
    a. Insulin
    b. Glucagon
    c. Ghrelin
    d. Somatostatin

27. Tertiary hypercortisolism may result from:
    a. Interleukin stimulation of CRH
    b. A functional adrenocortical tumor
    c. A functional pituitary corticotropic tumor
    d. Genetic amplification of the *POMC* gene

28. A gain-of-function mutation in the type 3 deiodinase may cause:
    a. Elevated blood T_3 levels
    b. Suppressed T_4 synthesis
    c. Elevated iodine uptake curve
    d. Suppressed TSH levels

29. With respect to cardiovascular function, hyperthyroidism causes:
    a. Increased inotropy and increased peripheral resistance
    b. Increased inotropy and decreased peripheral resistance
    c. Decreased inotropy and increased peripheral resistance
    d. Decreased inotropy and decreased peripheral resistance

30. Iodide is transported into the colloid by:
    a. Sodium/iodide symporter (NIS)
    b. Thyroid-specific iodotyrosine deiodinase
    c. Thyroid peroxidase
    d. Pendrin

31. How would acute chemical inhibition of thyroid peroxidase affect the iodine uptake curve?
    a. Decreased initial uptake, then plateau over 24 hr
    b. Normal initial uptake, with loss of iodine within 24 hr
    c. Increased initial uptake, with loss of iodine within 24 hr
    d. Increased initial uptake, then plateau over 24 hr

32. Maternal blood thyroid hormone levels in late pregnancy can be characterized as:
    a. Elevated total T_4, normal free T_4
    b. Elevated total T_4, elevated T_4
    c. Normal total T_4, normal T_4
    d. Normal total T_4, elevated T_4

33. In an individual with iodine deficiency–induced goiter and signs of cold intolerance and a decreased heart rate, one would expect to find the following circulating hormone levels:
    a. High TSH and high T_3
    b. High TSH and low T_3
    c. Low TSH and high T_3
    d. Low TSH and low T_3

34. In an individual with Graves disease–induced goiter and signs of heat intolerance and an elevated heart rate, one would expect to find the following circulating hormone levels:
    a. High TSH and high T_3
    b. High TSH and low T_3
    c. Low TSH and high T_3
    d. Low TSH and low T_3

35. A thyroid hormone receptor not bound to T_3 is located:
    a. In the cytoplasm
    b. Within the plasma membrane
    c. In the nucleus
    d. Within the endoplasmic reticulum membrane

36. During exercise, epinephrine and norepinephrine act to:
    a. Increase muscle glycogenolysis
    b. Increase hepatic glycolysis
    c. Decrease adipocyte lipolysis
    d. Decrease hepatic ketogenesis

37. A clinical sign or symptom of adrenocortical insufficiency (Addison disease) is:
    a. Puffy, flushed face ("moon face")
    b. Skin hyperpigmentation
    c. Increased skin bruisability
    d. Hyperglycemia

38. A congenital null mutation of CYP11B1 would result in:
    a. Sodium wasting
    b. Hyperglycemia
    c. Masculinization of a female fetus
    d. Atrophy of adrenal cortex

39. One treatment for hypertension is the use of aldosterone receptor antagonists (e.g., spironolactone). A side effect of this treatment can be:
    a. Cardiac hypertrophy
    b. Hyperkalemia
    c. Metabolic alkalosis
    d. Edema

40. Glucocorticoid analogs are used at high levels to suppress inflammation. A side effect of this treatment can be:
    a. Adrenocortical hypertrophy
    b. Hypoglycemia
    c. Skin darkening
    d. Osteoporosis

41. Cortisol is prevented from interacting with the mineralocorticoid receptor (MR) in the distal nephron through the action of:
    a. Cortisol-binding protein
    b. 11β-hydroxysteroid dehydrogenase type 2
    c. 17β-hydroxysteroid dehydrogenase type 1
    d. Serum and glucocorticoid-regulated kinase (SGK)

42. Aldosterone resistance (type 1 pseudohypoaldosteronism) can be due to an inactivating mutation in:
    a. Glucocorticoid receptor
    b. Epithelial sodium channel (ENaC)
    c. 11β-hydroxysteroid dehydrogenase type 2
    d. Aquaporin-2

43. The basis for the generation of millions of genetically distinct gametes in a gonad is called:
    a. Independent assortment
    b. Genetic recombination
    c. Disjunction
    d. Euploidy

44. Phenotypic gender is directly regulated by:
    a. XX or XY sex chromosomes
    b. Reproductive tract differentiation
    c. Sex steroids
    d. Gonadal differentiation

45. The primary source of endogenous estradiol in a postmenopausal woman is the peripheral conversion of androgens made by:
    a. The remaining few follicles
    b. The ovarian stroma
    c. The adrenal cortex
    d. The adipose tissue

46. Congenital deficiency of 5α-reductase type 2 may lead to the following in a male:
    a. Ovarian differentiation of the gonad
    b. Poorly developed seminal vesicle
    c. Persistence of Müllerian duct derivatives
    d. Poorly developed prostate gland

47. A mutation that renders the FSH receptor constitutively active would result in:
    a. Elevated blood testosterone levels
    b. Low blood LH levels
    c. Elevated blood inhibin levels
    d. Low androgen–binding protein (ABP) in the seminiferous tubule

48. Administration of an exogenous androgen can result in:
    a. Elevated sperm production
    b. Elevated blood LH levels
    c. Elevated hematocrit (polycythemia)
    d. Elevated proteolysis in muscle

49. The Sertoli cell performs the following functions, *except:*
    a. Regulates sperm development up to full motility
    b. Expresses androgen-binding protein
    c. Maintains blood-testis barrier
    d. Expresses receptors for both FSH and testosterone

50. Congenital deficiency of 17β-hydroxysteroid dehydrogenase (HSD) type 3 in a 46,XY individual would result in the following:
    a. Lack of pubic hair in the adult
    b. Breast development at puberty
    c. Precocious penile and testicular growth at puberty
    d. Development of oviducts and uterus

51. DHT binds to the:
    a. Estrogen receptor
    b. DHT receptor
    c. Androgen receptor
    d. Prostate-specific antigen (PSA)

52. Upregulation of penile cyclic GMP phosphodiesterase would result in the following within the vascular smooth muscle in the helicine arteries:
    a. Increased tone
    b. Increased nitric oxide levels
    c. Increased intracellular Ca^{2+}
    d. Increased cyclic GMP

53. Emission refers to sperm moving into the:
    a. Vas deferens
    b. Spongy urethra
    c. Epididymis
    d. Prostatic urethra

54. Testosterone has the following effect on the liver:
    a. Upregulates LDL receptor
    b. Increases VLDL production
    c. Increases ApoA1 expression
    d. Activates AMP kinase (AMPK)

55. In the late follicular phase, the LH receptor is expressed on:
    a. Theca cells only
    b. Granulosa cells only
    c. Theca and granulosa cells
    d. Theca, granulosa cells, and the oocyte

56. During the secretory phase of the uterus, progesterone induces:
    a. Inactivation of estradiol to estrone
    b. Proliferation of predecidual cells
    c. Myometrial contractions
    d. Release of matrix metalloproteases from stroma

57. The *ovarian reserve* is a collective term for:
    a. The number of preovulatory follicles
    b. The number of primordial follicles
    c. The ovarian stroma
    d. The number of oogonia

58. During her annual examination, a patient tells her gynecologist that she has noticed increased facial hair and acne. Ultrasound imaging of the ovaries reveals the presence of multiple "cysts," and the diagnosis of polycystic ovary syndrome (PCOS) is made. The patient's BMI is 32, indicating obesity. In this individual, the probable root cause of her PCOS is:
    a. Elevated estradiol production
    b. Hyperinsulinemia
    c. Peripheral conversion of estrone to androgens
    d. Elevated circulating FSH

59. In the two-cell model of ovarian steroidogenesis, theca cells primarily produce:
    a. Estradiol
    b. Progesterone
    c. Testosterone
    d. Androstenedione

60. A key factor in the selection of a dominant follicle is high expression of which receptor?
    a. FSH receptor
    b. Androgen receptor
    c. LH receptor
    d. Progesterone receptor

61. During the early luteal phase, the following process occurs:
    a. Increase in FSH secretion
    b. Upregulation of CYP19-aromatase in granulosa cells
    c. Meiotic completion and formation of the second polar body
    d. Selection of a dominant follicle

62. The steroidogenic pathway of the mature corpus luteum is characterized by very low expression of:
    a. CYP19-aromatase
    b. CYP17 (17-hydroxylase)
    c. 3β-Hydroxysteroid dehydrogenase (3β-HSD)
    d. 17β-Hydroxysteroid dehydrogenase (17β-HSD; activating isoform)

63. The inability of the cumulus-oocyte complex to enter the female reproductive tract may be caused by an infection or inflammation of:
    a. The isthmus of the oviduct
    b. The ampulla of the oviduct
    c. The intramural portion of the oviduct
    d. The infundibulum of the oviduct

64. The priming of the endometrium by estrogen refers to:
   a. Development of vascular lacunae
   b. Induction of progesterone receptors
   c. Rapid proliferation of all cell types
   d. Expression of pinopods by the surface epithelial cells

65. The primary signal for the LH surge is:
   a. Increased frequency of GnRH pulses by hypothalamic GnRH neurons
   b. Decreased inhibin B production from both ovaries
   c. Persistently high blood levels of estradiol from the dominant follicle
   d. Rapid downregulation of the GnRH receptors on the gonadotropes

66. Sperm undergo the process of capacitation as they:
   a. Are stored in the tail of the epididymis
   b. Become adhered to the oviduct
   c. As they pass through the cervical mucus
   d. In the vagina just after ejaculation

67. An infertile couple undergo in vitro fertilization. Although the husband ejaculates several hundred million sperm, with greater than 50% normal phenotype, they fail to fertilize eggs retrieved from the wife's ovaries after intracytoplasmic sperm injection. This observation suggests an insufficiency of:
   a. Surface hyaluronidase (PH-20) expression
   b. Binding to ZP3
   c. PLCζ
   d. Sperm hyperactivation

68. The "window of receptivity" refers to:
   a. The desire on the part of the woman to have sex
   b. The adherent endometrium at midluteal phase
   c. The duration of a viable cumulus-oocyte complex in the oviduct
   d. The time of increased thickness of cervical mucus

69. The primary function of the endometrial lacunae and associated vessels is to:
   a. Capture hCG from the implanting embryo
   b. Provide nutrition and oxygen to the implanting embryo
   c. Deliver ovarian hormones to the implanting embryo
   d. Induce the differentiation of syncytiotrophoblasts around the implanting embryo

70. In humans, the placental barrier in the mature placenta includes the following cell types:
   a. Syncytiotrophoblast, fetal endothelial cell
   b. Maternal endothelial cell, syncytiotrophoblast, fetal endothelial cell
   c. Syncytiotrophoblast, cytotrophoblast, fetal endothelial cell
   d. Cytotrophoblast, fetal endothelial cell

71. In a fetus carrying a null mutation in the gene encoding StAR protein, the following would be observed during the third trimester:
   a. Maternal progesterone levels would be very low
   b. Maternal estriol levels would be very low
   c. Amniotic ACTH levels would be very low
   d. Maternal cortisol levels would be very low

72. In a fetus carrying a null mutation in the liver *CYP3A7* gene encoding 16-hydroxylase, maternal blood would show an absence of:
   a. Progesterone
   b. Estradiol
   c. Estriol
   d. Estrone

73. Transient gestational hyperthyroidism is due to:
   a. Deficiency in the placental type 1 deiodinase
   b. Induction of hypothalamic TRH by elevated levels of progesterone
   c. Cross-reaction of hCG with the TSH receptor
   d. Estradiol-induced hypertrophy and hyperplasia of thyroid epithelial cells

74. Reversible vision problems may be experienced by some women during late pregnancy. This is due to an enlarged pituitary gland that presses on the optic nerves. Pituitary enlargement is caused by:
   a. Estrogen-induction of lactotrope size and number
   b. Progesterone-induced edema within the sella turcica
   c. GnRH-induced growth of gonadotropes
   d. hCG-induced growth of thyrotropes

75. One factor that assists the mother in increasing her volume (for the umbilical circulation, growing fetus, and enlarging amniotic sac) is:
   a. Progesterone inhibition of antinatriuretic factor (ANF)
   b. hCG inhibition of ADH
   c. Estrogen induction of liver angiotensinogen
   d. Increased threshold for thirst

76. Lactational amenorrhea is similar to clinical amenorrhea and infertility due to:
   a. Elevated ovarian androgens
   b. Hyperprolactinemia
   c. An oxytocin-producing tumor
   d. Cessation of GnRH neuronal pulsatility

77. Tamoxifen is used to treat invasive breast cancer (after surgery and radiation). The mechanism of tamoxifen's action is:
   a. Inhibition of CYP19-aromatase
   b. Competitive inhibition of the progesterone receptor
   c. Increased inactivation of circulating estradiol
   d. Competitive inhibition of the estrogen receptor

78. Maternal cortisol levels increase during pregnancy and contribute to:
    a. Increased prolactin production by the pituitary gland
    b. Increased maternal tidal volume
    c. Increased maternal insulin levels
    d. Increased production of cortisol-binding protein by the liver
79. Fetal cortisol rises significantly just before term. This is due to a positive feedback between cortisol and placental:
    a. CRH
    b. Progesterone
    c. Estrogen
    d. hPL
80. Extravillous cytotrophoblasts perform the following function during the first trimester:
    a. Induction of decidual cells to form the basal plate
    b. Phagocytosis of dead cells
    c. Conversion of spiral arteries
    d. Formation of a layer of the amniodecidual membrane

ANSWERS TO COMPREHENSIVE MULTIPLE-CHOICE EXAMINATION

1. d	17. b	33. b	49. a	65. c
2. c	18. a	34. c	50. b	66. b
3. b	19. c	35. c	51. c	67. c
4. a	20. c	36. a	52. a	68. b
5. d	21. b	37. b	53. d	69. a
6. a	22. c	38. c	54. b	70. a
7. d	23. d	39. b	55. c	71. b
8. b	24. b	40. d	56. a	72. c
9. d	25. c	41. b	57. b	73. c
10. c	26. c	42. b	58. b	74. a
11. d	27. a	43. a	59. d	75. c
12. b	28. c	44. c	60. a	76. b
13. a	29. c	45. c	61. c	77. d
14. c	30. d	46. c	62. b	78. c
15. c	31. b	47. c	63. d	79. a
16. a	32. a	48. c	64. b	80. c

C APPENDIX

Abbreviations and Symbols

αGSU	alpha glycoprotein subunit
β-hCG	hormone-specific β-subunit of hCG
β-TSH	β-Thyroid-stimulating hormone
3β-HSD	3β-hydroxysteroid dehydrogenase
11β-HSD2	11β-hydroxysteroid dehydrogenase
17β-HSD	17β-hydroxysteroid dehydrogenase
AA	amino acid
ABP	androgen-binding protein
ACE	angiotensin-converting enzyme
Ach	acetylcholine
ACTH	adrenocorticotropic hormone (corticotropin)
ADH	antidiuretic hormone
AIS	androgen insensitivity syndrome
ALS	acid-labile subunit
AMH	antiMüllerian hormone
ANP	atrial natriuretic peptide
APO	apoprotein
AR	androgen receptor
ARE	androgen-response element
ATP	adenosine triphosphate
BAT	brown adipose tissue
bFGF	basic fibroblast growth factor
BMP-15	bone morphogenetic protein-15
BMR	basal metabolic rate
Ca^{2+}	calcium phosphate
CaMKII	Ca^{2+}-calmodulin-dependent protein kinase-II
cAMP	cyclic adenosine monophosphate
CaSR	Ca^{2+}-sensing receptor
CBG	corticosteroid-binding globulin (also *transcortin*)
CCK	cholecystokinin
CDK1	cyclin-dependent kinase-1
CETP	cholesterol ester transfer protein
cGMP	cyclic guanosine monophosphate
CGRP	calcitonin gene–related peptide
CNS	central nervous system
COMT	catechol-*O*-methyltransferase
COX-2	cyclooxygenase-2

CPT-1/CPT-2	carnitine-palmitoyl transferase
CREB protein	cAMP-response element–binding protein
CRH	corticotropin-releasing hormone
CSF	cytostatic factor
CYP11β	11β-hydroxylase
CYP21β	21β-hydroxylase
CYP	cytochrome P-450 monooxidase gene
DAG	diacylglycerol
DBP	vitamin D–binding protein
DHEAS	dehydroepiandrosterone sulfate
DHT	dihydrotestosterone
DI	diabetes insipidus
DIT	diiodotyrosine
DM	diabetes mellitus
DNA	deoxyribonucleic acid
DOC	deoxycorticosterone
DOPA	dihydroxyphenylalanine
ECL	enterochromaffin-like (cell)
ED	erectile dysfunction
EGF	epidermal growth factor
EnaC	epithelial Na^+ channel
ENS	enteric nervous system
ER	estrogen receptor
ERE	estrogen-response element
FAS	fatty acid synthase (complex)
FBHH	familial benign hypocalciuric hypercalcemia
FDA	Food and Drug Administration
FFA	free fatty acid
FGF-23	fibroblast growth factor-23
FSH	follicle-stimulating hormone
Gα	Gα-subunit
Gβ/γ	Gβ-subunit dimer
G-6-P	glucose-6-phosphate
GAG	glycosaminoglycan
GDF-9	growth differentiation factor-9
GEF	guanine nucleotide exchange factor
GFR	glomerular filtration rate

GH	growth hormone		MIT	monoiodotyrosine
GHRH	growth hormone–releasing hormone		MMC	migrating myoelectric complex
GHS	growth hormone secretogogue		MODY	mature onset of diabetes of the young
GH-V	growth hormone variant-V		MPF	maturation-promoting factor
GI	gastrointestinal		MR	mineralocorticoid receptor
GIP	gastroinhibitory peptide		MRE	mineralocorticoid-response element
GLUT	glucose transporter		MIS	Müllerian-inhibiting substance
GnRH	gonadotropin-releasing hormone		MPF	maturation-promoting factor
GPCR	G-protein–coupled receptor		mRNA	messenger RNA
GPCR3	G-protein–coupled receptor-3		NCX	sodium-calcium exchanger
GR	glucocorticoid receptor		NO	nitric oxide
GRE	glucocorticoid-response element		OHSS	ovarian hyperstimulation syndrome
GRK/RTK	GPCR kinases		OPG	osteoprotegerin
GRP	gastrin-releasing peptide		OxPhos	oxidative phosphorylation
GTP	guanosine nucleotide triphosphate		P_{CO_2}	partial pressure of carbon dioxide
GVBD	germinal vesicle breakdown		PCOS	polycystic ovarian syndrome
HAD	histone diacetylase		PEPCK\t	PEP carboxykinase (phosphoenolpyruvate carboxykinase)
HAT	histone acetyltransferase			
Hb A_{1c}	hemoglobin A_{1c}		PFK1	phosphofructokinase-1
hCG	human chorionic gonadotropin		PGE_2	prostaglandin E_2
HCO_3^-	bicarbonate ion		$PGF_{2\alpha}$	prostaglandin $F_{2\alpha}$
hCS	human chorionic somatomammotropin		PHEX	phosphate-regulating gene with homologies to endopeptidases on the X chromosome
HDL	high-density lipoprotein			
HPA	hypothalamus-pituitary-adrenal		P_i	phosphate
hPL	human placental lactogen		PI3K	phosphatidylinositol-3-kinase
HRE	hormone-response element		PIP_3	phosphatidylinositol 3,4, 5-triphosphate
HSD	hydroxysteroid dehydrogenase			
HSL	hormone-sensitive lipase		PKA	protein kinase A
ICSI	intracytoplasmic sperm injection		PKB	protein kinase B
IDL	intermediate-density lipoprotein (particles)		PKG	protein kinase G
			PLCζ	phospholipase Cζ
IGF	insulin-like growth factor		PMCA	plasma membrane calcium ATPase
IGF-I	insulin-like growth factor-I		PMS	premenstrual syndrome
IGFBP	insulin-like growth factor–binding proteins		PNMT	phenylethanolamine-N-methyl transferase
IP_3	inositol 1,4,5-triphosphate		P_{O_2}	partial pressure of oxygen
IR	insulin receptor		POMC	proopiomelanocortin
IRS	insulin receptor substrate		PPARγ	peroxisome proliferator-activated receptor-γ
IUD	intrauterine device			
IVF	in vitro fertilization		PR	progesterone receptor
LDL	low-density lipoprotein		PRE	progesterone-response element
LH	luteinizing hormone		PRF	prolactin-releasing factor
LPD	luteal phase deficiency		PRL	prolactin
LPL	lipoprotein lipase		PSA	prostate-specific antigen
MAO	monoamine oxidase		PTH	parathyroid hormone
MAP	mitogen-activated protein kinase (also ERK)		PTHrP	parathyroid hormone–related peptide
MAPK	mitogen-activated kinase		PTU	propylthiouracil
MC2R	melanocortin-2 receptor		PVH	paraventricular hypothalamus
MCsF	monocyte colony-stimulating factor			

PVN	paraventricular nuclei	T_3	triiodothyronine
RAIU	radioactive iodide uptake	T_4	thyroxine
RANKL	receptor activator of NF-KB ligand	TBG	thyroxine-binding globulin
RAS	renin-angiotensin system	TCA	tricarboxylic acid (cycle)
RDS	respiratory distress syndrome	TGF	transforming growth factor
RGS	regulators of G-protein signaling	TGF-β	transforming growth factor-β
RIA	radioimmunoassay	TG	thyroglobulin
RNA	ribonucleic acid	TGs	triglycerides
ROMK channel	renal outer medullary K^+ channel	TNF-α	tumor necrosis factor-α
ROS	reactive oxygen species	TPO	thyroid peroxidase
rT_3	reverse T_3	TR	thyroid hormone receptor
RTK	receptor tyrosine kinase	TRE	thyroid hormone–response element
SERM	selective estrogen receptor modulator	TRH	thyrotropin-releasing hormone (also *thyroid-releasing hormone*)
SHBG	sex hormone–binding globulin	T/S	thyroid/serum (ratio)
SIADH	syndrome of inappropriate secretion of antidiuretic hormone	T/S[I]	thyroid/serum (measured with radioactive iodide)
SOCS	suppressor of cytokine signaling	TSA	thyroid-stimulating antibody
SON	supraoptic nuclei	TSAb	thyroid-stimulating antibody (abnormal)
SRBEP-1C	sterol regulatory–binding element protein-1C	TSH	thyroid-stimulating hormone (also called *thyrotropin*)
SRY	sex-determining region Y	TTR	thyroxine-binding prealbumin
StAR protein	steroidogenic acute regulatory protein	TZD	thiazolidinedione
STAT	signal transducers and activator of transcription	VDR	vitamin D receptor
		VEGF	vascular endothelial growth factor
SUR	ATP-binding subunit	VLDL	very-low-density lipoprotein
$t_{1/2}$	half-life	VMA	vanillylmandelic acid
T1DM	type 1 diabetes mellitus	WAT	white adipose tissue
T2DM	type 2 diabetes mellitus		

Note: Page numbers followed by "f" indicate figures, "t" indicate tables, and "b" indicate boxes.